The Production
of Speech

Edited by
Peter F. MacNeilage

With 90 Figures

Springer-Verlag
New York   Heidelberg   Berlin

Peter F. MacNeilage
Departments of Linguistics and Psychology
The University of Texas at Austin
Austin, Texas 78712, U.S.A.

Library of Congress Cataloging in Publication Data
Main entry under title:
The Production of speech.
  Papers presented at a conference on the production of speech, held at the University of
Texas at Austin, on April 28–30, 1981, sponsored by the Center for Cognitive Science,
and other bodies.
  Bibliography: p.
  Includes index.
  1. Speech—Physiological aspects—Congresses.
I. MacNeilage, Peter F. II. University of Texas at Austin. Center for Cognitive
Science.
QP306.P693 1983 612'.78 82-19246

Typeset by Ampersand, Rutland, Vermont
Printed and bound by Halliday Lithograph, West Hanover, Massachusetts
Printed in the United States of America

9 8 7 6 5 4 3 2 1

ISBN 0-387-90735-1 Springer-Verlag New York Heidelberg Berlin
ISBN 3-540-90735-1 Springer-Verlag Berlin Heidelberg New York

Preface

This monograph arose from a conference on the Production of Speech held at the University of Texas at Austin on April 28–30, 1981. It was sponsored by the Center for Cognitive Science, the College of Liberal Arts, and the Linguistics and Psychology Departments. The conference was the second in a series of conferences on human experimental psychology: the first, held to commemorate the 50th anniversary of the founding of the Psychology Department, resulted in publication of the monograph *Neural Mechanisms in Behavior,* D. McFadden (Ed.), Springer-Verlag, 1980.

The choice of the particular topic of the second conference was motivated by the belief that the state of knowledge of speech production had recently reached a critical mass, and that a good deal was to be gained from bringing together the foremost researchers in this field. The benefits were the opportunity for the participants to compare notes on their common problems, the publication of a monograph giving a comprehensive state-of-the-art picture of this research area, and the provision of enormous intellectual stimulus for local students of this topic.

The conference also provided an opportunity to honor Dr. Franklin Cooper, former President of Haskins Laboratories, who delivered the opening address at the conference, for his important research contributions to this area, his influence in fostering development of the area and, for want of a better phrase, his monumental good-citizenship. This purpose of the conference gave the present author (P.F.M.) particular pleasure, as the six-year period he had spent on the staff at Haskins Laboratories was the major formative influence on his thinking about speech production.

The area of speech production is a multidisciplinary one: contributors to this volume range from neurophysiologists to linguists and include experimental psychologists, electrical engineers, otolaryngologists, speech scientists, and students of motor skill. This diversity, though clearly an advantage in the attempt to understand such a complex topic, results in problems of comprehension for the outsider, as the different approaches have different motivations and metatheories which are often tacit. In the following paragraphs I will briefly review the various contributions to the monograph, with the particular intention of providing an explicit statement of the motivation underlying the work.

The first part of the monograph addresses the topic of Control Processes in Speech Production; the central concern here is with the means by which the movements of speech production are organized. Paradoxically, the first chapter of this section is not about speech at all. Dr. Bizzi was invited to the conference because of his important work on the general question of how voluntary movements are controlled, a question fundamental to the understanding of speech production. His work on voluntary movements of monkeys suggests that, for certain visually controlled head–eye and arm movements, control takes the form of a preprogrammed process that sets final position "as an equilibrium point resulting from the interaction of agonist and antagonist muscles." An analogy is made with a pair of adjustable springs acting across a hinge: it is noted that this position-setting operation is not step-like but more in the form of a time-dependent trajectory. In addition, differences between the behavior of normal and de-afferented monkeys lead Bizzi to emphasize "the great importance of afferent feedback in updating and adjusting the execution of learned motor patterns when posture is changed." Bizzi avails himself of simple tasks and a degree of experiment control and intervention not possible for speech researchers. While the implications of these results in speech control remain to be established, the incisiveness of this work and its provocativeness for theories of speech motor control ensure its relevance in the present context.

We first turn to speech itself in Chapter 2, by Sawashima and Hirose, and we immediately come face to face with the complexity of the speech production process. There are two particular sources of complexity in this case: first, the inaccessibility of laryngeal structures to direct observation has restricted our understanding of their operation even in common speech patterns; second, the impression of complexity is enormously magnified when one addresses, as do these authors, the range of possibilities of laryngeal function exploited by the world's languages (Ladefoged's Chapter 8 has a similar effect). The current focus of concern for laryngeal function in speech is more on *what* occurs during speech than on how the events are controlled. Workers at the Research Center for Logopedics and Phoniatrics of the University of Tokyo, including these authors, have played the foremost role in the elucidation of laryngeal function during speech, and this review is the most authoritative at present available on this topic.

In speech production research, much attention has been given to modelling the process, i.e., simulating some aspect of output with a limited number of control parameters. Despite the complexity of laryngeal function just discussed, Fujisaki, in Chapter 3, reports considerable success in modelling fundamental frequency contours of Japanese speakers and singers. Input to the model consists of an utterance command, associated with the characteristic F_0 declination during an utterance, and a binary accent command associated with the binary (high or low) pitch accent applied to each mora of an utterance (a mora is roughly equivalent to a syllable). Commands "are assumed to be smoothed separately by the low pass characteristics of their respective control mechanisms, each being approximated here by a critically damped second-order linear system." Fujisaki also makes an initial attempt to interpret his output functions in terms of the biomechanical properties of the larynx.

Kent (Chapter 4) is a representative of what could be called the traditional or standard approach to the theory of speech production. His concern is with the segmental organization of speech (i.e., with vowels and consonants). He summarizes approaches to the central question: given that there is an underlying, relatively context-free segmental level and an observable surface level where context dependence is ubiquitous (e.g., in coarticulation), how does one characterize these two levels and their relations, and in particular can there be a simple characterization of context-dependent phenomena? In a thorough examination of this question he finds the answer to be inconclusive, but convincingly suggests that we can broaden our perspective on this question by looking more carefully at speech development, speech pathology, and even the unusual case of a person who talks backwards.

Oller and MacNeilage (Chapter 5) enquire further into an avenue suggested by Kent. They review the evidence on the acquisition of segmental forms by children. It is now well-accepted that children begin language use with a small, universally preferred subset of segmental forms and syllable structures already displayed in their babbling repertoires, and gradually work towards the achievement of adult forms by about age 4. They point out that, at present, the nature of these segmental patterns and their development seems to be determined more by constraints on production capabilities than by constraints on perception or internal representation. In a pilot study they explore the possibility that bite-block techniques, which have been used so successfully to demonstrate the extreme versatility of the adult control mechanism, might be used to tell us more about the nature of speech development, especially beyond the age at which basic segmental production is correct.

Of the contributors to this volume, Shattuck-Hufnagel (Chapter 6) is alone in focusing on the nature of the relatively context-free underlying level of segmental representation assumed in traditional views of speech production. She reviews and adds to a model presented in her earlier publications, which is derived primarily from analyses of speech errors. In this model, serial ordering of segments is accomplished by a scan-copy mechanism that scans representations of words selected for an utterance and copies these representations into a matrix of canonical syllable or morpheme structures arising from suprasegmental properties of the utterance. In addition to further development of her views on the nature of segmental and suprasegmental representation derived from spontaneous speech errors, Shattuck-Hufnagel presents studies of experimentally elicited speech errors, hoping for an ultimate convergence of evidence from spontaneous and elicited errors, and hoping that the obvious disadvantages of each method taken alone will be cancelled by the other, while the advantages of each will be additive.

In the final chapter in this section (Chapter 7), Kelso, Tuller and Harris offer a new perspective on the control of speech production from the standpoint of what has come to be called Action Theory, a general approach to the coordination of movement of all kinds. They assert that the solution to the fundamental problem of movement control—the reduction of the internal degrees of freedom of the control system—involves the formation of coordinative structures, which are "fundamental groupings of muscles, often spanning several joints, which are constrained to act as a unit." Rejecting other approaches such as those based on "closed-loop servomechanism accounts," and "the formal machine metaphor of central programs," with which traditional theories of speech production tend to be aligned, they attempt to explicate the coordinative structure concept in terms of "dynamic principles that have their groundings in homeokinetic physics and dissipative structure (dynamic pattern) theory." They aim to show "that real systems (as opposed to formal machines) consist of ensembles of coupled and mutually entrained oscillators and that coordination is a natural consequence of this organization."

The second part of the monograph considers what can be called constraints on the design of speech sound systems. The basic question here is that of why the sound patterns of languages take the form that they do. The first chapter, by Ladefoged (Chapter 8), is in a way preliminary to this question. As is clear from this chapter we are probably not yet even at the point where the sound *inventories* of the world's languages are properly documented, let alone their patterns of combination within languages. Ladefoged's chapter, presented from the standpoint of traditional articulatory phonetics, is probably the most comprehensive summary of the speech production possibilities in the world's languages currently available. Two implications Ladefoged draws from his analysis are of particular interest: first, perceptual distinctiveness apparently needs to be considered along with production constraints in accounting for the natural patterns of sound contrasts chosen by languages. This important consideration tends to be overlooked in a monograph on speech production; second, classifications of sounds couched in standard (or even new) descriptive terms or distinctive-feature terms must be supplemented by detailed phonetic investigations in order to give a valid indication of the capabilities of the speech production mechanism.

In Chapter 9, Ohala continues his own productive tradition of attempting to explain phonological phenomena in terms of "the real world constraints—physical, physiological, psychological, and social—within which language is used." In this chapter he focuses on aerodynamic properties of speech, and considers their consequences for a number of well-known aspects of sound patterns of languages: preferred segment types, constraints on voicing–devoicing of stops, constraints on voicing in fricatives, frication and devoicing of glides and vowels, blocking of devoicing and affrication by nasalization, stop consonant epenthesis, and conditions on nasal prosody. As a result of this type of work, an increasing number of speech production phenomena are becoming intelligible in terms of the forces that motivate them, rather than appearing as arbitrary elements of sound substance.

Lindblom (Chapter 10) attempts to provide an explanation for a well-known truism: that speech production involves a least-effort principle, or a tendency towards ease of articulation. Using a modelling approach, he finds evidence for two physiologically based conditions of articulation: (1) a synergy constraint governing static spatial relations among articulators in situations involving coarticulation—extreme articulation positions are avoided; (2) a rate constraint resulting in articulatory undershoot in conditions of reduced segment duration. He observes that both processes operate as if "governed by a power constraint limiting energy expenditure per unit time," a constraint he finds to be widespread in forms of motor control other than speech. In the second part of the chapter he reviews assimilation phenomena and coarticulatory contingencies in syllable structure providing further evidence for the power constraint. Lindblom's work, together with Ohala's, is representative of a small group of functionalists who attempt to derive linguistic elements and processes deductively from an extralinguistic base, in contrast to the more common formal approach within linguistics, in which linguistic elements and processes are postulated axiomatically.

Stevens (Chapter 11), like the other authors in this section, is concerned with extralinguistic bases for the form of speech sound systems. But he is distinct from the others in beginning with a strong hypothesis about the role of distinctive features in speech, that "each feature is represented in the sound wave as a unique acoustic property to which the auditory system responds in a distinctive way." In an illustration of his thesis Stevens provides three bodies of data: (1) studies of speech production suggesting that articulatory targets are chosen to maximize signal distinctiveness by favoring configurations in which slight variations in precise positioning have a minimal effect on the signal; (2) acoustic analysis studies seeking evidence for invariant acoustic properties of a feature in different contexts; and (3) psychoacoustic studies and studies of auditory physiology supporting a role of properties of the reception system in determining what will be a distinctive input.

In Chapter 12, in the first of two perspectives on our topic, Mark Liberman addresses an issue crucial to the future development of speech production theory. This issue is the divergence between the approaches of phonologists, attempting to understand sound patterns of languages from the standpoint of an autonomous linguistics tradition (an approach not represented in this volume), and the phonetician, who attempts to account for the observable form of speech from the standpoint of biology and physics. Liberman argues that each of these two approaches could profit from an infusion of traditions from the other, with phonology using more phonetic (and psycholinguistic) evidence to constrain the choices among their various systems of abstract representations, and phonetics paying more attention to the form of the abstract representations which must be central to any explanatory attempts. As an illustration of what Liberman regards as the optimal hybrid approach he reviews his work on intonation: this approach, he argues, was demanded by the nature of the problem, and was in a sense allowed by the absence, in approaches to intonation, of an accepted pretheoretical phonetic symbol system. On the other hand, the presence of such a system in more traditional areas of enquiry (primarily at the segmental level) has allowed the phoneticians and the phonologists, in Liberman's opinion, each to ignore the concerns of the other.

Cooper's concluding chapter is a personal perspective on speech research based on the author's 35 years of experience. In the "retrospective" at the beginning of Chapter 13, he briefly reviews some aspects of the early history of speech research, ranging widely over linguistic, phonetic, acoustic, and engineering contributions. Then he presents a case history of the process by which he and Haskins Laboratories became interested in speech production research from a desire to test implications of the motor theory of speech perception. In the second part of the chapter, Cooper considers some current research problems and reflects on various approaches to them. From this chapter one gets a sense of the enormous progress we have made in technical aspects of speech research but also a sense of fundamental theoretical questions which remain to be answered.

It is to be hoped that this volume will provide the reader not only with an overview of this field of research but also with some sense of the excitement and intrigue that exists in this rapidly developing area. If so, the efforts of the contributors will be well rewarded.

Austin, Texas   PETER F. MACNEILAGE
January, 1983

Contents

List of Contributors

EMILIO BIZZI

Department of Psychology, Massachusetts
Institute of Technology, Cambridge,
Massachusetts 02139, USA

FRANKLIN S. COOPER

Haskins Laboratories, 270 Crown Street,
New Haven, Connecticut 06510, USA

HIROYA FUJISAKI

Department of Electrical Engineering,
University of Tokyo, 731 Hongo,
Bunkyo-Ku, Tokyo, Japan

KATHERINE S. HARRIS

Haskins Laboratories, 270 Crown Street,
New Haven, Connecticut 06510, USA

HAJIME HIROSE

Research Institute of Logopedics and
Phoniatrics, Faculty of Medicine,
University of Tokyo, 731 Hongo,
Bunkyo-Ku, Tokyo, Japan

R. D. KENT

Human Communications Laboratories,
Boys Town Institute for Communication
Disorders in Children, 555 North 30th
Street, Omaha, Nebraska 68131, USA

J.A. SCOTT KELSO

Haskins Laboratories, 270 Crown Street,
New Haven, Connecticut 06510, USA

PETER LADEFOGED

Department of Linguistics, University of California at Los Angeles, Los Angeles, California 90024, USA

M. Y. LIBERMAN

Bell Laboratories, 600 Mountain Avenue, Murray Hill, New Jersey 07974, USA

BJÖRN LINDBLOM

Department of Linguistics, Stockholm University, Fack S-10691, Stockholm, Sweden

PETER F. MACNEILAGE

Departments of Linguistics and Psychology, University of Texas at Austin, Austin, Texas 78712, USA

JOHN J. OHALA

Department of Linguistics, University of California at Los Angeles, Los Angeles, California 90024, USA

D. KIMBROUGH OLLER

Mailman Center for Child Development, University of Miami, P.O. Box 016820, Miami, Florida 33101, USA

MASAYUKI SAWASHIMA

Research Institute of Logopedics and Phoniatrics, Faculty of Medicine, University of Tokyo, 731 Hongo, Bunkyo-Ku, Tokyo, Japan

STEFANIE SHATTUCK-HUFNAGEL

Research Laboratory of Electronics, Massachusetts Institute of Technology, Cambridge, Massachusetts 02139, USA

KENNETH N. STEVENS

Research Laboratory of Electronics, Massachusetts Institute of Technology, Cambridge, Massachusetts 02139, USA

BETTY TULLER

Haskins Laboratories, 270 Crown Street, New Haven, Connecticut 06510, USA

Part I
Control Processes in Speech Production

Chapter 1

Central Processes Involved in Arm Movement Control

Emilio Bizzi

I. Introduction

The mechanism whereby the central nervous system (CNS) controls, simultaneously, the large number of degrees of freedom of the multijoint
musculoskeletal system has long been one of the major questions in motor
physiology. This incredibly complex task must be dependent upon "rules"
which permit original and creative motor solutions to problems such as reaching
for objects in a structured space. As a step toward understanding these rules, a
number of investigators have studied relatively simple motions involving a
limited number of joints (Asatryan & Feldman, 1965; Bizzi, Polit, & Morasso,
1976; Cooke, 1979; Kelso & Holt, 1980). The results have indicated some of
the processes that subserve these movements and have given us a picture of the
elementary building blocks from which more complex movements may be
constructed. Several points have emerged from these investigations. First, it has
become apparent that the forces that control the muscles result from
"commands" that are, to a great extent, precomputed in some part of the CNS.
These observations are based on studies made in deafferented animals that have
demonstrated open-loop reaching (Bizzi et al., 1976; Polit & Bizzi, 1979; Taub,
Goldberg, & Taub, 1975). Second, recent investigations have convincingly
demonstrated that muscles, to a first approximation, can be thought of as
behaving like tunable springs (Rack & Westbury, 1974). In fact, springs and
muscles have a fundamental property in common: they produce force as a
function of length (Feldman, 1966; Partridge, 1979; Rack & Westbury, 1974).

These findings have suggested some possible control strategies whereby the CNS takes advantage of the mechanical properties of the muscles.

In this chapter I will discuss the foregoing points by examining the results obtained from monkeys performing visually evoked head and arm movements. In general, the questions of open-loop control and the role of feedback during movements were studied in intact animals that were later deprived of sensory feedback. In addition, both intact and sensory deprived animals were subjected to various force disturbances. The combination of these two approaches has allowed us to make some inferences on the way in which the CNS controls movement.

II. Experiments and Results

I will review first the results obtained by applying a constant-torque load to the head. When this type of load was applied, a constant degree of head undershoot was observed. In the intact animal, while a constant load was being applied there was an increase in electromyographic (EMG) activity, presumably due to an increase in muscle spindle and tendon organ activity. As shown in Figure 1-1, in spite of these changes in the flow of proprioceptive activity the head reached its "intended" final position *after* the constant load was removed. In fact, the final head position was equal (on average) to that reached when the load had not been applied, which suggests that the program for final position was maintained during load application and was not readjusted by proprioceptive afferents generated during the movement, but is preprogrammed. It should be noted that the load disturbances were totally unexpected and that the monkeys were *not* trained to move their head to a certain position, but chose to program a head movement together with an eye movement in order to perform a visual discrimination task (Bizzi, 1974; Bizzi, Kalil, & Tagliasco, 1971; Bizzi et al, 1976).

In a second set of experiments Bizzi, Polit, and Morasso (1976) examined the effect of stimulating proprioceptors only during the dynamic phase. To this end they used as a stimulus a load that modified the trajectory but did not represent a steady-state disturbance. This was done by using an inertial load. As a result of the sudden and unexpected increase in inertia during centrally initiated head movement, the following changes in head trajectory, relative to unloaded movement, were observed: an initial slowing down of the head, followed by a relative increase in velocity (due to the kinetic energy acquired by the load being transmitted to the decelerating head) that culminated in an overshoot; finally, the head returned to the intended position (Fig. 1-2).

The changes in head trajectory brought about by the sudden and unexpected increase in head inertia induced corresponding modifications in the length and tension of neck muscles. The agonist muscles were, in fact, first subjected to

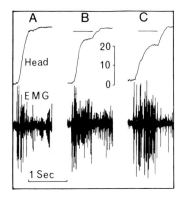

Figure 1-1. Typical visually triggered head movements in chronically vestibulecto-mized monkey to appearance of target at 40° but performed in total darkness. A shows an unloaded movement. In B, a constant-force load (315 g/cm) was applied at the start of the movement, resulting in an undershoot of final position relative to A despite an increase in EMG activity. In C, a constant-force load (726 g/cm) was applied. Note that the head returns to the same final position after removal of the load. Vertical calibration in degrees; time marker is 1 sec; EMG recorded from left splenius capitis. (From Bizzi et al., 1976.)

increased tension because the application of the load slowed down the process of muscle shortening; then the shortening of the same muscles was facilitated during the overshoot phase of the head movement induced by the kinetic energy of the load. Such loading and unloading did, of course, provoke the classical muscle spindle response (presumably mediated by group IA and group II afferent fibers) which, in turn, affected the agonist EMG activity. Figure 1-2B shows that there was first a greater increase in motor unit discharge during muscle stretch than would have occurred if no load were applied, followed by a sudden decrease in activity at the beginning of the overshoot phase. Therefore, during a head movement, an unexpected inertial load induced a series of waxing and waning proprioceptive signals from muscle spindles, tendons, and joints, but the *intended head position* was eventually reached, even in the complete absence of other sensory (visual and vestibular) cues. This observation, together with those on the effect of constant-torque loads, suggests that the central program establishing final head position is not dependent on a readout of proprioceptive afferents generated during the movement, but instead is pre-programmed.

   To provide a further test of the hypothesis that final position is pre-programmed, Bizzi et al. (1976) investigated how chronically vestibulectomized monkeys reached final head position without visual feedback when they were deprived, in addition, of neck proprioceptive feedback. Following the un-expected application of a constant-torque load at the beginning of a visually triggered movement, the posture attained by the head was short of intended final position. After removal of the constant torque, the head attained a position that was found to be equal to the one reached by the head in the no-load case. These results indicate that the head motor system behaved qualitatively in the same way both before and after deafferentation with respect to head position.

I believe that the results of these experiments contribute to our understanding of the mechanism whereby movement is terminated and a newly acquired position is maintained. If one assumes that the "program" for head movements and posture specifies a given level of alpha motoneuron activity to both agonist and antagonist muscles, and that the firing of these neurons will determine a particular length–tension curve in each muscle, then it must be concluded that the final resting position of the head is determined by the length-tension properties of all of the muscles involved. This hypothesis explains both the head undershoot when a constant load is applied and the attainment of the intended final head position following the removal of the load, as shown in Figures 1-1 and 1-2, respectively.

In a complementary set of experiments involving arm movements, Polit and Bizzi (1979) extended the previously described findings on the final position of the head. Adult rhesus monkeys were trained to point to a target light with the forearm and to hold the arm in that position for about 1 sec in order to obtain a reward (Figure 1-3). The monkey was seated in a primate chair, and its forearm was fastened to an elbow apparatus that permitted flexion and extension of the forearm about the elbow in the horizontal plane. A torque motor in series with

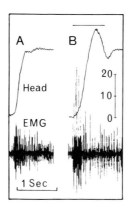

Figure 1-2. Typical head responses of a chronically vestibulectomized monkey to sudden appearance of target at $-40°$. A represents an unloaded movement, whereas in B a load of approximately six times the inertia of the head was applied at the start of the movement, as indicated by the force record. Both movements were performed in total darkness, the light having been turned off by the increase in EMG (splenius capitis). Peak force exerted by the monkey is approximately 750 g/cm; head calibration is in degrees; time marker is 1 sec. (From Bizzi et al., 1976.)

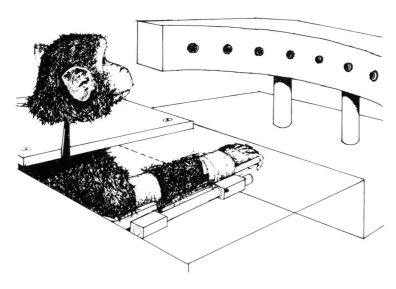

Figure 1-3.   Monkey set up in arm apparatus. Arm is strapped to splint, which pivots at elbow. Target lights are mounted in perimeter arc at 5° intervals. During experimental session, the monkey was not permitted to see its arm, and the room was darkened. (From Polit & Bizzi, 1979.)

the shaft of this apparatus was used to apply positional disturbances to the arm. The experiments were conducted in a dark room to minimize visual cues; at no time during an experiment was the animal able to see its forearm. At random times, the initial position of the forearm was displaced. In most cases, the positional disturbance was applied immediately after the appearance of the target light and was stopped just prior to the activation of the motor units in the agonist muscle. Hence, when the motor command specifying a given forearm movement occurred, the positional disturbance had altered the length of the agonist and antagonist muscles, and the proprioceptive stimulation resulting from this disturbance had altered their state of activation. In spite of these changes, the intended final arm position was always reached; this was true whether the torque motor had displaced the forearm farther away from, closer to, or even beyond the intended final position. There were no significant differences among the final positions achieved in these three conditions. Naturally, the attainment of the intended arm position in this experiment could be explained by assuming that afferent proprioceptive information modified the original motor command. However, the results of previous work on final head position suggest an alternative hypothesis: The motor program underlying arm movement specifies, through the selection of a new set of length–tension curves, an equilibrium point between agonists and antagonists that correctly positions the arm in relation to the visual target. To investigate this hypothesis, Polit and

Bizzi (1979) retested the monkey's pointing performance after it had undergone a bilateral C_1–T_3 dorsal rhizotomy. They could elicit the pointing response very soon after the surgery (within 2 days in some of the animals). The forearm was again displaced (at random times) immediately after the appearance of the target light and released just prior to the activation of motor units in the agonist muscles. Even though the arm was not visible to the animal and the proprioceptive activity could not reach the spinal cord, the arm reached its intended final position "open loop" (a fact corroborated by lack of any sign of reflex response or reprogramming in the EMG activity). For each target position, t tests were performed to test for differences between the average final position of movements in the undisturbed and the disturbed conditions. No significant differences were found.

These findings, together with those derived from head movement experiments, suggest that arm and head movements depend on neural patterns that are programmed prior to movement initiation. What is being preprogrammed is a process that is capable of controlling final head and arm position as an equilibrium point resulting from the interaction of agonist and antagonist muscles. This view may be illustrated by reference to a simple mechanical analogue. Assume that the muscles moving a body segment can be represented by a pair of springs acting across a hinge in the agonist–antagonist configuration. If the CNS were to specify a new length–tension relationship for one of the springs, movements would occur until a new equilibrium point of the two opposing springs was reached. However, the specification of a new set of length-tension settings does not occur in a steplike fashion. In fact, recent experimental evidence addressed to the question of the time course of the neural signal executing the transition from an initial to a final posture has demonstrated the existence of a gradually changing control signal during arm movement performed at moderate speed (Bizzi, Accornero, Chapple, & Hogan, 1982).

III. Conclusion

The experimental evidence that has been summarized here indicates that for certain visuomotor responses the "commands" to the musculature are preprogrammed. What is being specified by these commands is a trajectory as well as a final position. Whether the process underlying final arm position and the process specifying movement duration and velocity can be thought of as parallel and relatively independent processes or as a single process specifying, in time, a series of positions remains to be ascertained.

A second goal of these studies was to develop some perspectives on the role of afferent feedback during voluntary movements (Bizzi et al., 1976; Bizzi, Dev, Morasso, & Polit, 1978; Polit & Bizzi, 1979). The studies of the deafferented animal showed that the successful execution of forearm programs released by target presentation was contingent on the animal's knowing the position of its arm relative to its body. Whenever the usual spatial relationship between the animal and the arm apparatus was changed or a constant-bias load was applied, the monkey's pointing response was inaccurate. The intact monkeys, in contrast, were able to compensate quickly for any variations in their accustomed position with respect to the arm apparatus. The dramatic inability of the deafferented monkey to execute accurate pointing responses in an unusual postural setting or when a constant-bias load was applied underscores the great importance of afferent feedback in updating and adjusting the execution of learned motor patterns when posture is changed. These findings emphasize the widespread influence and importance of afferent impulses in the control of voluntary movement. They suggest that, in addition to contributing to the classical spinal and supraspinal reflex loops, which may servo-assist movement (Marsden, Merton, & Morton, 1976a, 1976b; Vallbo, 1973; Wilson, 1961), provide a small contribution to load compensation (Allum, 1975; Bizzi et al., 1978; Conrad, Matsunami, Meyer-Lohmann, Weisendanger, & Brooks, 1974), and/or linearize muscle properties (Nichols & Houk, 1973, 1976), the afferent system may affect, in a manner that is not yet understood, a reorganization of the central processes that are released when targets are presented. It is perhaps of interest to comment that although servo assistance or load compensation can occur during a single centrally driven movement, the postulated reorganization has a longer time scale, encompassing a few movements.

Acknowledgments. This research was supported by National Institute of Neurological Disease and Stroke Research Grant NSO9343, National Institute of Arthritis, Metabolism and Digestive Diseases Research Grant AM 26710, and National Eye Institute Grant EYO2621.

References

Allum, J. H. J. Responses to load disturbances in human shoulder muscles: The hypothesis that one component is a pulse test information signal. *Experimental Brain Research*, 1975, *22*, 307–326.

Asatryan, D. G., & Feldman, A. G. Biophysics of complex systems and mathematical models. Functional tuning of nervous system with control of movement or maintenance of a steady posture. I. Mechanographic analysis of the work of the joint on execution of a postural task. *Biophysics*, 1965, *10*, 925–935.

Bizzi, E. The coordination of eye–head movement. *Scientific American*, 1974, *231*, 100–106.

Bizzi, E., Accornero, N., Chapple, W., & Hogan, N. Arm trajectory formation in monkeys. Experimental Brain Research, 1982, 46, 139–143.

Bizzi, E., Dev, P., Morasso, P., & Polit, A. The effect of load disturbances during centrally initiated movements. *Journal of Neurophysiology*, 1978, *41*, 542–556.

Bizzi, E., Kalil, R. E., & Tagliasco, V. Eye–head coordination in monkeys: Evidence for centrally patterned organization. *Science*, 1971, *173*, 452–454.

Bizzi, E., Polit, A., & Morasso, P. Mechanisms underlying achievement of final head position. *Journal of Neurophysiology*, 1976, *39*, 435–444.

Conrad, B., Matsunami, C., Meyer-Lohmann, J., Wiesendanger, M., & Brooks, V. B. Cortical load compensation during voluntary elbow movements. *Brain Research*, 1974, *81*, 507–514.

Cooke, J. D. Dependence of human arm movements on limb mechanical properties. *Brain Research*, 1979, *165*, 366–369.

Feldman, A. G. Functional tuning of the nervous system during control of movement or maintenance of a steady posture. III. Mechanographic analysis of the execution by man of the simplest motor tasks. *Biophysics*, 1966, *11*, 766–775.

Kelso, J. A. S., & Holt, K. G. Exploring a vibratory system's analysis of human movement production. *Journal of Neurophysiology*, 1980, *43*, 1183–1196.

Marsden, C. D., Merton, P. A., & Morton, H. B. Servo action in the human thumb. *Journal of Physiology, London*, 1976, *257*, 1–44. (a)

Marsden, C. D., Merton, P. A., & Morton, H. B. Stretch reflexes and servo actions in a variety of human muscles. *Journal of Physiology, London*, 1976, *257*, 531–560.(b)

Nichols, T. R. & Houk, J. C. Reflex compensation for variations in the mechanical properties of a muscle. *Science*, 1973, *181*, 182–184.

Nichols, T. R., & Houk, J. C. The improvement in linearity and the regulation of stiffness that results from the actions of the stretch reflex. *Journal of Neurophysiology*, 1976, *39*, 119–142.

Partridge, L. D. Muscle properties: A problem for the motor controller physiologist. In R. E. Talbott & D. R. Humphrey (Eds.), *Posture and movement*. New York: Raven Press, 1979.

Polit, A., & Bizzi, E. Characteristics of motor programs underlying arm movements in monkeys. *Journal of Neurophysiology*, 1979, *42*, 183–194.

Rack, P. M. H., & Westbury, D. R. The short range stiffness of active mammalian muscle and its effect on mechanical properties. *Journal of Physiology, London*, 1974, *240*, 331–350.

Taub, E., Goldberg, I. A., & Taub, P. Deafferentation in monkeys: Pointing at a target without visual feedback. *Experimental Neurology*, 1975, *46*, 178–186.

Vallbo, Å. B. The significance of intramuscular receptors in load compensation during voluntary contractions in man. In R. B. Stein, K. G. Pearson, R. S. Smith, & J. B. Redford, (Eds.), *Control of posture and locomotion*. New York: Plenum, 1973.

Wilson, D. M. The central nervous control of flight in a locust. *Journal of Experimental Biology*, 1961, *38*, 471–490.

Chapter 2

Laryngeal Gestures in Speech Production

MASAYUKI SAWASHIMA and HAJIME HIROSE

I. Introduction

This chapter describes the physiological mechanisms of laryngeal gestures for various phonetic distinctions in speech production. An orientation toward the basic laryngeal gestures is presented in Section II, and detailed experimental data are discussed in Section III.

II. Basic Laryngeal Gestures

The framework of the larynx consists of four different cartilages: the epiglottis, thyroid, cricoid, and arytenoid cartilages. The thyroid and cricoid cartilages are connected by the cricothyroid joint. The movements of this joint change the length of the vocal fold. Movements of the arytenoid cartilage on the surface of the cricoarytenoid joint contribute to the abduction–adduction of the vocal fold. Abduction of the vocal fold also results in an increase in the vocal fold length. Studies of the functional anatomy of the cricoarytenoid joint in human larynges (Sonesson, 1958; von Leden & Moore, 1961; Frable, 1961; Takase, 1964) have revealed that the main part of the joint movement is a rotating motion (abduction–adduction) of the arytenoid cartilage around the longitudinal axis of the joint. Other possible movements of the arytenoid are a small degree of sliding motion along the longitudinal axis of the joint and a rocking motion with a fixed point at the attachment of the posterior cricoarytenoid ligament. In some classical textbooks a rotating motion of the arytenoid around its vertical axis has been described; however, this kind of joint movement is quite unlikely. The results of these studies have been summarized elsewhere (Sawashima, 1974).

Movements of the cricothyroid and cricoarytenoid joints are controlled by the intrinsic laryngeal muscles. Elongation of the vocal fold is achieved by contraction of the cricothyroid muscle. Movements of the arytenoid cartilage and the resultant abduction–adduction of the vocal fold are controlled by the abductor and adductor muscles. The posterior cricoarytenoid muscle is the only abductor muscle, while the other three—the interarytenoid, lateral crico-arytenoid, and thyroarytenoid muscles—are the adductor muscles. Contraction of the cricothyroid muscle may also result in a small degree of glottal abduction. The vocalis muscle, which is the medial part of the thyroarytenoid muscle, contributes to the control of the effective mass and stiffness of the vocal fold rather than to abduction–adduction movements.

The layer structure of the vocal fold edge described by Hirano (1975) is shown in Figure 2-1. As can be seen in the figure, the vocal fold consists of the mucosa epithelium, the lamina propria, and the vocalis muscle. In the lamina propria, the superficial layer is the loose connective tissue, and the intermediate and deep layers correspond to the vocal ligament. Based on this layer structure, Hirano proposed a structural model of the vocal fold. In his model, the vocal fold consists of three structures—cover, transition, and body—each having different physical or mechanical properties. The cover includes the mucosa epithelium and the superficial layer of the lamina propria; the transition includes the intermediate and the deep layers; and the body includes the vocalis muscle. To simplify the model, we may consider the transition as part of the body.

Hirano proposed this cover–body model in order to explain variations in the mode of vocal fold vibration with different laryngeal adjustments and with various pathological conditions. Contraction of the cricothyroid muscle elong-ates the vocal fold, its effective mass being decreased. Because of the elongation of the vocal fold, the stiffness of both the cover and body increases. This is the situation of the vocal fold for phonation in the falsetto or the light register. Contraction of the vocalis muscle, in contrast, shortens the vocal fold, its effective mass being increased. Stiffness of the body increases while that of the cover decreases. Contraction of the vocalis muscle in combination with the cricothyroid usually takes place for phonation in the chest or the heavy register. Thus the difference in the model of vocal fold vibration between the falsetto and the chest registers can be accounted for by the different conditions of the cover and the body.

The entire larynx is supported by the extrinsic laryngeal muscles, of which the

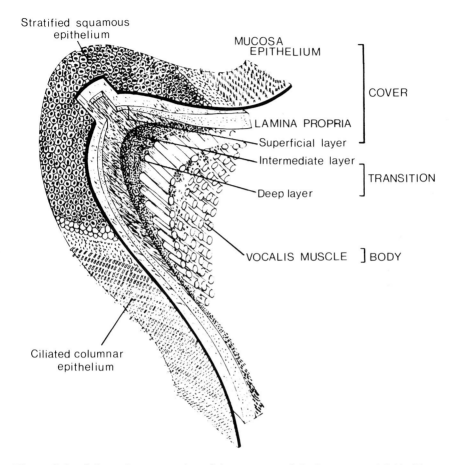

Figure 2-1. Schematic presentation of the structure of the human vocal fold. (From Hirano, 1975.)

suprahyoid and infrahyoid muscles form the important members. These muscles contribute to the up and down movements of the larynx, as well as to articulatory adjustments such as jaw opening. Whether or not these muscles are the primary contributors to the control of phonation is still to be examined.

The basic features of the laryngeal adjustments may be summarized as follows:

1. abduction–adduction of the vocal folds;
2. constriction of the false vocal folds and other supraglottic laryngeal structures;
3. changes in the length and thickness of the vocal fold;
4. up and down movements of the larynx.

A. Abduction–Adduction of the Glottis

This type of adjustment is used for the distinction of respiration versus phonation, as well as for the voiced versus voiceless distinction during speech production. The vocal folds are fully abducted with an increase in the activity of the posterior cricoarytenoid muscle for deep inspiration. For quiet respiration, the extent of the glottal opening is approximately half that for deep inspiration. This vocal fold position is known as the intermediate position. The activities of both the abductor and adductor muscles are minimal in the case of quiet respiration.

For normal phonation, the vocal folds are in the adducted position and are set vibrating by transglottal air flow. In this position, a narrow spindle-shaped gap is usually seen in the membranous portion of the glottis before the vocal folds start to vibrate, as shown in Figure 2-2. There is an increase in the activity of the adductor and vocalis muscles, coupled with a decrease in the activity of the posterior cricoarytenoid (abductor) muscles. The cricothyroid muscle is also activated for phonation. The transglottal air flow may also generate vocal fold vibration with the glottis open to a certain extent. The resultant voice is the breathy voice or murmur.

The general picture of the glottal condition in the abduction–adduction dimension during speech is that the glottis is closed or nearly closed for voiced sounds whereas it is open for voiceless sounds, the extent of the glottal opening varying with different phonemes and phonological environments. An example of the glottal opening and closing movements for an utterance of a Japanese word /keikei/ in a frame sentence is shown in Figure 2–3 (Sawashima, Hirose & Yoshioka, 1976). It is seen that for the word-initial [k] there is a fairly large extent of glottal opening, although the glottal aperture is smaller than in the case of respiration. The distance between the tips of the arytenoid cartilages provides a good measure of the degree of glottal opening. For the word-medial [k], the glottal aperture is observed to be noticeably smaller than that for the word-initial [k].

Some languages, such as Korean, Chinese, and Hindi, show a phonemic distinction between aspirated and unaspirated voiceless stops. The time course of glottal width for aspirated and unaspirated voiceless stops in Fukienese, a dialect of southern China, is shown in Figure 2-4 (Iwata, Sawashima, Hirose, & Niimi, 1979). In the figure, the abscissa indicates the time axis and the ordinate the glottal width. The vertical line near the middle of the time axis is the time point of the oral release. In the aspirated stops there is a great degree of glottal opening, and the peak glottal width is reached near the time of the oral release. For the unaspirated stops, the glottis is also open but the size of the glottal aperture is far smaller. Furthermore, the glottis is closed or nearly closed at the oral release.

The abduction–adduction of the glottis is mainly controlled by the posterior cricoarytenoid (abductor) and interarytenoid (adductor) muscles respectively

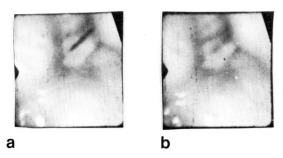

a   **b**

Figure 2-2. Glottal views at the phonatory position immediately before (a) and after (b) the onset of vocal fold vibration.

(Hirose & Gay, 1972; Hirose & Ushijima, 1978; Hirose, Yoshioka, & Niimi, 1978). The time course of glottal width and integrated electromyographic (EMG) curves of the two muscles for the [s] of the Japanese word /iseH/ in a frame sentence uttered by two subjects are shown in Figure 2-5a. Figure 2-5b shows the same display for the voiceless sound sequence [siss] in /siQseH/ where the vowel /i/ between the word-initial [s] and the medial [ss] is unvoiced. There is a clear reciprocal pattern in the activity of the two muscles— suppression of the interarytenoid (INT) muscle and activation of the posterior cricoarytenoid (PCA) muscle—for glottal opening corresponding to the voice-

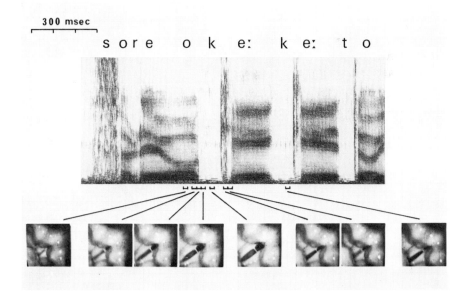

Figure 2-3. Selected frames of a laryngeal film and a sound spectrogram of the utterance /keikei/ in a frame sentence. (From Sawashima et al., 1976.)

oral release

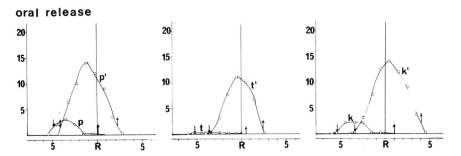

Figure 2-4. Time curves of glottal width for aspirated and unaspirated stops in Fukienese. (From Iwata et al., 1979.)

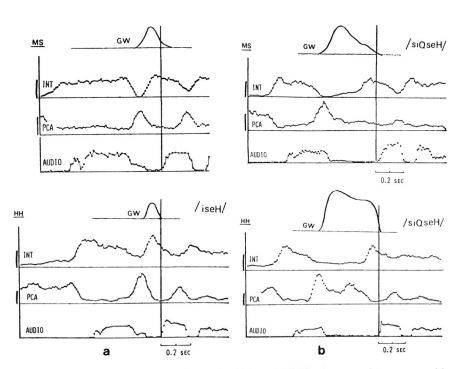

Figure 2-5. The time course of glottal width and EMG patterns of interarytenoid (INT) and posterior cricoarytenoid (PCA) muscles for the [s] of /iseH/ (a) and the [sʲss] of /siQseH/ (b). (From Sawashima et al., 1978.)

less sounds. Contrary to the voiceless sounds, there is an exactly reverse pattern—activation of the INT and suppression of the PCA—for the voiced segments where the glottis is closed. For both subjects, it is seen that the extent as well as the time course of the glottal width is well represented by the activity patterns of the two muscles, although there seems to be some subject-to-subject variation in the relative extent of the contribution of these muscles.

The voiced–voiceless distinction is achieved by control of the glottal conditions in combination with the aerodynamic conditions at the glottis. Figure 2-6 shows transillumination traces for the syllables containing voiced and voiceless sounds in Japanese in a frame sentence. Abduction–adduction of the vocal folds as well as the presence or absence of vocal fold vibration can be observed in each trace. It is noted that the intervocalic /h/ is voiced in spite of a considerable degree of glottal opening. In the /h/ here, there is no constriction in the vocal tract, and the resulting fast air flow through the glottis enables the vocal fold to maintain vibration. For the medial [t] of /te²te/, in contrast, the vocal fold vibration ceases immediately after the oral closure in spite of a very small glottal opening. The oral closure prevents the air from passing through the glottis. Thus the extent of the glottal opening itself is not necessarily a crucial condition for the cessation of the vocal fold vibration. A gradual cessation of the vocal fold vibration in [s] may also reflect the aerodynamic condition at the glottis caused by the oral constriction. The aerodynamic effect on the vocal fold vibration with the closed glottis is also observable in voiced consonants. For [d], there is a decrease in both the amplitude and frequency because of the oral

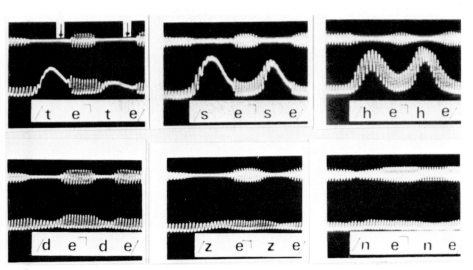

Figure 2-6. Photoelectric glottograms for Japanese consonants. Lower trace: glottogram; upper trace: oscillogram. Bar = 200 msec.

closure. For [n], however, no such change is observable because the nasal passage is open for the air flow.

B. Constriction of the False Vocal Folds and Other Supraglottic Laryngeal Structures

A typical example of supraglottic laryngeal constriction with the glottis open is observed in whispered phonation, as shown in Figure 2-7 (Weitzman, Sawashima, Hirose, & Ushijima, 1976). Here, an adduction of the false vocal folds takes place with a decrease in the size of the anterior–posterior dimension of the larynx cavity. This type of laryngeal constriction becomes more exaggerated for the strong, so-called stage whispering. This particular gesture for whispering is considered to contribute to the prevention of the vocal fold vibration by the transglottal air flow, as well as to facilitate the generation of turbulent noise in the larynx cavity.

The physiological mechanism behind supraglottic laryngeal constriction is not clear. There seems to be no systematic study on this type of laryngeal adjustment. Our experiences with laryngeal EMG indicate that in whispering there is a greater activity of the lateral cricoarytenoid muscle as compared with normal phonation. This might be related to supraglottic laryngeal constriction. An increase in the activity of the PCA to a certain extent combined with a decrease in INT activity also appears to characterize whispered phonation. This

[i]   [u]   [i]   [u]

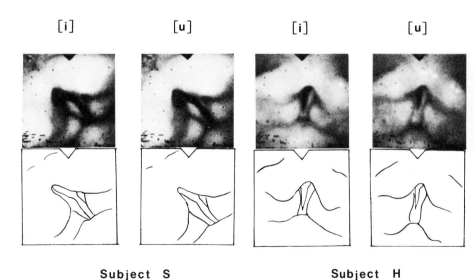

Subject   S   Subject   H

Figure 2-7. Laryngeal pictures for whispered vowels.

should account for the glottal abduction in whispering. The activity of the cricothyroid (CT) muscle is observed to be suppressed for whispering.

Supraglottic laryngeal constriction with the closed glottis is typically observed for the glottal stop, as can be seen in Figure 2-8. The figure shows the laryngeal view for the glottal stop as the syllable-final applosive sound in Fukienese (Iwata et al., 1979). This type of gesture is also observable for the syllable-final stops in English (Fujimura & Sawashima, 1971). The gesture prevents the air from the lung from passing through the glottis. The lateral cricoarytenoid muscle also appears to show a high degree of activity for this particular gesture.

A lesser degree of supraglottic laryngeal constriction with the glottis closed may be considered to characterize the gesture known as "laryngealization," as pointed out by Gauffin (1977). Figure 2-9 shows laryngeal pictures for sustained phonations in different pitches and intensities. The pictures suggest

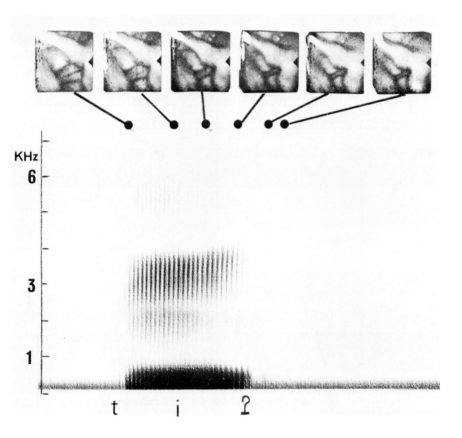

Figure 2-8.   Selected frames of a laryngeal film and a sound spectrogram for the utterance [ti?] in Fukienese.

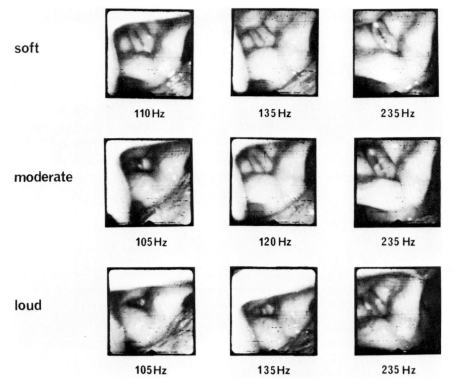

Figure 2-9. Laryngeal pictures for sustained phonations in different pitches and intensities.

that in addition to the elongation or thickening of the vocal folds, the supraglottic laryngeal constrictions may also contribute to vocal pitch control, especially for producing a loud voice with low pitch.

C. Changes in the Length and Thickness of the Vocal Folds

A good example of this type of adjustment is the control of vocal pitch, F_0, during voicing. F_0 control at the larynx is considered to be achieved mainly by controlling the effective mass and the stiffness of the vocal folds. Among the intrinsic muscles, possible candidates contributing to these controls are the cricothyroid and the vocalis muscles. Figure 2-10 shows the EMG curves of these two muscles for stepwise F_0 changes during sustained phonation in the chest register (Sawashima, Gay, & Harris, 1969). The activity of both muscles increases for raising pitch and decreases for lowering pitch. As mentioned earlier, contraction of the cricothyroid muscle elongates the vocal folds. The

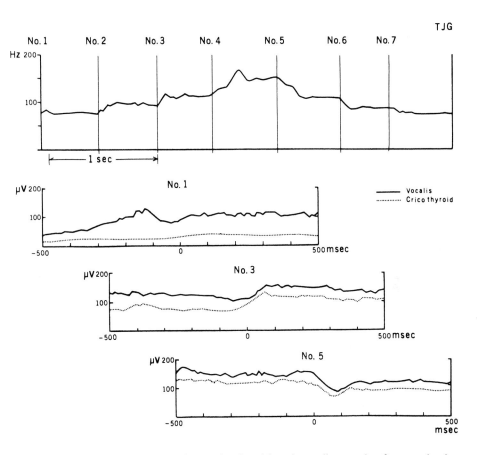

Figure 2-10. EMG patterns of the cricothyroid and vocalis muscles for sustained phonation in stepwise change in F_0.

results are a decrease in the effective mass and an increase in the stiffness of both the body and the cover. Contraction of the vocalis muscle results in a thickening of the vocal folds, their effective mass being increased. The stiffness of the body increases while that of the cover decreases.

In the chest register, a rise in vocal pitch is characteristically achieved by contractions of both muscles. The most noticeable difference in muscle control between the chest and the falsetto registers is observed in the activity of the vocalis muscle, as shown in Figure 2-11 (Sawashima et al., 1969). In the falsetto, as compared to the chest voice, there is a marked decrease in the EMG level in the vocalis, accompanied by a slight decrease in CT activity. The difference in the muscle control between the two registers results in a difference in the physical conditions of the cover and body of the vocal folds, which is reflected in the mode of vocal fold vibration. The laryngeal views and the

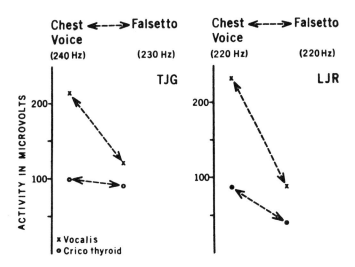

Figure 2-11. EMG levels of the cricothyroid and vocalis muscles for phonations in the chest and falsetto registers.

transillumination traces of the glottal vibrations for the two registers are contrasted in Figure 2-12.

In speech, the CT is the only muscle that is uniquely related to F_0 changes, as shown in Figure 2-13. At the bottom of the figure, two different F_0 contours for the sentences /i ⌐ zininaru/ and /izi ⌐ ninaru/ are illustrated. In the upper part of the figure are shown the EMG patterns of the cricothyroid (CT), the sterno-hyoid (SH), and the sternothyroid (Sth) muscles for the two sentences. The activity of the sternothyroid also appears to be correlated to F_0 lowering in this case. The problem concerning the participation of the extrinsic laryngeal muscles, especially for pitch lowering, is discussed in Section II.

Stiffening or slackening of the vocal folds associated with the voicing distinction has been proposed by Halle and Stevens (1971). According to their proposal, stiffening of the vocal folds takes place for voiceless consonants, and slackening for voiced consonants. In this problem too, the activity levels of the CT and vocalis may provide good physiological correlates of stiffening/slackening controls. Experimental data so far obtained indicate that this problem still needs to be examined, as discussed in Section II.

D. Up and Down Movements of the Larynx

This type of adjustment is typically seen in the action of swallowing, as well as very often during speech with vocal pitch control and voiced–voiceless distinction. But the contribution of these movements to the phonetic distinctions

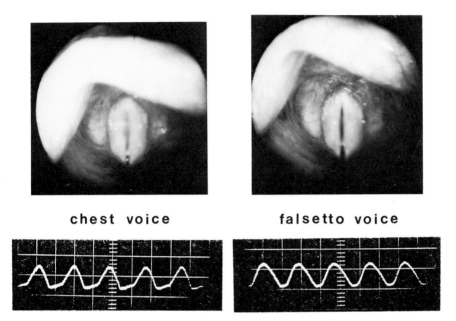

chest voice   **falsetto voice**

Figure 2-12. Laryngeal views and photoelectric glottograms for chest and falsetto voices.

still needs to be examined, except for specific adjustments such as the elevation of the larynx for the ejective sound and the lowering of the larynx for generating or maintaining the vocal fold vibration with the vocal tract closed.

III. Laryngeal Articulatory Adjustments

The basic laryngeal mechanisms are considered to consist of three different postures of the larynx, that is, those for breathing, phonation, and airway protection. These postures are also widely used in the production of different languages as glottal adduction–abduction gestures or the glottal stop gesture. The principal mechanism underlying adduction–abduction is reciprocal activation of the adductor and abductor groups of the larynx.

The reciprocal activity pattern between the two groups of laryngeal muscles has been revealed by recent electromyographic studies combined with fiber-optic observation. In particular, the posterior cricoarytenoid (PCA) is found to be important for the active vocal fold abduction for those speech sounds produced with an open glottis (Hirose, 1976). The reciprocity between the PCA and the adductors has been observed for different languages, including American English, Japanese, Danish, and French.

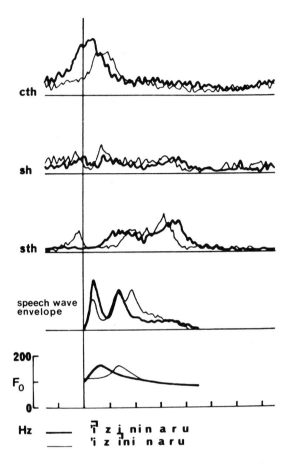

Figure 2-13. Laryngeal EMG patterns and F_0 contours for utterances of /i⌐ zininaru/ and /izi⌐ ninaru/. (From Simada & Hirose, 1971.)

Figure 2-14 shows an example of averaged EMG curves of the interarytenoid (INT), the adductor, and the PCA, for a pair of test words /əpʌp/ and /əbʌp/ produced by an American English speaker (Hirose & Gay, 1972). It can be seen that PCA activity is suppressed for the voiced portion of the test words, whereas it increases for the production of the intervocalic voiceless stop /p/ as well as for the word-final /p/. On the other hand, the INT shows a reciprocal pattern when compared with that of the PCA in that its activity increases for the voiced portion and decreases for the voiceless portion of the test words.

The glottal opening gesture and its timing were further observed in more complicated phonetic conditions in American English. For example, a recent study on American English clusters like /sk/ sequences revealed interesting findings (Yoshioka, Löfqvist, & Hirose, 1979). Figure 2-15 compares /sk/

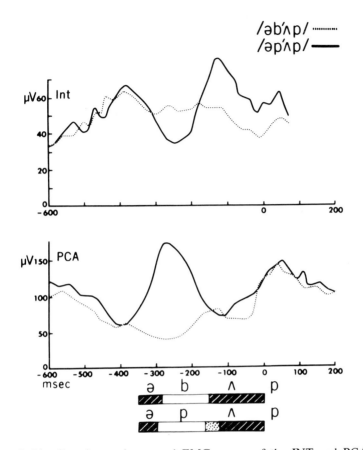

Figure 2-14. Superimposed averaged EMG curves of the INT and PCA for the utterances /əpʌp/ (——) and /əbʌp/ (· · ·). The lineup point (zero on the abscissa) indicates voice offset of the stressed vowel.

sequences in different phonetic conditions represented by three utterance types: "I may scale," "My ace caves," and "I mask aid." Note that there are two distinct peaks in the PCA activity curve for the /sk/ sequence when a word boundary intervenes, where the glottal width curve also shows two separate peaks.

This type of reciprocal control of the laryngeal muscles associated with glottal adduction–abduction gestures has been found not only in the typical voiced–voiceless contrast but also in more complex phonetic conditions. As an extreme example, one of our previously reported data on laryngeal adjustment for a five-way distinction in labial stops produced by an American phonetician is shown in Figure 2-16, in which the activities of the PCA and INT are compared among five phonetic types: voiced inaspirates, implosive voiced

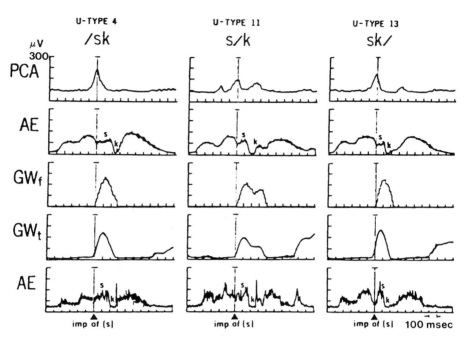

Figure 2-15. Averaged EMG of the PCA, (top trace) averaged audio envelopes (AE), representative plots of glottal width using fiber optics (GW_f), corresponding glottograms (GW_t) and unaveraged audio envelopes for three utterance types: "I may scale" (type 4), "My ace caves" (type 11), and "I mask aid" (type 13). (From Yoshioka et al., 1979.)

inaspirates, voiced aspirates, voiceless aspirates, and voiceless inaspirates (Hirose, Lisker, & Abramson, 1972). Each stop type was embedded in a nonsense trisyllabic word t^hikiCV, where C stands for each type of stop and V for /i/, /a/, and /u/. The zero on the time axis marks the lineup point for averaging, which was taken at the implosion of each stop closure. For each type, three curves are superimposed, each of which represents one of the three different vowels in the word-final position. It can be seen that regardless of the difference in the final vowels, the three curves for each stop show similar contours. Further, it must be noted here that, except for the variation relevant to the phonetic difference among the labial stops, the contours of the five different types are quite similar. This would indicate that the pattern of activity of each of the two muscles for the carrier portion of the test utterance is constant, irrespective of the difference in the embedded labial stops.

It can also be seen that PCA activity increases for the following three labial stop types: voiced aspirates, voiceless aspirates, and voiceless inaspirates, while corresponding INT suppression can also be seen for these three types. Further,

PCA   **INT**

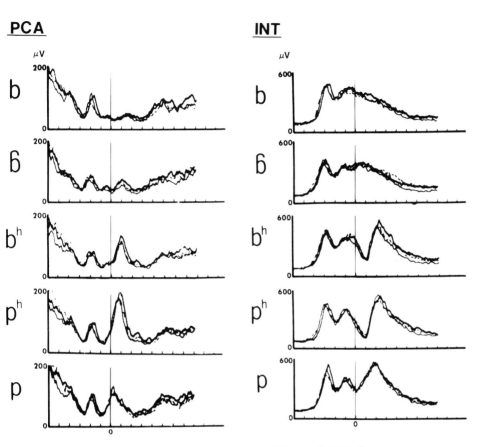

Figure 2-16. Averaged EMG curves of the PCA and INT for test utterances containing five phonetically different labial stops embedded word-medially. A nonsense word "tʰikiCV" is used as a test utterance, where C stands for a labial stop and V is either /i/, /a/ or /u/. For each stop type, three curves are superimposed, each of which represents a different vowel carrier following the stop consonant.

for the three types, analysis of a fiber-optic movie taken separately in the same subject reveals separation of the arytenoids corresponding to stop production.

Thus the degree of glottal abduction appears to be controlled by activation of the PCA associated with the INT and other adductor suppression. For glottal adduction, the lateral cricoarytenoid (LCA) in this subject appeared to provide supplementary adduction control. Similar findings were also obtained in other experimental conditions. As Dixit (1975) claimed and other anatomical studies have suggested, the action of the INT alone does not seem to fully adduct the vocal fold. Rather, it may be plausible to consider that the INT provides the finer adjustments of the glottal aperture for various speech sounds, possibly with supportive action of the LCA, once the larynx has been geared to "speech mode" by the activation of all the adductors and the suppression of the PCA.

Figure 2-17 shows the relationship between the pattern of PCA activity and the time course of the glottal width measured at the vocal processes of the three stop types showing arytenoid separation (Hirose, 1977b). The curves are lined up at the articulatory release taken as time 0 on the abscissa, and durations of oral closure and aspiration are also illustrated. It is shown in this figure that there is a good agreement not only in degree but also in timing between PCA activity and the opening gesture of the glottis. Thus, we must fully realize that, in addition to the control of the degree of glottal adduction–abduction dimension, the control of laryngeal timing is also quite essential in phonetic realization of different types of consonants. As explicitly discussed by Abramson (1977), various languages of the world make extensive use of the timing of the valvular action of the larynx relative to supraglottal articulation in order to distinguish classes of consonants, although certain nonlaryngeal features such as pharyngeal expansion may also be linked with laryngeal timing.

One may argue that these results were not obtained from a native speaker of the specific language. However, our subsequent analysis of the laryngeal behavior in the speaker of a comparable language, such as Hindi, has generally confirmed these findings. Recent fiber-optic studies by Benguerel and Bhatia have also confirmed that the timing of glottal gestures relative to the oral release clearly distinguishes among the three stop types of Hindi discussed earlier.

The contribution to the voicing distinction of each intrinsic laryngeal muscle other than the PCA and INT is not completely understood as yet. Figure 2-18 shows an example of averaged EMG curves of the thyroarytenoid (VOC), LCA, and CT for the production of a Swedish labial stop pair /p/ versus /b/ in different phonetic environments, where we can compare voiced and voiceless as well as long and short contrasts (Hirose, 1977a). As can be seen, both the VOC and LCA are more clearly suppressed for short and long voiceless consonants, given in the left half of the figure, when compared to their voiced counterparts. This would indicate that, at least in this case, these adductors are involved in the voicing distinction. It can also be seen that CT suppression is less marked for voiceless consonants than for voiced.

Figure 2-19 compares the patterns of EMG suppression of the INT, VOC, LCA, and CT for the consonantal segments of Japanese test words in which voiced and voiceless stops and fricatives placed in both word-initial and word-medial positions were considered for paired comparison (Hirose & Ushijima, 1978). For each muscle, the leftmost point indicates the value of the averaged EMG peak for the vowel segment preceding the consonant, which is unanimously taken as 100%. The EMG value for the consonantal segment is plotted along the right side of each figure, again with the peak value for the preceding vowel taken to be 100%. The figure shows that INT suppression is consistently more marked for voiceless than for voiced cognates if the comparison is made in the same phonetic environment. On the other hand, the degree of suppression of the LCA and VOC appears to be different depending

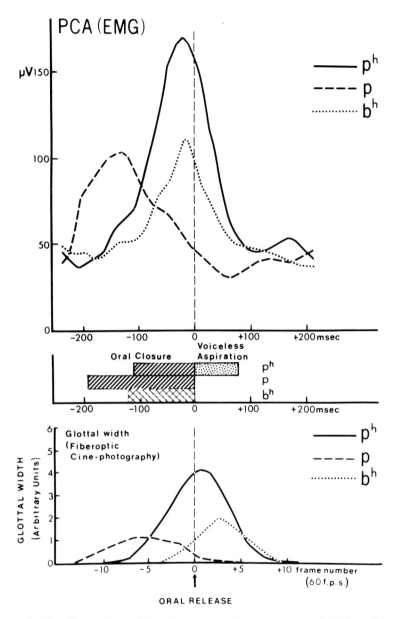

Figure 2-17. Comparison of the time courses between averaged PCA activity and glottal opening gesture. All curves are lined up at the oral release.

primarily on the phonetic environment and not on voicing distinction. In the same environment, suppression appears to be more marked in the VOC than in the LCA. Suppression of the CT is not remarkable in the word-medial position, whereas in the word-initial position it is generally more marked for the voiced cognates (Hirose & Ushijima, 1978).

As suggested by Dixit (1975), the CT can contribute to the increase in tension of the vocal fold, which might eventually be relevant for eliminating voicing. In this sense, it might be plausible to consider the relatively high CT activity in the production of a voiceless consonant in certain cases as one possible factor in enhancing voicelessness. However, this is not always the case. Our studies on American English, French, and Hindi did not confirm the CT contribution to voicelessness, and in the case of Danish, a relatively high activity of the CT was seen for voiced /h/, which was produced with an open glottis. Thus, the interpretation of the apparent high CT activity in certain consonantal segments is still unresolved and further investigation is warranted.

It has been pointed out that another dimension independent of glottal adduction–abduction must be taken into consideration in the case of laryngeal control relating to specific phonetic phenomena (Hirose, 1977b). An example is

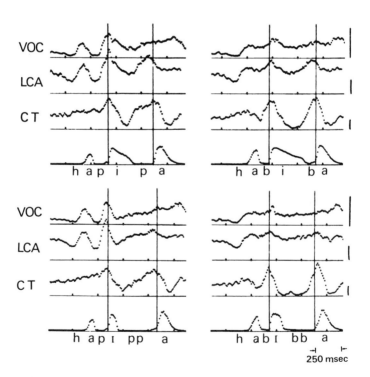

Figure 2-18.   Averaged EMG curves of the VOC, LCA, and CT of a Swedish subject for test words comparing voiced–voiceless and short–long consonant pairs (Cal. 100 μV).

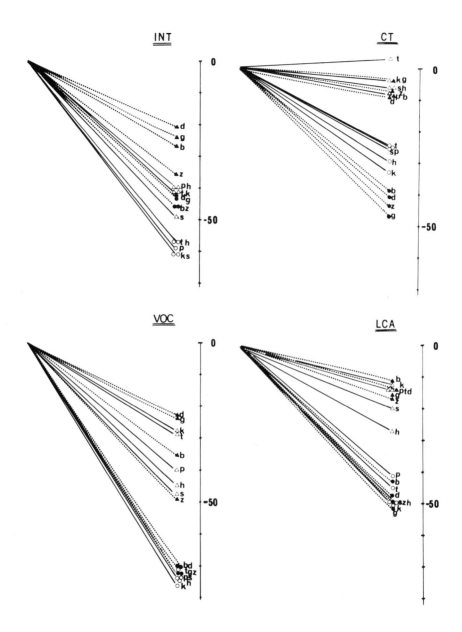

Figure 2-19. The degree of suppression of averaged EMG activity of four different muscles around the obstruents in the test utterances. Word initial: O voiceless; --- ● voiced. Word medial: △ voiceless; ---▲ voiced.

the Korean forced stop, which has been known to be accompanied by distinct, sharp activation of the VOC, as shown in Figure 2-20 (Hirose, Lee & Ushijima, 1974). Represented here are the averaged EMG curves of the VOC and CT for the production of Korean nonsense words (CV) preceded by a carrier sentence /ikəsi/, where C stands for three types of stops and V for /i/, /a/, and /u/. Here again, difference in the postconsonantal vowel does not yield any discernible variation in EMG patterns for each consonant type.

Recently we had an opportunity to perform an additional EMG study on a native Korean phonetician asked to produce three types of Korean stops. It was confirmed in this case too that the VOC showed higher activity immediately before the articulatory release of forced-type stops when compared to the other types of stops, although the activation of the VOC in this case is not so sharp as illustrated in Figure 2-20. A similar type of VOC activity is also found in the case of the Danish *stød*. Whether this mode of contraction is necessary for a relatively fast-response voice trigger mechanism is still open to discussion, but the dimension of tension control of the vocal fold seems to be another important correlate of laryngeal adjustment.

Our recent fiber-optic studies on applosives (unreleased plosives) in the

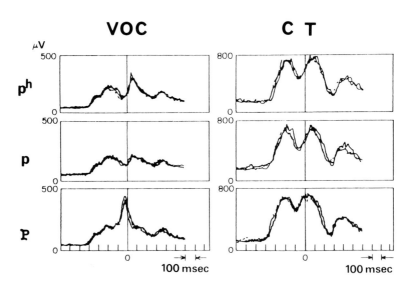

Figure 2-20. Averaged EMG curves of the VOC and CT for the three bilabial stops of Korean in word-initial position in a test sentence "ikəsi CVita," where C stands for a labial stop and V is either /i/, /a/ or /u/. In each type, three curves are superimposed for the postconsonantal vowels. The 0 on the abscissa marks the lineup for the averaging, which corresponds to the stop release.

word-final position in Fukienese, a dialect of southern China, revealed interesting findings on laryngeal adjustment (Iwata et al., 1979). In the production of isolated applosives, there was observed a closed glottis without glottal vibration accompanied by the glottalization gesture, which was represented by a rapid adduction of the false vocal folds immediately after the oral closure.

Selected frames of the laryngeal views for a typical sample of the isolated form are shown in Figure 2-21, where the closed glottis without vibration is observed for the syllable-final /t/ produced by a native speaker of Fukienese. Immediately after implosion, a rapid adduction of the false vocal fold can be seen. The curve in the lower part of the figure indicates the distance between the two false vocal folds; this distance reaches a minimum point at about 100–120 msec after the implosion. It is assumed that the syllabic ending may be signified by the glottalization in the syllable ending as a demarcating signal. This demarcating signal, however, is often less marked in sentences or phrases, under the influence of phonetic conditions like speech tempo or following segments, and final applosives may be assimilated to the following segments, although a considerable individual difference does exist on this point.

The principal mechanism for pitch change is to increase or decrease the longitudinal tension of the vocal fold, and the function of the CT is certainly related to this mechanism. In particular, the increase in longitudinal tension and stretch of the vocal fold is obtained by CT activation. However, the mechanism of pitch lowering is not so straightforward as compared to the case of pitch elevation. As for the contribution of the strap muscles to pitch lowering, their activities often appear to be a response to, rather than the cause of, a change in conditions, lacking the lead in time in relation to physical effects of pitch change.

Figure 2-22 shows examples of EMG curves of the LCA, CT, and SH for single tokens of isolated two-mora words in Japanese, in four different accent types found in the Kinki dialect (Sugito & Hirose, 1978). It is obvious that CT activation is related to pitch rise with some lead in time. As for pitch drop, the decrease in CT activity and increase in SH appear to correlate with the F_0 contour, particularly in types A and B. However, in type A there is an obvious time lag between the onset of decline in CT activity and the start of an increase in SH activity. Thus, SH seems to play a role in assisting or enhancing the sharp pitch descent seen in these cases, but it is not likely that SH acts as the primary pitch lowerer. A similar claim was made by Collier (1975) regarding Dutch intonation control with respect to laryngeal adjustments.

It is also interesting to note that there is SH activation before the voice onset only for the so-called low-start types: types B and C. This increase in SH activity has also been found in other cases, by Atkinson (1978) for example, and taken as an indication of the SH's role in preparing the larynx for the speech mode in certain specific cases. This topic seems to need further investigation.

The physiological correlates of stress seem very complex in nature. As the so-called extra-energy theory suggests, extra energy can be applied to the stressed

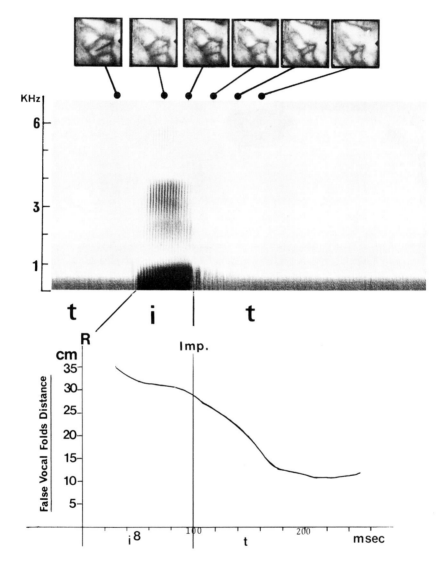

Figure 2-21. Selected frames of the glottal view for [tit′] in the isolated form with the wide-band spectrogram and the pitch contour.

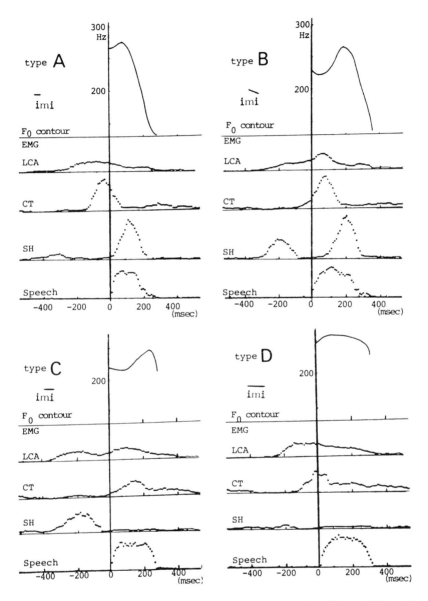

Figure 2-22. Integrated and smoothed EMG curves of the LCA, CT, and SH, and F_0 contours, for single tokens of two-mora words in Japanese in four different accent patterns found in Kinki dialect. A vertical bar indicates the onset of voicing.

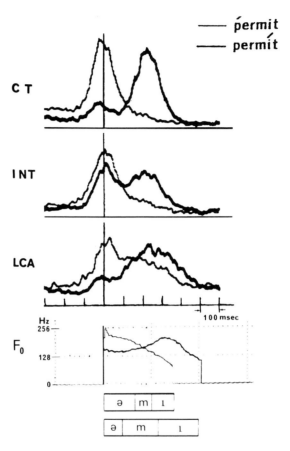

Figure 2-23. Averaged EMG curves of the CT, INT, and LCA, and pitch contours, for the pair *pérmit* and *permít* produced by an American English speaker.

vowel. Also, as many acoustic and perceptual studies have revealed, a rise in pitch appears to be one of the most important correlates of stress.

Figure 2-23 compares averaged EMG curves of the CT, INT, and LCA together with F_0 contours for the words *pérmit* and *permít* produced by a native speaker of American English. It is obvious that the CT activity pattern closely relates to pitch contour in this case also. In addition, it can be seen that the other two muscles also appear to be activated for the production of stress. Of course, other physiological factors must be taken into consideration when we interpret the results shown in this figure. For example, the INT shows increasing activity for the initiation of utterance, and LCA activation can be related partly to the tendency toward the glottal stop gesture for the final /t/. In any case, however, it is not easy to conclude whether the general tendency toward the increase in activity of these muscles is related simply to the rise in pitch, or whether it is to be regarded as evidence of extra effort.

IV. Conclusion

In the foregoing, we have presented several topics related to laryngeal control in speech. We believe that the human larynx is not simply an organ of phonation, but serves as an important organ for speech articulation. It is expected that future research will further unravel the role of the human larynx in both phonation and articulation.

Acknowledgments. The work reported in this chapter was supported in part by a Grant-in-Aid for Cooperative Research (No. 337040) and a Grant-in-Aid for Scientific Research (No. 448322, 557392) from the Japanese Ministry of Education, Science and Culture.

References

Abramson, A. S. Laryngeal timing in consonant distinction. *Phonetica*, 1977, *34*; 295–303.

Atkinson, J. E. Correlation analysis of the physiological factors controlling fundamental voice frequency. *Journal of the Acoustical Society of America*, 1978, *63*; 211–222.

Benguerel, A-P., & Bhatia, T. K. Hindi stop consonant: An acoustic and fiberscopic study (to be published).

Collier, R. Physiological correlates of intonation patterns. *Journal of the Acoustical Society of America*, 1975, *58*; 249–255.

Dixit, R. P. *Neuromuscular aspects of laryngeal control: With special reference to Hindi.* Unpublished doctoral dissertation, University of Texas at Austin, 1975.

Frable, M. A. Computation of motion of cricoarytenoid joint. *Archives of Oto-laryngology*, 1961, *73*; 551–556.

Fujimura, O., & Sawashima, M. Consonant sequences and laryngeal control. *Ann. Bull.Research Institute of Logopedics and Phoniatrics*, 1971, 5, 1–6.

Gauffin, J. Mechanism of larynx tube constriction. *Phonetica*, 1977; *34*; 307–309.

Halle, M. & Stevens, K. N. A note on laryngeal features. *Quarterly Progress Report Research Laboratory Electronics*, MIT., 1971, *101*; 198–213.

Hirano, M. Phonosurgery: Basic and clinical investigations. *Otologia Fukuoka*, 1975, *21*; Suppl. 1. (In Japanese.)

Hirose, H. Posterior cricoarytenoid as a speech muscle. *Ann. Otology, Rhinology and Laryngology*, 1976, *85*; 334–343.

Hirose, H. Electromyography of the larynx and other speech organs. In M. Sawashima, & F. S. Cooper (Eds.), *Dynamic aspects of speech production.* Tokyo: University of Tokyo Press, 1977. (a)

Hirose, H. Laryngeal adjustments in consonant production. *Phonetica*, 1977, *34*; 289–294. (b)

Hirose, H., & Gay, T. The activity of the intrinsic laryngeal muscles in voicing control: Electromyographic study. *Phonetica*, 1972, *25*; 140–164.

Hirose, H., Lee, C. Y., & Ushijima, T. Laryngeal control in Korean stop production. *Journal of Phonetics*, 1974, *2*; 145–152.

Hirose, H., Lisker, L., & Abramson, A. Physiological aspects of certain laryngeal features in stop production. *Haskins Laboratories Status Report on Speech Research*, 1972, *SR-31/32*; 183–191.

Hirose, H., & Ushijima, T. Laryngeal control for voicing distinction in Japanese consonant production. *Phonetica*, 1978, *35*; 1–10.

Hirose, H., Yoshioka, H., & Niimi, S. A cross language study of laryngeal adjustment in consonant production. *Ann. Bull. Research Institute of Logopedics and Phoniatrics*, 1978, *12*; 61–71.

Iwata, R., Sawashima, M., Hirose, H., & Niimi, S. Laryngeal adjustments of Fukienese stops: Initial plosives and final applosives. *Ann. Bull. Research Institute of Logopedics and Phoniatrics*, 1979, *13*; 61–81.

Sawashima, M. Laryngeal research in experimental phonetics. *Current Trends in Linguistics*, 1974, *12*; 2303–2348.

Sawashima, M., Gay, T., & Harris, K. H. Laryngeal muscle activity during vocal pitch and intensity changes. *Haskins Laboratories Status Report on Speech Research*, 1969, *SR-19/20*, 211–220.

Sawashima, M., Hirose, M., & Niimi, S. Glottal conditions in articulation of Japanese voiceless consonants. *Proceedings of the 16th International Congress on Logopedics and Phoniatrics*, 1974, pp. 409–414.

Sawashima, M., Hirose, H., & Yoshioka, H. Abductor (PCA) and adductor (INT) muscles of the larynx in voiceless sound production. *Ann. Bull. Research Institute of Logopedics and Phoniatrics*, 1978, *12*; 53–60.

Simada, Z., & Hirose, H. Physiological correlates of Japanese accent patterns. *Ann. Bull. Research Institute of Logopedics and Phoniatrics*, 1971, 5 ,41–49.

Sonesson, B. Die funktionelle Anatomie des cricoarytenoidgelenkes. *Zeitschrift für Anatomie und Entwicklungsgeschichte*, 1958, *121*; 292–303.

Sugito, M., & Hirose, H. An electromyographic study of Kinki accent. *Ann. Bull. Research Institute of Logopedics and Phoniatrics*, 1978, *12*; 35–52.

Takase, S. Studies on the intrinsic laryngeal muscles of mammals: Comparative anatomy and physiology. *Otologia Fukuoka*, 1964, 10; Suppl. 1. (In Japanese.)

von Leden, H., & Moore, P. The mechanism of the cricoarytenoid joint. *Archives of Otolaryngology*, 1961, *73*; 541–550.

Weitzman, R. S., Sawashima, M., Hirose, H., & Ushijima, T. Devoiced and whispered vowels in Japanese. *Ann. Bull. Research Institute of Logopedics and Phoniatrics*, 1976, *10*; 61–80.

Yoshioka, H., Löfqvist, A., & Hirose, H. Laryngeal adjustments in the production of consonant clusters and geminates in American English. *Haskins Laboratories Status Report on Speech Research*, 1979, *SR-59/60*, 127–151.

Chapter 3

Dynamic Characteristics of Voice Fundamental Frequency in Speech and Singing

HIROYA FUJISAKI

I. Introduction

In many of the Indo-European languages (Öhman, 1967; Isačenko & Schädlich, 1966; 't Hart, 1966; Maeda, 1974; Vaissière-Maeda, 1980) as well as in the Japanese language (Fujisaki & Nagashima, 1969), the contour of the voice fundamental frequency (henceforth F_0 contour) plays an important role in transmitting not only linguistic information but also nonlinguistic information such as naturalness, emotion, and speaker idiosyncrasy. Because of difficulties in accurate analysis and in quantitative description, the relationships between the linguistic–nonlinguistic information and the F_0-contour characteristics have not been fully clarified. The elucidation of these relationships requires, first, the selection of characteristic parameters that are capable of describing the essential features of an F_0 contour, and second, a method for extracting these parameters from an observed F_0 contour. In other words, an analytical formulation (i.e., a model) of the control process of voice fundamental frequency is indispensable for the quantitative analysis and linguistic interpretation of F_0-contour characteristics.

It is widely recognized that the F_0 contours of words and sentences are generally characterized by a gradual declination from the onset toward the end of an utterance, on which are superimposed local humps corresponding to word accent and the like. Most of the models that have been proposed for the interpretation of F_0-contour characteristics, however, are based on a rather crude approximation of the contour on a linear scale of fundamental frequency, and fall short of the explanatory power to deal precisely and quantitatively with the contribution of the various factors involved in the formation of an F_0 contour. This chapter summarizes the author's approach to this problem, and presents models developed for the analysis and interpretation of word and sentence intonation as well as of pitch control in singing. Although the data presented here relate exclusively to Japanese, the approach has been found to be valid for English, too.

II. Fundamental Frequency Contour of Isolated Words

A. Formulation of the Model

The word prosody found in many dialects of spoken Japanese is characterized essentially by binary patterns of subjective pitch associated with each mora (i.e., each unit of metric timing; a mora is usually equal to, but sometimes smaller than, a syllable). The existence of such pitch patterns constitutes the *word accent*, and a specific pitch pattern is called an *accent type* (Fujisaki & Nagashima, 1969; Fujisaki & Sudo, 1971a, 1971b; Fujisaki & Sugito, 1978; Hirose, Fujisaki, & Sugito, 1978). Each dialect is characterized by its own accent system, that is, system of word accent types peculiar to a dialect or a group of dialects. For example, the accent system of the Tokyo dialect is characterized by the following constraints: (1) the subjective pitch invariably displays a transition, either upward or downward, at the end of the initial mora; and (2) an upward transition can be followed by a downward transition, but not vice versa, within a word. The type with a "high" final mora is further divided into two types, depending on whether or not the high pitch is carried over to the following particle. Thus the total number of accent types of n-mora words is $n + 1$ in the Tokyo dialect. On the other hand, the accent system of the Osaka dialect is characterized by a different set of constraints, which yield $2n - 1$ accent types for n-mora words, with a few exceptions in one- and two-mora words.

While the prosodic information intended by the speaker and perceived by the listener is thus discrete and binary, the contour of the voice fundamental frequency is continuous both in time and in frequency. As illustrated by the example of an isolated utterance of the word /ame/ shown in Figure 3-1, an F_0 contour generally displays a smooth rise and decay in the vicinity of the "accented" mora, superimposed on a baseline that initially rises and then gradually decays toward the end of an utterance regardless of the accent type. Thus the observed F_0 contour can be considered as the response of the phonatory system to a set of suprasegmental commands: the (word) utterance command and the accent command. The utterance command is for the utterance of the entire word and produces the *baseline* component, whereas the accent command is for the realization of a specific accent type and produces the *accent* component of an F_0 contour. We assume that both commands are discrete and

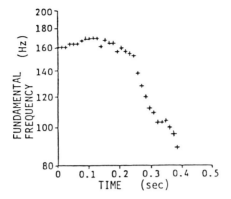

Figure 3-1.   An example of a measured F_0 contour of the word /ame/ ("rain") in the Tokyo dialect. The plus signs represent fundamental frequencies interpolated at intervals of 12.8 msec.

binary. Comparison of F_0 contours uttered by a number of speakers at various pitch ranges also suggests that the formulation of the F_0 contour characteristics will be much simpler if stated in terms of a logarithmic scale rather than in terms of a linear scale of voice fundamental frequency.

These considerations have led us to the functional model of Figure 3-2 for the generation process of an F_0 contour of a word spoken in isolation. Binary commands for utterance and accent are assumed to be smoothed separately by the low-pass characteristics of their respective control mechanisms, each being approximated here by a critically damped, second-order linear system. The outputs of these two mechanisms (i.e., the baseline component and the accent component) are combined to control the fundamental frequency of glottal oscillations through a nonlinear mechanism. Thus the F_0 contour, $F_0(t)$, of a word can be expressed by

$$\ln F_0(t) = \ln F_{min} + A_u[G_u(t - T_0) - G_u(t - T_3)]$$
$$+ A_a[G_a(t - T_1) - G_a(t - T_2)], \tag{1}$$

where

$$G_u(t) = \alpha t \exp(-at)u(t), \qquad u(t) = \text{unit step function},$$

and

$$G_a(t) = [1 - (1 + \beta t)\exp(-\beta t)]u(t)$$

respectively indicate the step response function of the corresponding control mechanism to the utterance and accent commands; F_{min} is the lower limit of fundamental frequency below which vocal fold vibration cannot be sustained in the glottis of a speaker; A_u and A_a respectively denote the amplitude of the utterance and accent command; T_0 and T_3 respectively denote the onset and end

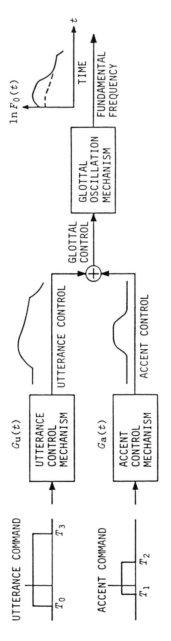

Figure 3-2. A functional model for the process of generating an F_0 contour of a word; conversion of utterance and accent commands into an actual F_0 contour.

of the utterance command, while T_1 and T_2 respectively denote the onset and end of the accent command.

B. Experimental Results

The validity of a model can be tested by its ability to approximate observed F_0 contours. For this purpose, F_0 contours were analyzed for a number of utterances of various accent types produced by speakers of the Tokyo and the Osaka dialects.

The F_0 contour analysis involves the extraction of fundamental frequency followed by feature extraction from the F_0 contour. The fundamental periods are detected pitch-synchronously by a method based on short-term auto-correlation analysis and peak detection. These fundamental periods are con-verted to fundamental frequencies, which are further interpolated to produce F_0 contours uniformly sampled at intervals of 12.8 msec. The parameters of the above-mentioned model are determined by minimizing the mean square error between the extracted F_0 contour and that of the model on a logarithmic scale.

Figure 3-3 illustrates examples for each of the four accent types of /ame/ uttered by a male speaker who has a good command of both the Tokyo and Osaka dialects. The plus signs indicate the F_0 contour measured at intervals of 12.8 msec; the solid curve represents the best approximation given by the model; and the stepwise waveform indicates schematically the timing of the binary accent command. The validity of the model has been widely de-monstrated by analysis of F_0 contours of words with various numbers of morae, uttered by speakers of both the Tokyo and Osaka dialects.

III. Fundamental Frequency Contour of Sentences

A. Extension of the Word Model

The sentence prosody of spoken Japanese has acoustic manifestations in the voice fundamental frequency and the duration of pauses and segments, as well as in the tempo of an utterance. Although all three are important and somewhat interrelated, we shall be concerned here only with the fundamental frequency contour.

Observation of F_0 contours of various declarative sentences of the Tokyo dialect indicates that a sentence F_0 contour displays local humps superimposed on a smoothly decaying baseline. Each local hump corresponds to a word or a word compound (which behaves like a word with a single accent type), and the humps may or may not differ in their height. The baseline may be interrupted and resumed at major syntactic boundaries. Except for these points, however,

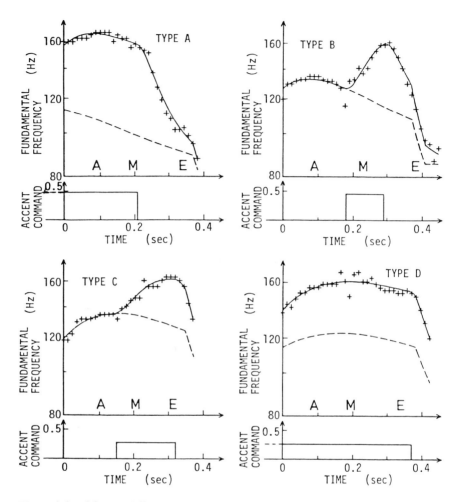

Figure 3-3. Measured F_0 contours and their best approximations in utterances of four word accent types of /ame/. The dashed lines indicate the baseline component, while the stepwise waveform represents the timing and the amplitude of the accent command.

the general characteristics of sentence F_0 contours are found to be essentially similar to those of words, and suggest that the model for word F_0 contours can be extended to sentences. Instead of a single utterance command for the baseline component, we may assume a phrase command for each of the major syntactic phrases. These phrase commands are again assumed to take the form of a step function, but their amplitudes, denoted by A_{pi}, may not necessarily be equal for all the phrase components. Likewise, the accent commands are also assumed to be step functions, but their amplitudes, denoted by A_{aj}, may vary from one accent component to another. Thus the F_0 contour of a sentence can be expressed by

$$\ln F_0(t) = \ln F_{\min} + \sum_{i=1}^{I} A_{pi} [G_{pi}(t - T_{0i}) - G_{pi}(t - T_{3i})]$$
$$+ \sum_{j=1}^{J} A_{aj}[G_{aj}(t - T_{1j}) - G_{aj}(t - T_{2j})], \qquad (2)$$

where

$$G_{pi}(t) = \alpha_i t \exp(-\alpha_i t)u(t), \qquad u(t) = \text{unit step function},$$

and

$$G_{aj}(t) = [1 - (1 + \beta_j t) \exp(-\beta_j t)]u(t),$$

respectively indicate the step response function of the corresponding control mechanism to the phrase and accent commands. The α_i's and β_j's are expected to be fairly constant within a sentence, or among utterances of an individual speaker. I and J are the number of phrase and accent commands, T_{0i} and T_{3i} denote the onset and end, respectively, of the ith phrase command, while T_{1j} and T_{2j} denote the onset and end, respectively, of the jth accent command. In the absence of respiratory pauses within a spoken sentence, the offset times T_{3i} for all phrase commands are assumed to be identical for all i's within an utterance. On the other hand, the accent commands are constrained not to overlap each other.

B. Experimental Results

A set of 10 declarative sentences, each consisting of voiced segments only and ranging in length from 8 to 24 morae, were selected. Utterances of these sentences by three male speakers of the Tokyo dialect were recorded and analyzed. For the purpose of this study, these utterances were made without respiratory pauses within a sentence.

Figure 3-4 illustrates results of one sample each from the three sentences:

(a) /aoinoewaaru/ ("There is a picture of hollyhocks");
(b) /aoiaoinoewaaru/ ("There is a picture of blue hollyhocks");
(c) /aoiaoinoewajamanouenoieniaru/ ("There is a picture of blue hollyhocks in a house on a mountain").

The measurement of the voice fundamental frequency was made at intervals of 12.8 msec, but the plus signs indicate the measured F_0 contour only at every 3 points. The curve displayed as a solid line represents the best approximation given by the model, and the curve displayed as a broken line indicates the baseline component estimated at the same time. The analysis clearly indicates the existence of partial rephrasing at the boundary between the subject phrase and the predicate phrase in the case of sentence (c). The stepwise waveforms at

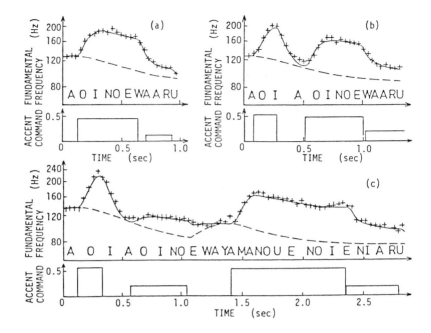

Figure 3-4. Measured F_0 contours and their best approximations in (a) /aoinoewaaru/, (b) /aoiaoinoewaaru/, and (c) /aoiaoinoewajamanouenoieniaru/. The broken lines represent the phrase component, while the stepwise waveform represents the timing and the amplitude of the accent commands.

the bottom of each panel schematically indicate the timing and the amplitude of the accent commands. The values of the parameters, obtained from the analysis of the three utterances by one speaker, are listed in Table 3-1.

The timing parameters for the accent commands naturally vary widely from one sentence to another, since they reflect the lexical information of each of the constituent words. On the other hand, parameters such as α_i and β_j are found to remain fairly constant, since they characterize the dynamic responses of a subject's glottal control mechanism to phrase and accent commands. The amplitude A_{aj} of the accent command is seen to be distributed over two distinct ranges of values: one from 0.46 to 0.56, and the other from 0.13 to 0.22. This result may reflect the discrete (binary) character of accentuation.

These results also suggest that the approximation by the present model to an F_0 contour may not be seriously impaired by constraining all the α_i's and β_j's to remain constant, and by allowing only two values for the A_{aj}'s. Analyses of F_0 contours under these constraints have actually been conducted, and the results tend to confirm the validity of this simplication.

The relationships between the sentence length n and the parameters of the simplified model are shown in Figures 3-5 and 3-6. As seen from Figure 3-5, the

Table 3-1. Parameter of Sentence F_0 Contours Extracted by Finding the Best Approximations to the Observed F_0 Contours

Sentence	F_{min} (Hz)	i	T_0 (sec)	T_3 (sec)	A_p	α (sec^{-1})	j	T_1 (sec)	T_2 (sec)	A_a	β (sec^{-1})
(a)	83	1	− .21	1.01	1.18	3.3	1	.13	.64	.46	20.5
8 morae							2	.71	.93	.13	20.8
(b)	84	1	− .21	1.42	1.20	3.6	1	.08	.27	.54	21.2
11 morae							2	.51	1.00	.49	20.5
							3	1.02	1.34	.20	20.0
(c)	76	1	− .19	2.87	1.50	3.0	1	.12	.33	.56	24.0
20 morae		2	1.07	2.87	.80	3.2	2	.57	1.05	.20	26.0
							3	1.41	2.36	.52	24.0
							4	2.36	2.81	.22	23.5

influences of sentence length n on parameters α and β are quite small, indicating that the apparent slow declination in longer sentences can be well explained by the existence of "rephrasing" at major syntactic boundaries. The results in Figure 3-6 indicate that the influence of n on the amplitude parameters A_p and A_a is also quite small. Furthermore, the ratio of the two values obtained for the amplitudes of the accent commands does not vary appreciably with n, suggesting that the amplitude is controlled in a binary way to show either presence or absence of emphasis, at least as far as the present speech samples are concerned.

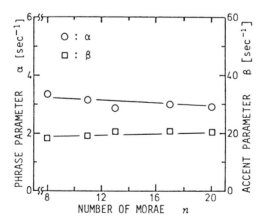

Figure 3-5. Parameters α, β of phrase and accent components versus number of morae n in a sentence.

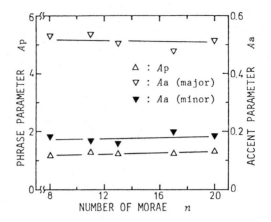

Figure 3-6. Amplitude of phrase and accent components versus number of morae n in a sentence.

IV. Pitch Control in Singing

A. Aim of the Study

The voice fundamental frequency is no less important in singing than in speech, but its role is obviously different. The difference lies in the following points:

1. A singer (at least in classical music) is expected to sustain the mean fundamental frequency at a constant value over the time interval of a note, whereas a speaker is never expected to do so during an utterance in speech.
2. Hence, there is no F_0 declination within a note, whereas F_0 declination is quite common in speech.
3. A singer is asked to control the rate of F_0 transition from one note to another according to the specified manner of performance, whereas the rate is never consciously controlled in speech.

Thus the study of F_0 control in singing is of interest in its own right, but is also relevant to the study of F_0 control in speech, since it involves the same control mechanisms as are used in speech production.

B. Experiment

The material for study consisted of a number of two-note sequences sung with the vowel [a] in various manners of performance (i.e., in various degrees of articulation of the two notes). They were (a) a note with an *appoggiatura*, (b) two notes sung *staccato*, (c) two notes sung *non legato*, (d) two notes sung *legato*, and (e) two notes sung as a *portamento*. Since, however, the two notes sung *staccato* are generally separated by a silent gap of considerable duration, they were omitted from the subsequent analysis. The subjects were two females with a similar range and quality of voice. One (subject MT) was a voice trainer with 10 years of professional training in singing, and the other (subject YS) was a student at a music conservatory with 3 years of training in singing. The pitches of the two notes were selected to suit the voice range of the singers, and the intervals were either a musical fourth (A_4–D_5) or an octave (D_4–D_5). The sequences were produced in both directions, upward and downward. Each sequence was repeated several times in three-quarter time with metronome (M.M.) setting of 100, except in the case of the *portamento*, where the beat was approximately M.M. 80. These sequences were sung at three levels of volume: forte (*f*), mezzo piano (*mp*), and pianissimo (*pp*). A minimum of five samples were collected for each of the conditions and subjects. For the sake of comparison, speech materials were also recorded. These were isolated utterances of two words in the Tokyo dialect of Japanese: /ame/ "candy" and /ame/ "rain." These two words possess an identical phonemic structure but differ in the accent type manifested mainly in their F_0 contours, the former being the "low–high" type and the latter being the "high–low" type.

The technique for fundamental frequency extraction was the same as that adopted for speech, but the data were interpolated at intervals of 10 msec. The extraction of characteristic parameters of an F_0 contour also followed the same line as that for F_0 contours of spoken words, but the model was modified to suit the observed data by suppressing the utterance component and by removing the "critical-damping" constraint on the form of F_0 transition. If we assume a step function for the shape of the command to switch notes, the F_0 contour of a two-note sequence can be represented by

$$\ln F_0(t) = \ln F_i + (\ln F_f - \ln F_i)f(\beta, \gamma, t)u(t), \tag{3}$$

where

$$
\begin{aligned}
f(\beta, \gamma, t) \\
&= 1 - (\cos\beta\sqrt{1-\gamma^2}\,t + \frac{\gamma}{\sqrt{1-\gamma^2}}\sin\beta\sqrt{1-\gamma^2}\,t)\exp(-\beta\gamma t), \\
&\qquad\qquad\qquad\qquad\qquad\qquad\qquad\qquad\qquad\quad \text{for } \gamma < 1, \\[4pt]
&= 1 - (1+\beta t)\exp(-\beta t), \qquad\qquad\qquad\qquad \text{for } \gamma = 1, \\[4pt]
&= 1 + (\cosh\beta\sqrt{\gamma^2-1}\,t + \frac{\gamma}{\sqrt{\gamma^2-1}}\sinh\beta\sqrt{\gamma^2+1}\,t)\exp(-\beta\gamma t), \\
&\qquad\qquad\qquad\qquad\qquad\qquad\qquad\qquad\qquad\quad \text{for } \gamma > 1,
\end{aligned}
$$

and $u(t)$ denotes the unit step function, F_i and F_f respectively denote the initial and final values of the transition, and β and γ are parameters characterizing the second-order linear system. The origin of the time axis is selected at the onset of transition.

Although it is possible to measure such characteristics as the rise and fall times directly from an F_0 contour, the formulation above gives us more insight into the underlying mechanism of pitch control. Parameters such as β and γ can be obtained from a measured F_0 contour by finding its best approximation given by the equations above, which can then be used to determine the rise and fall times. For the sake of comparison with the published results by Ohala and Sundberg (1979), we adopt here the same definition of the rise–fall time as in their studies. Namely, the rise–fall time is defined as the time required for the pitch to change from 1/8 to 7/8 of the total range of transition.

Figure 3-7 illustrates one example each of pitch transitions across the interval of a fourth (A_4–D_5) in the sung material of subject MT produced mezzo piano under eight different conditions, that is, upward and downward transitions sung at four different degrees of articulation (*appoggiatura, non legato, legato*, and *portamento*). The plus signs represent the F_0 contours measured at 10-msec intervals, while the curve in each panel indicates the best approximation based on Equation 3.

Quite naturally, the rate of pitch change is seen to vary to a large extent with the degree of articulation, and also to vary with the direction, that is, a downward transition is faster than an upward transition, especially in *appoggiatura* and in *non legato*. The F_0 contours are clearly underdamped in these fast transitions, whereas they are almost critically damped in normal and slower transitions (*legato* and *portamento*).

Table 3-2 lists the mean values of β and γ averaged over several samples of each of the eight conditions, obtained from the analysis of the material sung by MT, together with the mean rise–fall times τ^* defined in the preceding section and calculated from β and γ. For the sake of comparison, parameter values obtained from the speech material are also listed. Analysis of materials sung at different levels indicated that in most cases changes in the volume do not appreciably affect the rate of transition.

All the foregoing results were obtained from the analysis of materials sung by MT, but the results for subject YS also showed similar tendencies.

C. A Physiological–Physical Interpretation

Our studies on F_0 contours of both speech and singing have proved the essential validity of:

1. the functional formulation of the dynamic characteristics of pitch control on a logarithmic scale of fundamental frequency; and
2. the approximation of the F_0 contour in terms of the response characteristics of a second-order linear system.

Although these results were obtained empirically, an interpretation will be presented on the basis of some theoretical considerations and published data on the physical properties of skeletal muscles.

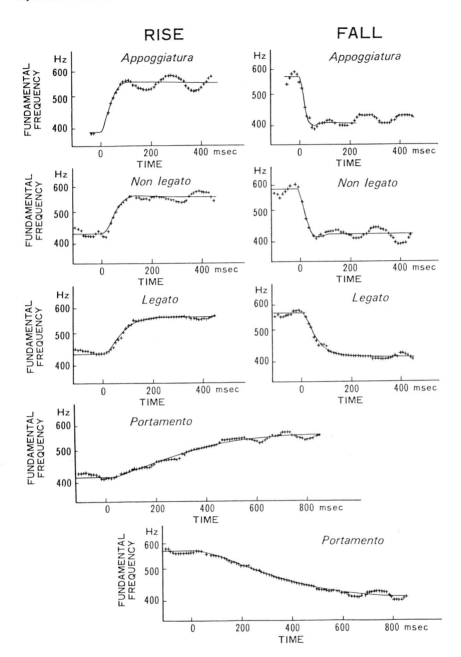

Figure 3-7.   Analysis of F_0 contours in singing. Typical results obtained from samples of two-note sequences separated by an interval of a fourth (subject **MT**).

Table 3-2. Characteristic Parameters and Rise–Fall Times of F_0 Contours in Singing and in Speech[a]

	Rise			Fall		
	β (sec^{-1})	γ	τ^* (msec)	β (sec^{-1})	γ	τ^* (msec)
Appoggiatura	40	.76	54	75	.50	20
Non legato	38	.85	67	57	.77	38
Legato	27	.85	91	33	.94	87
Portamento	6.8	.95	419	6.9	.93	409
Speech	18	1.00	167	18	1.00	171

[a] The results for singing are from two-note sequences separated by an interval of a fourth (subject MT).

The closeness of approximation of (logarithmic) F_0 contours by our model strongly suggests that the logarithmic fundamental frequency may actually reflect the mechanical motion of an element in the laryngeal mechanism which, from the point of view of pitch control, can be approximated by a second-order linear system. More specifically, we present the following hypotheses and show evidence supporting these hypotheses.

Hypothesis 1: The logarithmic fundamental frequency varies linearly with the displacement of a point in the laryngeal structure.

Hypothesis 2: The displacement of the point reflects the mechanical motion of a mass element connected with stiffness and viscous resistance elements.

Supporting evidence for Hypothesis 1 can be found in the stress–strain relationship of muscles. The following experimental relationship has been known to apply between the tension T and the elongation x of skeletal muscles in general (Buchthal & Kaiser, 1944; Sandow, 1958):

$$T = a[\exp(bx) - 1] \tag{4}$$

In the present study, we regard x as the elongation of the vocalis muscle due mainly to the displacement of its anterior end. If $\exp(bx) \gg 1$, Equation 4 can be approximated by

$$T = a \exp(bx). \tag{5}$$

On the other hand, the frequency of vibration of elastic strings as well as of membranes with simple structures varies generally in proportion to the square root of their tension (Slater & Frank, 1933). This relationship will hold even for the vibration of the vocal fold, which can be regarded as an elastic membrane to a first-order approximation. Thus

$$F_0 = c_0\sqrt{T}. \tag{6}$$

From Equations 5 and 6 we obtain

$$\ln F_0 = \frac{b}{2}x + \ln(\sqrt{a}c_0), \tag{7}$$

where, strictly speaking, c_0 also varies slightly with x, but the overall dependency of $\ln F_0$ is primarily determined by the first term on the right-hand side of Equation 7.

Hypothesis 2 can be supported by the analysis of the mechanical properties of the laryngeal structure whose major elements are shown in Figure 3-8. If we adopt a coordinate fixed with the cricoid cartilage (and the trachea, which is connected more or less tightly with the cricoid), the thyroid cartilage can be regarded as one major mass element supported by two stiffness elements (the cricothyroid and vocalis muscles) and rotating around the cricothyroid joint with a viscous resistance. The two stiffness elements are also accompanied by viscous resistances that represent their interval losses. If we denote the angular displacement of the thyroid by θ, its rotation can be described by the following equation of motion:

$$I\ddot{\theta} + R\dot{\theta} + (c_1 K_1 + c_2 K_2)\theta = \tau(t), \tag{8}$$

where I represents the moment of inertia, R represents the combined viscous loss, K_1 and K_2 represent the stiffness of the cricothyroid and vocalis muscles, and $\tau(t)$ represents the torque caused by the contraction of the cricothyroid muscle. Since the anterior end of the vocalis muscle is fixed at a point on the thyroid cartilage, the following relationship holds approximately between x and θ for small angular displacement of the thyroid cartilage:

$$x = c_3 \theta. \tag{9}$$

For a unit step forcing function $u(t)$, x can be given by

$$x = c_4 f(\beta, \gamma, t)u(t), \tag{10}$$

where $f(\beta, \gamma, t)$ is the same as in Equation 3, and

$$\beta = \sqrt{\frac{c_1 K_1 + c_2 K_2}{I}}, \qquad \gamma = \frac{R}{2\sqrt{I(c_1 K_1 + c_2 K_2)}}.$$

Equations 7 and 10 with initial and final conditions will lead to Equation 3.

As one of the possible ways to control the rate of F_0 transition, we may assume that only the stiffness of the related laryngeal muscles is changed. In this case, a hyperbolic relationship is expected to hold between β and γ. This may actually be the main cause for the strong negative correlation between measured values of β and γ in Table 3-2, although their relationship is not exactly hyperbolic.

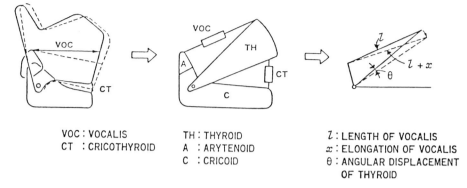

VOC : VOCALIS   TH : THYROID l : LENGTH OF VOCALIS
CT   : CRICOTHYROID   A   : ARYTENOID x : ELONGATION OF VOCALIS
                       C   : CRICOID θ : ANGULAR DISPLACEMENT
                                                  OF THYROID

Figure 3-8. Successive stages of simplification of the essential structure of the larynx.

On the other hand, differences in the rate for upward and downward transitions can be explained by referring to the stress–strain relationship of Equation 4. The incremental stiffness, as given by $\partial T/\partial x$, is obviously greater at larger values of x. Since the initial value of x is greater in the downward transitions, the stiffness is greater and hence produces a larger value of β than in the upward transitions.

References

Buchthal, F., & Kaiser, E. Factors determining tension development in skeletal muscle. *Acta Physiologica Scandinavica*, 1944, *8*, 38–74.

Fujisaki, H., & Nagashima, S. A model for synthesis of pitch contours of connected speech. *Annual Report, Engineering Research Institute (University of Tokyo)*, 1969, *28*, 53–60.

Fujisaki, H., & Sudo, H. A model for the generation of fundamental frequency contours of Japanese word accent. *Journal of the Acoustical Society of Japan*, 1971, *27*, 445–453.(a)

Fujisaki, H., & Sudo, H. Synthesis by rule of prosodic features of connected Japanese. *Proceedings of the 7th International Congress of Acoustics*, 1971, *3*, 133–136.(b)

Fujisaki, H., & Sudo, H. A generative model for the prosody of connected speech in Japanese. *Conference Record, 1972 Conference on Speech Communication and Processing, IEEE-AFCRL*, 1972, 140–143.

Fujisaki, H., & Sugito, M. Analysis and perception of two-mora word accent types in the Kinki dialect. *Journal of the Acoustical Society of Japan*, 1978, *34*, 167–176.

Hirose, K., & Fujisaki, H. Acoustical features of fundamental frequency contours of Japanese sentences. *Proceedings of the 10th ICA*, 1980, *2*, AL-9.2.

Hirose, K., Fujisaki, H., & Sugito, M. Acoustic correlates of word accent in English and Japanese. *Transactions of the Committee on Speech Research, Acoustical Society of Japan*, 1978, S78–41.

Isačenko, A. V., & Schädlich, H. J. Untersuchungen über die deutsche Satzintonation. *Studia Grammatica*, 1966, *7*, 7–67.

Maeda, S. A characterization of fundamental frequency contours of speech. *Quarterly Progress Report, Research Laboratory of Electronics, MIT*, 1974, *114*, 193–211.

Ohala, J., & Ewan, W. Speed of pitch change. *Journal of the Acoustical Society of America*, 1973, *53*, 345(A).

Öhman, S. Word and sentence intonation: A quantitative model. *Speech Transmission Laboratory Quarterly Progress and Status Report (Stockholm)*, 1967, *2–3*, 20–54.

Sandow, A. A theory of active state mechanisms in isometric muscular contraction. *Science*, 1958, *127*, 760–762.

Slater, J. C., & Frank, N. H. *Introduction to theoretical physics*. New York: McGraw-Hill, 1933.

Sundberg, J. Maximum speed of pitch changes in singers and untrained subjects. *Journal of Phonetics*, 1979, *7*, 71–79.

't Hart, J. Perceptual analysis of Dutch intonation features. *I. P. O. Annual Progress Report*, 1966, *1*, 47–51.

Vaissière-Maeda, J. La structuration acoustique de la phrase française. *Annali della Scuola Normale Superiore di Pisa* (Ser. III), 1980, *10*(2), 529–560.

Chapter 4

The Segmental Organization of Speech

R. D. KENT

I. Introduction

I take *segmental organization* to mean the description of speech patterns in terms of units that are not further divisible within the limits of a particular method of analysis. This definition is broader (more evasive, perhaps) than others in the literature. For example, Fujimura and Lovins (1978, p. 107) defined the segment as a "phonetic unit that constitutes an integrated event—an organized set of articulatory gestures or auditory cues—in a temporal flow of speech." Conventionally, segmental organization is taken to mean the organization of speech according to a sequence of phonetic or, more rarely, syllabic pieces. Segmental organization often is described acoustically by a kind of segmental decomposition; that is, demarcation of time intervals in which each interval has either a uniform acoustic structure (say, frication for /s/) or an articulatory–acoustic integrity (say, formant transitions between consonants and vowels). Principles of acoustic segmentation have been described by Dukel'skiy (1965) and Fant (1973) among others. An example of acoustic segmentation derived from spectrograms is shown in Figure 4-1. Segments are depicted in temporal profile for 10 young adults, each reciting four times the sentence "I took a spoon and a knife." Although the details of timing vary across speakers, and across utterances by the same speaker, an overall similarity in relative temporal structure can be seen. Acoustic segmentation is not without its difficulties, but it generally can be done with a fairly high reliability. However, segmentation of a lateral-view cinefluorographic film of speech requires different criteria, adapted to multiarticulator movement patterns, and meets with greater uncertainty in segment demarcation.

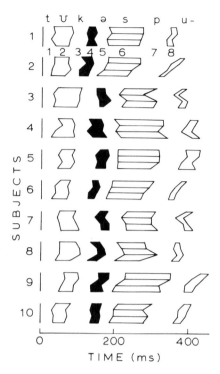

Figure 4-1. Acoustic segmentation of the phrase *took a spoon* (from the sentence "I took a spoon and a knife) uttered four times each by 10 adults. The four replications by a talker are graphically enclosed to highlight the segments. The segments, identified by the horizontally oriented numbers, are as follows: (1) the period extending from the release burst of /t/ to the onset of voicing for /ʊ/; (2) the vocalic nucleus for /ʊ/; (3) stop gap for /k/; (4) release burst and following aspiration (if present) for /k/; (5) schwa vowel; (6) frication for /s/; (7) stop gap for /p/; and (8) interval from release burst for /p/ to onset of voicing for /u/. Individual talkers are identified by the vertically oriented numbers.

Suprasegmental organization might be defined as a residual, or everything that remains after the segmental organization is fully specified. However, some allowances would have to be made for the paralinguistic aspect of speech, that subcomponent that includes attitude, emotion, and other voice qualifications. Yet segmental and suprasegmental structure are not cleanly separated by a single slice of the experimental knife. Suprasegmental features or properties are not merely overlaid on segmental organization; rather they are intertwined with it. By analogy, segmental and suprasegmental organization are two threads of different color twisted to form a colorful braid. The two threads are not separated by a slice of the knife but by a gentle, and often tedious, unraveling. I am not trying to expound on the integration of segmental and suprasegmental properties, but only to indicate that I make no guarantee that I will not trespass on what another speech researcher would call suprasegmentals.

But what another person may call *suprasegmental*, I will call *prosodic*, for the reasons given by Gibbon (1976):

> There are slightly different connotations attached to the terms 'suprasegmental' and 'prosodic', however, the former presupposes segmental phonemic analysis, retaining Bloomfield's distinction between primary and secondary phonemes, whereas in the interpretations of other schools, prosodic features may be based in their own right on "observed general properties of auditory perception" (Pilch, 1968:97). The latter often applies in the actual practice of the 'suprasegmental' schools, most conspicuously, perhaps, in that of Pike . . . .; indeed, the 'suprasegmentals' are among the primary and most conspicuous cues for phonological and other linguistic structures. The terminology 'suprasegmental' does obscure the fact that suprasegmental features are themselves organized into many different kinds of segments. (p. 7)

II. Segments and the Treatment of Time

The phoneme or phonemic segment is a construct that is most properly defined in what Tatham (1970) has called *notional time*, that of phonology or the sequencing of segments. When this construct is used for explanation or prediction of events in *clock time*, the time in which we record muscle contractions, structural movements, and acoustic patterns, a difficult gap has to be bridged. The bridging of this gap seems to be a major part of the puzzle of coarticulation. The construct of the phoneme is historically linguistic in nature, but in the *Weltenschauung* of the contemporary speech researcher, this construct seems to have been broadened to include behavioral phenomena: patterns of articulation, errors in sequencing (see chapter 6), and performance of subjects in a raft of psychological experiments. Phonemes are useful in describing and explaining performance errors like those multiply evident in Figure 4-2. One of the intriguing aspects of the rather confused attempt at phonetic sequencing shown in this figure is that despite the misordering, all segments in the target utterance appear in the produced utterance.

One direction of psycholinguistics is investigation of the psychological reality of the phoneme. The phoneme, or something very similar to it, also appears in many studies of machine speech recognition and speech synthesis. If nothing else, the phoneme has come to serve a basic pragmatic function in speech research because it is the highly serviceable tool by which we describe our speech samples. The paradox of coarticulation is that its operational definition often hinges on a segment-oriented analysis of speech patterns. In a sense, coarticulation is defined as a failure to observe a transparent phonemic organization of speech.

The difficulty of bridging the gap between notional and clock time has been variously addressed. Kent, Carney, and Severeid (1974) concluded that binary-feature models of speech production are not satisfactory because, in general, "predicted statements about articulatory timing can offer no finer temporal

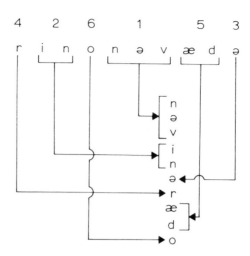

Figure 4-2. Sequencing errors in attempted production of *Reno, Nevada* by a normal talker. The misordering of the sequence is shown by the numbered pieces; for example, what should have been the initial consonant (/r/) of the intended utterance assumed fourth position in the misordered production. Note that each phonetic segment of the intended utterance is in fact produced in the error sequence.

resolution than that which characterizes the assumed input units" (p. 485). That is, the binary coding is fitted to the time intervals that correspond to phonemes. A part of the theory is missing: that part that accomplishes an interpretation of sequences of abstract units (notional time) into the clock time of motor and acoustic events. Similarly, Fowler (1980) concluded that extrinsic timing theories necessarily will fail to account for speech production. In a footnote, she defines an extrinsic timing theory as one in which

> the articulatory plan represents the serial ordering of features, segments or syllables—i.e., it represents their ordinal relationships along the time axis—but time is not taken to inhere in, or to be essential to, the specification of these production units. (p. 113)

III. Models of Segmental Organization in Speech

Many current models of speech production carry something of the character of a phoneme down to a level that looks suspiciously motoric. One sees frequent references to "motor commands by phoneme x" or other such segmentally tinged descriptions of motor behavior.

I will not attempt to review here the many solutions that have been proposed to account for the segmental organization of speech and the occurrence of coarticulation. Recent reviews of this subject include the papers of Kent and

Minifie (1977), Daniloff and Hammarberg (1973), and Fowler (1980). Rather, I will describe briefly some of the major directions that have been taken in an attempt to solve the problem. One point of comparison in examining the proposed solutions is the degree to which the inputs to the speech production model are imbued with allophonic detail. This consideration depends somewhat on the size of the presumed input units; for example, a model that operates on phoneme-sized segments will have a substantially different task than one that operates with syllabic input. Another point of comparison is the degree of reliance on table lookup, or retrieval of categorized control information. In some models, tables themselves seem to be taken almost as solutions. In other models, computational or generative operations are more important. A third point of comparison is the language of the model. Are the terms linguistic, articulatory, or motoric? Some models are developed almost entirely with a quasi-linguistic vocabulary.

A. The Extrinsic Allophone Model

An example of an allophonically detailed input unit is to define an extrinsic allophone by specifying the immediate bilateral context of an element. For example, in the theory proposed by Wickelgren (1969), the production units of speech are taken to be a rather large number of extrinsic allophones (elementary motor responses) of the form $_xy_z$ where the subscripts x and z represent the bilateral context of segment y. This theory has been criticized on several grounds, one of the most entertaining of which was computation of the number of extrinsic allophones that would need to be stored in the brain. The sum total then could be inserted in a rather rhetorical question, "Do you really think that the brain could store X units for the purpose of speech production?" If that number was not big enough to chill the heart or boggle the mind, it could be increased at will by pointing out that coarticulatory effects are not restricted to the immediate bilateral context and that something would have to be done with prosodic features, pipe speech, and pig Latin (see, e.g., Halwes & Jenkins, 1971). Most of the criticisms boil down to objections that this account is neither elegant nor parsimonious and that it does not have sufficient generality. Yet the idea survives, although it is perhaps more robust in speech perception than speech production. In a critique of three papers on machine-motivated models of speech perception, Norman (1980) wrote as follows in his paper entitled "Copycat Science or Does the Mind Really Work by Table Lookup?"

> The problem of acoustic–phonetic invariance is solved [in Klatt's model] by explicit storing of all possible combinations of sounds. The number of possible pronunciations that must be stored is large, but is still only in the few thousands. To my knowledge, this suggestion was first made by Wickelgren (1969), and I find it somewhat amusing to see this suggestion resurfacing, to see it being taken seriously, and to find that it is perhaps correct. I think Wickelgren too will be amused. (p. 389)

B. Binary-Feature Coding Models

One of the more popular models of speech articulation is one based on a binary-feature coding of phoneme-sized input units (Henke, 1966; Moll & Daniloff, 1971; Benguerel & Cowan, 1974). Most such models conceptualize an input unit as a vector or bundle of component features. (The infatuation with tables continues.) Speech articulation is governed by the particular feature values that obtain at a particular instant. Moreover, it usually is assumed that a feature can be anticipated, or assumed before its required appearance, as early as possible so long as the feature specification does not conflict with the requirements for preceding units. The range of anticipatory coarticulation is thus determined by the appearance of a contradictory feature specification in the phonetic string. Benguerel and Cowan (1974) described how this model might explain anticipatory lip rounding using the recoding levels shown in Figure 4-3. Line 1 gives the phonetic string: in this case an unrounded vowel V_u, six consonants (C), and rounded vowel V_r. The assigned (context-free) values of the lip-rounding feature are given in line 3: ($-$) for unrounded, (0) for unspecified, and ($+$) for rounded. A look-ahead operator or feature-spreading mechanism converts line 3 to the revised specifications in line 4. The modus operandi is to effect as early as possible in the string the next specified value of the feature in question. Because the consonants are unspecified with respect to lip rounding, this feature can be anticipated during their production. Consequently, as shown in line 5, the articulation of lip protrusion is assumed during the first /s/ in the consonant sequence, six sounds in advance of its mandatory appearance.

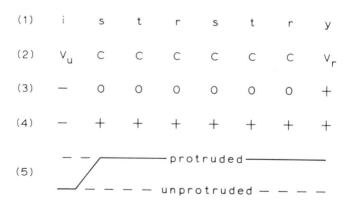

Figure 4-3. Levels of phonetic–articulatory recoding to show how a binary-feature description of lip protrusion, in conjunction with a look-ahead strategy, might account for anticipatory coarticulation of this feature. The phonetic string is described in lines 1 and 2; assigned (context-free) binary-feature values are given in line 3; feature values as reassigned by a look-ahead strategy are shown in line 4; and the schematic gesture of lip protrusion is depicted in line 5.

Shortcomings of the binary-feature coding models have been discussed by Kent et al. (1974), Kent and Minifie (1977), and Kunzel (1979). I will not repeat the arguments here except to say that these models do not satisfactorily predict the finer variations of articulatory timing. Because any predictions of movement timing are tied to a segmental input by means of the intervening feature coding, coarticulation occurs only as the result of feature spreading across *segments*.

C. Coarticulation Resistance Model

The idea of table look-up in speech behavior is given another expression by Bladon and Al-Bamerni (1976) and Bladon (1977). They propose that the various factors that determine the domain and direction of coarticulatory effects can be represented by a control principle of *coarticulation resistance* (CR). Bladon writes of CR as follows:

> The speech production mechanism is hypothesized to have continuous access to CR information, which can be considered to be initially stored linguistically as a scalar feature specification like any other—i.e., of the form [*n* CR]—and attaching to each allophone and boundary condition. Thus, for instance, English /h/ which is highly susceptible to coarticulation and English /O/ which is much more resistant, might be provided with specifications such as [1 CR] and [5 CR] respectively. The numerical value of the CR index is recomputed at a level of articulatory planning by what might be termed a CR compiler to take account of the wide range of constraints imposed by the factors surveyed in this paper. It is further suggested that coarticulation may proceed freely in either direction (left-to-right or right-to-left) in time, until impeded by a specification of CR on some segment.

In principle, this idea is similar to that of the feature-coding models of Henke (1966), Moll and Daniloff (1971), and Benguerel and Cowan (1974), but it replaces the binary-feature specification with a scalar. The primary disadvantage that I see in this model is that it does not do much to improve the prediction of events in clock time. The model appears to be designed to explain why allophonic variants differ in their accommodation of interactive articulatory forces; for example, why coarticulation is not tolerated equally by the dark syllabic [l], dark nonsyllabic [l], and clear nonsyllabic [l] of English Received Pronunciation.

D. Coproduction Models

Coarticulation also has been explained as the consequence of coproduction (Kozhevnikov & Chistovich, 1965; Öhman, 1966, 1967; Perkell, 1969; Fowler, 1980; Fowler, Rubin, Remez, & Turvey, 1980). Evidence of coproduction is seen in observations that articulatory adjustments for vowels may co-occur with the articulation of preceding consonant(s) and that consonantal gestures in VCV utterances apparently are superimposed on a vowel-to-vowel substrate gesture. As a mechanism of coproduction, it has been proposed that vowels and consonants are produced by different, though possibly overlapping, sets of muscles. The muscular distinction between these two classes supposedly finds empirical support in data on velocity, complexity, precision of movement, and anatomy (Perkell, 1969). Compared to consonants, vowels are said to have articulations that are slower, less complex, less precise in timing, and more reliant on the larger, slower extrinsic muscles that position the tongue body.

Fowler (1980) proposes to explain coarticulation as the result of the coproduction of consonants and vowels and of stressed and unstressed vowels. Thus, speech would be a continuous pattern of coproduction linkages. It is not clear from Fowler's description if this explanation works for the influence of consonants on preceding vowels or the influence of a stressed vowel on another stressed vowel. Any test of this model depends on a satisfactory description of the nesting of coordinative structures, that is, the functional organizations of muscles that define equivalence classes of movements (see Easton, 1972).

A fundamental principle in Fowler's formulation seems to be that co-production occurs for units that are quite different in their spatiotemporal properties, that is, units that are kinesiologically or motorically disjointed. Thus, she argues, as does Perkell (1969), that consonants and vowels have a number of distinguishing characteristics. Apparently, it is these differences in arti-culatory properties that permit coproduction of vowel and consonant. Fowler et. al. present the same argument, stating that because "for the most part, different muscles are involved in vowel and consonant production . . . .vowels and consonants can be, and are, coarticulated" (p. 414). But this approach leaves unexplained the many instances of coarticulation involving units or movements that are similar in articulation. For example, Bladon and Nolan (1977) have reported data showing frequent lingual coarticulation between consonants with canonically different tip and blade articulations. Coarticulations, then, could involve at least two major kinds of effects. First, we have the *apparent* coproduction of units that are minimally or slightly overlapping with respect to motor performance. Thus, in a VCV utterance, the consonant gesture may appear to be superimposed on an underlying diphthongal vowel articulation (Öhman, 1966). Second, there is an articulatory adaptation or accommodation between units that are highly similar in motor performance. An example here is the interaction of abutting blade and tip consonants.

Although much of the work on coarticulation has focused on positional differences observed in a quasi-steady state for a unit produced in different contexts, it is equally important that dynamic properties also show coar-ticulatory effects. A good example is the diphthong, which has an inherently dynamic articulatory correlate in the gradual movements of tongue or jaw or both. Figure 4-4 shows the articulation of the diphthong /aI/ in three different contexts, as recorded in a cinefluorographic film. Tongue movement is re-presented by two line segments that connect three markers attached to the lingual dorsum. Tongue motion is then shown as a plot of the marker positions at

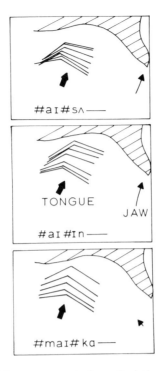

#aɪ#sʌ——

TONGUE

JAW

#aɪ#ɪn——

#maɪ#kɑ——

Figure 4-4. Tongue and jaw movements for articulation of diphthong /aɪ/ in three phonetic contexts. The range of jaw closing movement is shown by an arrow. Tongue-body articulation is shown by two line segments that connect three radiopaque markers attached to the midline of the tongue. The marker positions were recorded at intervals of 20 msec in a cinefluorographic film. Phonetic context is shown at the bottom of each panel; the number sign indicates a word boundary. The drawings show that both tongue and jaw movements vary with context.

20-msec intervals. Jaw movement is shown by an arrow, the length of which indicates the range of motion. Also shown for each panel is the phonetic context, in which the number sign represents a word boundary. The three panels show that the same phonemic segment, a segment defined by a *movement* rather than a steady state, is produced by quite different patterns of tongue and jaw articulation. Of particular interest is the result in the bottom panel where the diphthong is followed by the dorsal stop /k/. All three tongue points are involved in an elevating gesture, as though the diphthong is coproduced with a following stop. The blending of diphthongal and stop articulations is apparent at the first frame of movement. It seems likely that close examination of articulatory patterning will show many instances of apparent "coproduction." Moreover, this coproduction seems to occur not only because different muscles are used, but also when common muscles can be used to effect a movement parsimoniously adapted to the sequential articulation of two segments.

Models of speech articulation too often have neglected the biomechanical properties of the articulatory subsystems. Sussman and Westbury (1981) discuss this issue. The largest temporal ranges of coarticulation, whether measured in the notional time of phonetic segments or in clock time, have been observed for lip rounding and velopharyngeal opening, both of which are regarded as "sluggish" articulations by many speech researchers. In addition, these articulations simply do not exhibit as many changes in state or goal as do the articulations of the tongue. The extensive coarticulation for lip rounding and velopharyngeal opening might be explained in terms of coordinative structures by supposing that the muscle systems needed for their execution overlap to a rather small degree with those needed for more frequently occurring articulations. For example, lip rounding can be tolerated phonetically by a large number of sounds, and the articulation of rounding can be accommodated by other lip articulations such as bilabial closure. Similarly, nasalization can spread quite freely in English phonology, and velopharyngeal opening can accompany a variety of other articulations because the muscle systems overlap minimally.

IV. The Nature of Articulatory Variability

A straightforward articulatory interpretation of segmental organization is frustrated by two major classes of variability. First, the "same" sound (i.e., phoneme) is associated with a variety of articulatory configurations, depending on phonetic context, speaking rate, stress, and so on. An example is shown in Figure 4-5 for the prevocalic /r/. Tongue positions for the two major allophones of consonant /r/ (retroflexed and bunched) are shown at the top of the figure. Within these two major classes, however, there are still other variations. For example, the bottom of the figure shows that the bunched articulation can be relatively forward or central in the oral cavity, depending on the following vowel. Note also that the degree of lip protrusion and the position of the tongue root can vary across /r/ productions.

Another illustration of this type of variability is that as speaking rate is increased or as stress on a syllable is reduced, there is frequently a reduction in the range of individual articulatory movements. This reduction, commonly known as undershoot, is most easily demonstrated for vowels (Lindblom, 1963), but cinefluorographic studies reveal that a similar effect occurs for consonants, including obstruents. Kent (1970) and Kent and Moll (1972) presented evidence of tongue-body undershoot for the consonants /j/ and /z/. An example of the change in magnitude of displacement that can occur with increased speaking rate is shown in Figure 4-6. This graph shows the vertical position, as registered on a rectangular grid, of a radiopaque marker sutured to the undersurface of the velum during repetition of the syllable /t ʌ n/ at a slow and fast rate. The slow-rate production of about 2 repetitions per second is

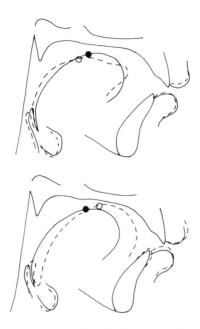

Figure 4-5. Articulations of prevocalic /r/. Shown at the top are the two major allophones: retroflex (broken line) and bunched (solid line). As shown at the bottom, tongue position varies even within an allophone: the bunched /r/ may be produced with a frontal or central tongue-body position.

represented by the open circles, and the fast-rate production of about 6 repetitions per second by the filled circles. The vertical displacement of the velar fleshpoint is diminished by about 60% at the faster rate. The reduction in rate affects both ends of the movement, that is, at the faster rate, the velum does not elevate as high for /t/ and it does not descend as low for /n/. The displacement plots also show that an increase in speaking rate does not necessarily lead to an increase in articulatory velocity. In fact, in this comparison, the highest velocity is observed for velar descent at the *slow* rate.

The second class of articulatory variability is that a given articulation may be timed differently with respect to other articulations that are taken to define the same speech sound (or segment). This variability is shown in Figure 4-7. This figure shows movement traces for the velum, tongue, and lips, as determined from lateral cinefluorography. The vertical lines indicate periods of oral closure. The articulations are for the test sentence "Next Monday morning bring three tents for the camping trip," for which a partial phonetic transcription appears at the bottom of the figure. The segments that are blacked in at the top are nasal consonants. Velar position during these segments varies considerably. Whenever the nasal consonant abuts an oral consonant, the velum actually is elevating *before and during* oral closure for the nasal. In some cases, as shown by the dashed vertical lines at the right side of the drawing, the gesture of velar

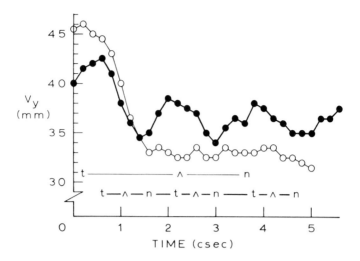

Figure 4-6. Vertical position of a radiopaque marker sutured to the undersurface of the velum during repetition of the syllable /tʌn/ at a slow rate (open circles) and fast rate (filled circles). Data were obtained by cinefluorography. Vertical displacement is about 60% less at the rapid rate than at the slow rate.

elevation begins almost simultaneously with the gesture of oral closure for the nasal consonant. The dashed line shows that the beginning of velar elevation in the top trace virtually coincides with the beginning of lip closure in the bottom trace. This timing pattern means that the velum is working to achieve a phonetic goal of nonnasal (-Nasal in binary-feature terms) while the oral articulator is just beginning to effect closure for the nasal segment. In the meantime, the tongue is still positioned for the /æ/ in *camping.* Figure 4-8 shows the divided attention of the speech motor executive: At the same instant, the tongue is held in a steady state for vowel /æ/, the lips are closing for the nasal /m/, and the velum is elevating to effect closure for the stop /p/.

Succession and Synchrony in Articulatory Planning

From movement analyses such as the foregoing, Kent et al. (1974) concluded that quite frequently in speech, "articulatory movements seem to be pro-grammed as coordinated structures so that movements of the tongue, lips, velum and jaw often occur in highly synchronous patterns" (p. 487). Kent and Minifie (1977) interpreted the sometimes overlapping and sometimes synchronous nature of speech articulation to mean that "articulations without immediate successional impact . . . are accommodated within the sequential pattern de-fined by the locally critical articulatory transitions" (p. 132). That is, some articulatory transitions determine the basic movement sequence that ensures

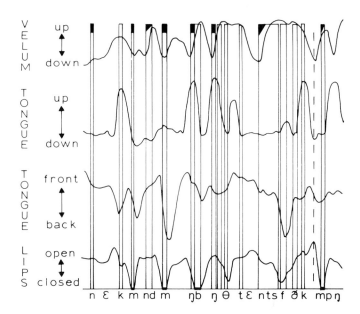

Figure 4-7. Movements of the velum, tongue, and lips recorded by lateral cine-fluorography during the sentence "Next Monday morning bring three tents for the camping trip." Movements of velum and tongue were recorded as displacements of radiopaque markers attached to these articulators. The segments blacked in at the top are nasal consonants. A partial phonetic transcription at the bottom of the illustration identifies major articulatory events. The dashed vertical line marks one example of nearly simultaneous movements of two articulators, in this case, velum and lips.

transmission of critical acoustic–phonetic cues. Other transitions are not locally critical and are subsumed in the plan as "state" variables that can be anticipated (or retained) without insult to phonetic integrity. In this view, an important factor in the conversion from phonological units to movement sequence is the specification of a plan of articulatory transitions. That is, transitions are more important in motor planning than are steady-state targets.

Of course, it is possible that synchronous patterns in articulation mean little, being perhaps mere accidents of a strategy that places no importance on their occurrence. But they are of potential significance if they do nothing more than mark certain points in time at which the powerful proclivity for overlapping of articulations is weakened. In addition, we have some limited evidence that synchronized movements can be seen in early speech development and in persons with certain neuromotor impairments of the speech mechanism. One example is shown in Figure 4-9. The articulatory patterns shown here were derived from a cinefluorographic film of a young boy with athetoid cerebral palsy. The position of the tongue, jaw, lip, and velum as recorded in several consecutive frames of the film are drawn in this composite to depict the nearly

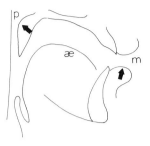

Figure 4-8. Cinefluorograph tracing of a frame in which the tongue is positioned for vowel /æ/, the lips are closing for nasal /m/, and velum is elevating for stop /p/. The articulations are for the word *camping*.

synchronous movements of these structures in the attempted production of /ata/ and /aga/. The gestures of tongue closure for /t/ and /g/ begin almost simultaneously with the closing motion of the jaw and the elevating motion of the velum. Normal adult speakers would, of course, close the velopharynx before the gesture of consonant closure is initiated.

In one sense, synchronous movements of the structures involved in a motor objective represent a simple or unrefined strategy of motor conttrol. The principle of "everything moves at once" might in fact be more common in

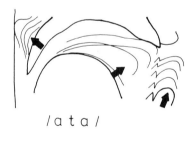

/ɑ t ɑ /

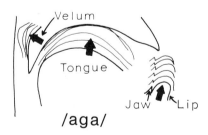

/aga/

Figure 4-9. Composite drawings obtained from cinefluorographic films of a cerebral-palsied child attempting the utterances /ata/ (top) and /aga/ (bottom). Positions of the articulators are shown at intervals of 40msec. For each utterance, movements of the tongue, velum, jaw, and lip begin and end at about the same time (i.e., they are nearly synchronous).

developing or impaired neuromotor systems than in a highly practiced and mature system. At least in the case of speech, fluent motor execution and a high event rate may depend on an overlapping of movements rather than synchronization of movements. I do not mean to imply that synchronized movements are unnecessary or undesirable, but only that exclusive reliance on the principle of "everything moves at once" does not seem to be the plan of speech articulation. Synchronous patterning may be a default principle that is overridden by phonetic and motor learning to yield the highly overlapping patterns that characterize rapid, fluent motor execution.

V. Segmental Organization in Backward Speech, Developing Speech, and Apraxia of Speech

I will now discuss some recent data pertaining to three areas that I believe to hold implications for the segmental organization of speech. The first of these might seem like a novelty experiment. It pertains to a fluent backward talker, that is, a speaker who can reverse phonetic strings quickly and quite accurately. The second area is speech development, which only recently has become the subject of detailed acoustic and physiological research. The third area is that of apraxia of speech, a neurologic communication disorder that frequently is described as an impairment of sequencing or motor programming of speech units.

A. Talking Backward

Recently, some Wisconsin colleagues and I (Cowan et al., 1982) had the opportunity to observe an individual with fluent backward speech. Upon being given a normal utterance, he could utter in simultaneous translation its backward counterpart, for example, [rʊtʃkɛl] for lecture [lɛktʃur]. One interesting aspect of this remarkable ability to reverse phonetic sequences is the extent to which the integrity of individual segments is maintained. Backward speech necessarily violates phoneme-sequencing constraints and certainly reduces the normal advantage of lexical access in a production task. Phonetic and acoustic analyses showed that the backward translation was not a mirror image of the forward string. Seldom was there reversal of on-glide and off-glide in diphthongs or diphthonglike sounds. For example, in the reversal of *continue* to /jutnitnak/, the diphthong or glide + vowel /ju/ was not reversed. Similarly, a diphthong such as /aI/ was not reversed to form /Ia/. Thus, *island* was reversed /dnalaI/. In this sense, some fairly strong evidence of phonemic integrity was observed. Phoneme-sized segments appeared to be convenient pieces for reversal of the utterance. A comparison of forward and backward speech by the speaker is shown in Figure 4-10. Spectrograms are displayed for the phrase *project to begin*, which was extracted from a sentence. The backward version /nɪgib ut tkɛjarp/ is shown at the bottom. Note that each word is reversed by a kind of backward play of its component phonemes. It thus appears that phonemes are as useful in talking backward as they seem to be in talking normally. Whether or not phonemes are real, they have an intuitive appeal to our backward talker, who was not linguistically sophisticated.

B. Speech Development: The Genesis of Segments

One major reason why data on speech development may be useful in understanding the segmental organization of speech is the possibility that young children have less extensive coarticulation than adult speakers. Although the data on this question are perhaps no more than suggestive, they invite more detailed studies of articulatory patterns in developing speech. One source of evidence is a recent study by Thompson and Hixon (1979), which showed that with increasing age, a greater proportion of speakers had nasal airflow beginning at the midpoint of the first vowel in /ini/. That is, anticipatory nasalization was observed more frequently with the older subjects. Kuehn and Tomblin (1974) reported in a cinefluorographic study of three children with articulation errors that there was "evidence of a limitation of certain dynamic properties of articulation, specifically with regard to the onset of anticipatory coarticulation."

Figure 4-11 shows further evidence that coarticulation is age dependent. Formant tracks for F_1 and F_2 (obtained from wide-band spectrograms) are shown for the production of the word *box* by three adults and three 4-year-old children. Notice that for the adults F_2 rises continuously during the vowel segment, apparently because these speakers anticipate the tongue-body elevation required for the velar stop (coproduction?). Thus, vowel and consonant articulation are blended together in the motor control of the tongue body. In contrast, the spectrograms for the children have a fairly well-defined steady state for the vowel; that is, the F_2 frequency stabilizes for a considerable interval of time. Our comparisons (Kent & Forner, 1980) also showed that the children had longer phonetic segment durations than the adults. One reason for the faster speaking rates of adults may be that their production patterns are more highly coarticulated, that is, more motorically fluent.

Differences in the temporal organization of adults' and children's speech also are shown in Figure 4-12, which depicts the F_2 frequency pattern during recitation of the words *saw you* in the sentence "We saw you hit the cat." The F_2 pattern is associated with the phonemic targets transcribed at the bottom of the illustration. Whereas the 4-year-old children exhibit a low–high–low F_2 pattern, with a low F_2 for the vowels /ɔ/ and /u/ and a high F_2 for the palatal /j/, the adults typically do not have an appreciable F_2 lowering for the /u/. Apparently, in rapid adult speech, the /u/ is not fully articulated (as compared with its isolated production), and the speaker anticipates the following /ɪ/ in *hit*.

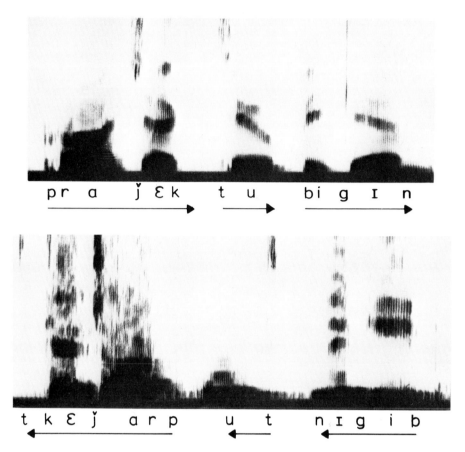

Figure 4-10. Wide-band spectrograms of a fluent backward talker saying the phrase *project to begin* forward (i.e., normally) at the top and backward (reversed) at the bottom. Speaking rate is nearly equivalent for the two conditions.

In articulatory terms, the adult speaker undershoots the /u/ target. The children are not as inclined to undershoot, and therefore a conspicuous F_2 lowering occurs for the /u/ target. Even when an adult does make a pronounced F_2 shift for /u/, as seen for the adult speaker at the bottom left, the time course of the formant-frequency shift is much faster than for the children.

The segmental influence appears to be much stronger in the children's speech than in the adults' speech. This result might be explained in motor terms by making a distinction between sequencing and phasing (Glencross, 1975). *Sequencing* refers to the temporal ordering of the units and *phasing* to the details of temporal structure aside from seriation of units. In development of a motor skill, mastery of sequencing is perhaps logically prior to mastery of phasing. Therefore, the motor patterns in children's speech tend to have a more segmental or discrete character than the motor patterns of adults. Phasing is

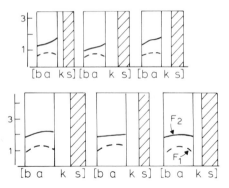

Figure 4-11. F_1 and F_2 patterns for the word *box* for (top) three young adults and (bottom) three 4-year-old children. Frequency in kilohertz is scaled on the ordinate. The three segments shown for each word are the voiced formant pattern for /b/ + /a/, the stop gap for /k/, and the combined noise segment for /k/ release + /s/ frication. Note the almost continuously rising second formant in the adults' productions in contrast to the flat, or steady-state, second formant in the children's productions.

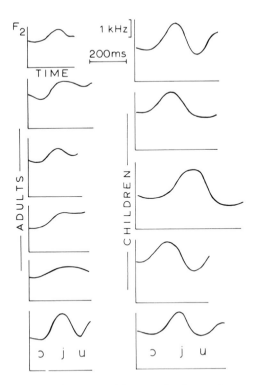

Figure 4-12. Trajectories of the second formant for the words *saw you* in the sentence "We saw you hit the cat." Results are shown for six adults and five children.

thus developmentally later than sequencing and serves to produce motor patterns that are rapid, efficient, and highly anticipatory. In a strategy dominated by sequencing, it is likely that synchronous movement patterns would occur relatively frequently, because motor control would reflect the discrete control of the motor executive. But as phasing is acquired, overlapping would increase and some movements that originally were part of a synchronous complex would be altered in timing to promote speed, efficiency, and anticipation—three factors that Bruner (1973) lists as criteria of motor skill learning.

It is clear from a number of investigations of children's speech that children are much more variable than adults in their articulatory patterns. However, the sources of the variability have not been isolated. One source of variability is the degree of refinement in motor execution needed to perform a certain phonetic goal. For example, we observed that 4-year-old children were more variable than older children and adults in controlling the durations of a variety of vowel and consonant segments in a simple sentence recitation task (Kent & Forner, 1980). It appeared that most of the variance could be represented as a continuous distribution of individual durations around a mean duration. In other words, the variation was unsystematic and might be regarded as "noise" in the neuromotor regulation of the speech movements.

Another source of variability appears to reflect basic segmental coding decisions and probably has a discontinuous distribution, or at least a distribution with distinct modes. An example is shown in the spectrogram of Figure 4-13, which shows two recitations by the same child of the words *took a spoon and* from the sentence "I took a spoon and a knife." The two utterances were obtained in the same recording session. In spectrogram A, the /p/ is produced as an aspirate but in spectrogram B it is produced as a nonaspirate. In both productions the /s/ preceding the /p/ was omitted. In this situation, the child must choose between two allophones of phoneme /p/. The aspirated /p/ is appropriate for English except when /p/ follows the fricative /s/. Thus, the aspirated [pʰ] in spectrogram A is phonologically correct given that /s/ was deleted, that is, /s/ was not present in the acoustic pattern. However, the unaspirated [p⁼] in spectrogram B also is phonologically correct *if* the child was attempting to produce the appropriate allophone for the intended context. Thus, spectrogram B shows that the child was adjusting the /p/ release to a preceding /s/ that was itself not acoustically evident.

The contrasting patterns in Figure 4-13 indicate that the child who is acquiring speech may have a phonological uncertainty related to segment or allophone selection. Additional data on patterns of this kind may give us a better understanding of whether children treat consonant clusters as segments in themselves or as combinations of segments. The occurrence of a word-initial unaspirated /p/, which is phonologically inadmissible in English, might be taken as evidence that the cluster is treated as a unit, for the lack of aspiration can be explained only by recognizing that the /p/ is part of a more complex phonological structure, even if that structure is not fully phonetically realized.

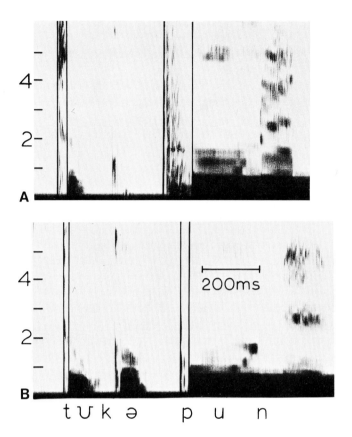

t ʊ k ə   p u   n

Figure 4-13. Wide-band spectograms of part of the sentence "I took a spoon and a knife" produced twice in the same recording session by a 4-year-old boy. Although /s/ is omitted both times, /p/ in *spoon* is realized allophonically as an aspirated stop in A but as a nonaspirated stop in B. The two spectrograms are evidence of allophonic variability in children's speech.

Although deletion of one segment in a cluster sometimes is taken as evidence that the child regards the cluster as consisting of isolatable segments, Barton, Miller, & Macken (1980) issue an appropriate caution concerning deletion as *prima facie* evidence for segment sequencing within clusters.

Young children typically fail to produce all the features of many adult phonemes, phonemes which are nevertheless uniformly treated as single units by phonologists. For example, recent work (Macken and Barton, 1980) has shown that at one stage in which English-speaking children produce both voiced and voiceless stop phonemes as voiceless and unaspirated, the children are in fact maintaining the phonological contrast. They do this not by means of aspiration as an adult would do, but rather by producing the voiceless stop phoneme with a slightly longer voice onset time than that used for the voiced stop. We can view the aspiration as being a component of the segment which is deleted. Similarly, the deletion of one member of a consonant cluster could simply be evidence for a phonologically unitary cluster being analyzed phonetically into components. (p. 106)

C. Verbal Apraxia: A Neuromotor Sequencing Disorder?

Of all the neuropathologies that affect speech and language, verbal apraxia (also called apraxia of speech) is even today one of the most controversial (Geschwind, 1975; Martin, 1974; Johns and LaPointe, 1975; Buckingham, 1979). LaPointe (1975) considered one of the most widely used definitions to be that of Deal and Darley (1972):

> an articulatory disorder resulting from impairment, as a result of brain damage, of the capacity to program the positioning of speech musculature and the sequencing of muscle movements for the volitional production of phonemes. The speech musculature does not show significant weakness, slowness or incoordination when used for reflex and automatic acts. Prosodic alterations may be associated with the articulatory problem, perhaps in compensation for it. (p. 634)

Many characteristics of the disorders have been described, but Johns and LaPointe (1976) list three as the most clinically salient (see also LaPointe, 1975):

1. Articulatory substitution errors predominate.
2. There are occurrences of initiation difficulty, characterized by stops, restarts, and repetitions of phones, syllables or whole words.
3. The error pattern is variable on repeated trials of the same word.

Shewan (1980) commented as follows on the general characteristics of verbal apraxia:

> Despite reported methodological and subject differences several consistent characteristics of verbal dyspraxia have emerged from the literature. (1) Verbal dyspraxia is distinct from the dysarthrias and from literal paraphasia. (2) Stimuli vary in their difficulty with a hierarchy of most to least difficult being consonant clusters, singleton consonants, and vowels. (3) Place of articulation is the feature most vulnerable to errors. (4) Phonemic substitutions are the predominant error type. (5) Errors increase with increasing syllabic length of stimuli. (p. 72)

The interpretation of verbal apraxia as a motor programming or sequencing disorder apparently is based on the observations that (a) errors are predominantly substitutions as opposed to omissions or distortions, (b) initiation difficulties are frequent, (c) the error pattern is highly variable, (d) place of articulation is more frequently in error than manner of articulation, and (e) error rate varies with phonetic complexity. However, Buckingham (1979) was critical of some of the terms used to describe apraxia of speech as an impairment of motor programming or seriation. Buckingham discussed definitional and observational difficulties associated with terms such as *programming, inco-*

ordination, and *selection*, and was especially critical of attempts to describe verbal apraxia as a motor disorder that affects phoneme selection and sequencing. He argued that because the phoneme is an abstract unit of linguistic analysis, it should not be incorporated as a construct in the motor programming of speech.

Canter, Burns, and Trost (1975) recognized two types of apraxic errors when they distinguished between "transitionalizing" between phonemes and the sequential ordering of phonemes. (A similar distinction, phasing versus sequencing, was introduced in the preceding discussion of speech development.) Thus, there might be two major types of disorder in temporal organization: disorders of sequential ordering and disorders of sequential flow. In summarizing the work on apraxia of speech in their Tokyo laboratory, Itoh, Sasanuma, Tatsumi, and Kobayashi (1979) concluded that the inconsistent articulatory errors in verbal apraxia are attributable to "an impairment of time programming for the appropriate phoneme rather than to a defect in selecting an appropriate phoneme" (p. 131).

Our preliminary acoustic analyses (Kent & Rosenbek, in press) seem to be in accord with Canter et al.'s (1975) suggestion that verbal apraxia involves a difficulty in "transitionalizing" as well as a difficulty in sequential ordering of segments. We have observed instances of mistiming of phonation: For example, voicing for a vowel begins during the frication segment for a preceding voiceless fricative. We also observed initiation difficulties in the form of false or labored starts. For example, a patient attempting to say *stealing* would say [steIpt] (pause) [stilIŋ]. Examples of segment substitutions were frequent. For example, a patient attempting to say *tornado* [torneIdo] said [dɔrneIro]. Our sample of subjects with apraxia of speech had a slow rate of speaking, with lengthening of phonetic segments, or marked pauses between syllables, or both.

Aside from initiation difficulties and frank articulatory errors such as substitutions and distortions, the most striking abnormality of the apraxic productions was distortion of the temporal organization of speech. Two types of temporal decomposition were sufficiently frequent in occurrence so as to deserve a descriptive label. We have called these two types *articulatory prolongation* and *syllable segregation* (Kent & Rosenbek, 1982; Kent & Rosenbek, in press). Articulatory prolongation is defined as a lengthening of transitional or steady-state components in an otherwise uninterrupted speech pattern. Syllable segregation is defined as temporal separation or isolation of the syllables in a syllabic series (other prosodic relationships among the syllables may or may not be disturbed).

One example of articulatory prolongation is illustrated in Figure 4-14, which shows spectrograms of the word *groceries* produced in sentence context by a normal and an apraxic speaker. The utterance for the apraxic subject is truncated during the final syllable for convenience of illustration; the full word is shown for the normal talker. The F_2 and F_3 trajectories are drawn on the spectrograms. Compared to the normal speaker, the apraxic speaker has a longer duration of utterance and a conspicuous lengthening of both transitional

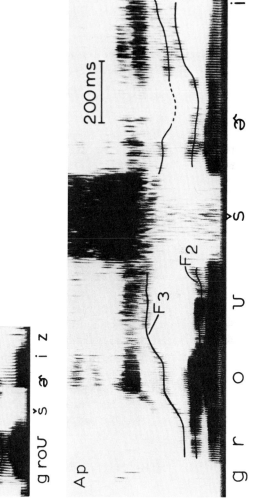

Figure 4-14. Wide-band spectrograms of the word *groceries* produced in sentence context by a normal speaker (N) and an apraxic speaker (Ap). The pattern for the apraxic subject is an example of segmental decomposition and segmental lengthening.

and steady-state segments. The first syllable in the apraxic pattern contains three fairly distinct steady-state segments joined by quasi-incremental transitions. The stair-step formant movements in the apraxic pattern contrast with the smooth formant movements in the normal pattern. Frication for /ʃ/ in the apraxic pattern is almost 300 msec in duration, about equal in duration to the final two syllables of the normal pattern.

Another example of this segmental decomposition is shown in Figure 4-15. The spectrogram shows an apraxic speaker's attempted production of the word *analysis*. The word duration was over 2 sec and individual phonetic segments often had durations of 200 msec or more. Furthermore, the spectrogram illustrates a tendency toward equalization of segment durations; for example, the segments for [n], [æ], [l], and [ʌ] have nearly equivalent durations. The overall picture, then, is one of lengthened and rather inflexible segment durations.

The other major kind of decomposition in verbal apraxia is one apparently based on syllable-sized units. An example is given in Figure 4-16, which shows wide-band spectrograms of a normal and apraxic production of the word *vegetables* uttered in the sentence, "In the summer they sell vegetables." Compared to the normal speaker, the apraxic speaker has much longer individual syllable durations and marked interruptions between syllables.

Syllable segregation often is manifest as an unusual temporal patterning of syllables and words in conversation or in reading. The spectrograms in Figure 4-17 are examples for two apraxic subjects. Both spectrograms represent partial productions of the target sentence "The shipwreck washed up on the shore." Individual syllables tend to be long in duration and widely separated from preceding and following syllables. Individual syllables also show articulatory prolongation; for example, the word *wreck* in pattern (a) has long formant transitions for the /r/ to /ɛ/ phonetic transition, a long stop gap for /k/, and an exaggerated release frication for /k/.

A speculative characterization of the widely spaced syllables in apraxia of speech is that the speaker expends considerable time in preparing or programming each syllable. Consequently, syllables are emitted at long intervals, sometimes with reduced prosodic cohesion. However, interpretation of the duration of intersyllabic breaks or pauses is filled with uncertainties. MacKay (1974) interpreted the interval between successive items in a repetition task to be a measure of programming complexity. Similarly, Sternberg, Monsell, Knoll, and Wright (1978) have interpreted their data on latency and duration of repeated sequences in a simple reaction time (RT) experiment in terms of response programming or subprogram retrieval. Klapp, Abbott, Coffman, Greim, Snider, and Young (1979) argued against such an interpretation, pointing out that "In the simple-RT case, the appropriate response is precued in advance of the signal which initiates the response so that programming can occur before rather than during the RT" (p. 100). A similar criticism might be made with respect to MacKay's interpretation of the interval

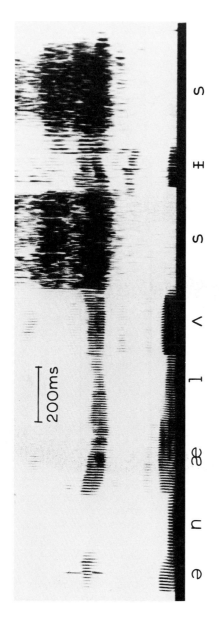

Figure 4-15. Wide-band spectrogram of the word *analysis* produced by an apraxic speaker. The spectrogram illustrates a segmental decomposition in which individual phonetic segments are markedly lengthened. There is a general tendency toward equal durations of segments. Note, for example, the durations of /n/, /æ/, /l/, and /ʌ/.

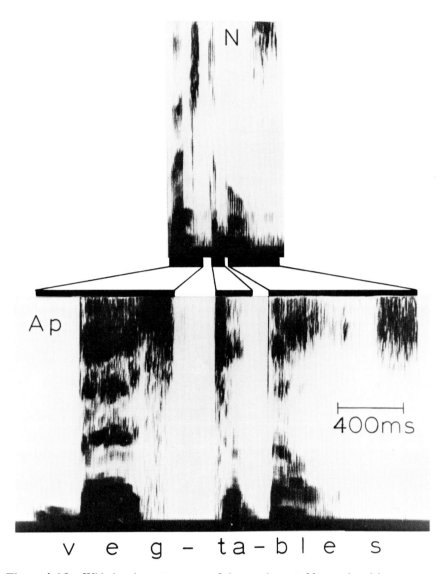

v e g – ta–b l e s

Figure 4-16. Wide-band spectrograms of the word *vegetables* produced in sentence context by a normal (N) and an apraxic (Ap) speaker. Note the greater syllable durations and intersyllable gaps in the apraxic pattern.

between repeated syllables as a measure of programming complexity. This interval may reflect something more akin to "read-out" time, that is, the time required to read out a program already prepared, rather than programming time per se. In the study of verbal apraxia, it may be as (or more) interesting to look at the location of pauses or prolongations as to measure the temporal magnitude of these effects.

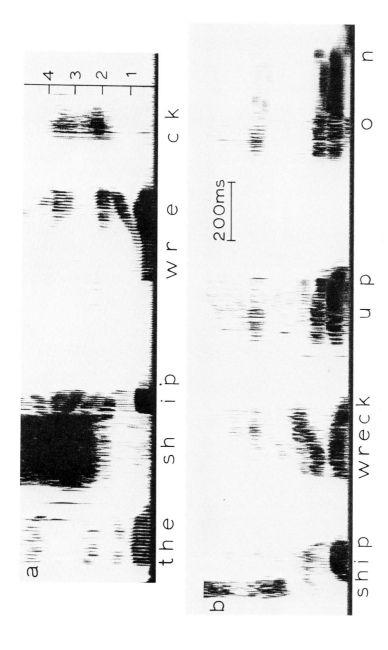

Figure 4-17. Wide-band spectrograms for two subjects with verbal apraxia, showing the effects of syllable segregation. Syllables tend to be lengthened and widely separated from neighboring syllables.

The apraxic errors in articulatory positioning and response sequencing might be explained by a theory of motor control of speech in which (1) temporal schemata (Semjen, 1977) regulate the sequencing of movements and (2) spatial targets are specified within a space coordinate system of the vocal tract. That is, generalized spatiotemporal schemata for speech articulation are learned and stored and individual motor programs are specified from these generalized schemata. Paillard (1960) noted that the disintegration of schemata might result in apraxic disorders in which the subject cannot plan an ordered motor sequence.

The spatiotemporal schema is a generalization by which various factors such as initial or current conditions, past experience, and desired outcome are considered in formulating response specifications for a particular, perhaps novel, motor performance (Schmidt, 1975). In the case of verbal apraxia, the subject might retain adequate movement control of the articulators for non-verbal functions, but suffer errors in speech movements because the spatio-temporal schemata peculiar to speech have deteriorated. As I have suggested elsewhere, "the schema is a means by which an abstract linguistic unit such as the phoneme can make contact with the physical events of articulatory control" (Kent, 1982).

A space coordinate system of the vocal tract has been proposed by MacNeilage (1970) and Sussman (1972). MacNeilage considered the space coordinate system to be part of a target-based model in which a phonological input is translated into a series of spatial target specifications. The targets "would result in a series of demands on a motor system control mechanism to generate movement command patterns which would allow the articulators to reach the specified targets in the required order" (MacNeilage, 1970, p. 189). A schema model of speech production might use targets defined within a space coordinate system as part of the information by which response specifications are generated. The errors of place of articulation in verbal apraxia might be taken to mean either that the subject's access to the space coordinate system is impaired or that the generalized spatiotemporal schema cannot reliably use the spatial information in generating response specifications. In this regard, Rosenbek, Wertz, and Darley (1973) reported that apraxics have depressed performance on tests of oral form identification, tasks that presumably require integration of kinesthetic and tactile information. In considering this deficit and the preference of verbal apraxics for the alveolar place of articulation in consonant substitutions, Klich, Ireland, and Weidner (1979) proposed that "place errors in apraxia of speech may be attributed to breakdowns in processes needed to use the space coordinate system for speech . . . [and that when] . . . such a breakdown occurs, speakers with apraxia of speech apparently restrict their articulatory activity to the more stable alveolar position" (p. 465).

Initiation errors in verbal apraxia might be explained as a general failure of the schema to specify motor commands given the intended motor response, the current state of the articulators, and experience in meeting similar demands. Substitution errors perhaps represent a default motor execution in which preference is given to the best established schema. Schemata for alveolars should be well established by virtue of the high frequency of occurrence of alveolar sounds in English. A related point is that Klich et al (1979) observed a greater frequency of occurrence of substitutions in the initial word position. They suggested that the word-position asymmetry in substitutions is related to the contextual sensitivity of initial consonants:

> For example, production of an initial consonant usually involves simultaneous articulatory adjustments for that consonant and for succeeding sounds (Öhman, 1966; Kent and Moll, 1969) whereas production of word-final post-vocalic consonants requires no anticipation of other speech sounds (MacNeilage and DeClerk, 1969). Since initial consonants therefore are accompanied by more complex encoding requirements, they may be associated with relatively more phonetic information. (p. 464)

Putting a schema perspective on this argument, one might suggest that the generation of response specifications is more complex for initial than medial or final consonants.

If it is assumed that schema also are used to evaluate a motor performance in terms of a comparison of the actual and predicted feedback (e.g., Schmidt's, 1975, recognition schema), a schema theory of speech production also might explain why persons with verbal apraxia sometimes have difficulty in correcting their errors. A deterioration of schemata could affect not only the generation of response specifications to perform an intended sequence, but also the derivation of error information to be used in correcting or adjusting the response specifications for future attempts.

VI. Conclusion

The literature is replete with speculations and arguments over the segmental organization of speech. Generally, the focus of both experiment and theory has been on fluent productions of normal talkers and, to a more limited extent, on the occasional errors (slips of the tongue) uttered by normal talkers. However, much less importance has been attached to developing speech in the child and to various speech disorders as fertile ground for both experiment and theory. Theories of segmental organization should be able to account not only for the well-informed utterances of the normal talker but also for the acquisition of speech by the child and for the systematic deterioration of speech that has been described for several disorders of communication. There is good reason to believe that speech is a complex recoding of a linguistic message into movements of the speech organs and the acoustic signal of speech. Furthermore, the nature of this recoding seems to be such as to obscure certain segmental properties in a way that is neither predicted nor explained by linguistic analyses per se. The obscuring occurs because of the demands of human performance in perception and production. Thus, for example, the study of speech articulation is not in itself a study of phonemic structure but is linked to such a study by the intervening processes of motor control and auditory perception. All of the major processes and influences must be considered in order to arrive at a sensible description of speech behavior. To study speech merely as a pattern of muscle contractions related to an observed movement sequence (as might be profitably applied to the study of locomotion) is as short-sighted as the complementary error of studying speech as a transparent expressive mode for any given linguistic theory. Speech has to be recognized as a motor skill but also as a mode of language expression.

References

Barton, D., Miller, R., & Macken, M. A. Do children treat clusters as one unit or two? *Papers and Reports on Child Language Development*, 1980, *18*, 105–137.

Benguerel, A. -P., & Cowan, H. A. Coarticulation of upper lip protrusion in French. *Phonetica*, 1974, *30*, 41–55.

Bladon, R. A. W. *Some control components of a speech production model.* Paper presented to International Phonetic Sciences Congress, Miami Beach, Fla., 1977.

Bladon, R. A. W. & Al-Bamerni, A. Coarticulation resistance of English /l/. *Journal of Phonetics*, 1976, *4*, 135–150.

Bladon, R. A. W. & Nolan, F. J. A videofluorographic investigation of tip and blade alveolars in English. *Phonetics*, 1977, *5*, 185–193.

Bruner, J. S. Organization of early skilled action. *Child Development*, 1973, *44*, 1–11.

Buckingham, H. W., Jr. Explanation in apraxia with consequences for the concept of apraxia of speech. *Brain and Language*, 1979, *8*, 202–226.

Canter, G., Burns, M., & Trost, J. *Differential phonemic behavior in anterior and posterior aphasic syndromes.* Paper presented to the 13th Annual Meeting of the Academy of Aphasia, Victoria, B.C., 1975.

Cowan, N., Leavitt, L. A., Massaro, D. W., & Kent, R. D. A fluent backward talker. *Journal of Speech and Hearing Research*, 1982, *25*, 48–53.

Daniloff, R. G., & Hammarberg, R. E. On defining coarticulation. *Journal of Phonetics*, 1973, *1*, 239–248.

Darley, F. L. *The classification of output disturbance in neurologic communication disorders.* Paper presented at the Annual Convention of the American Speech and Hearing Association, Chicago, Ill., 1969.

Deal, J. L., & Darley, F. L. The influence of linguistic and situational variables on phonemic accuracy in apraxia of speech. *Journal of Speech and Hearing Research*, 1972, *15*, 639–653.

Dukel'skiy, N. I. *Principles of segmentation of the speech stream.* Washington, D.C.: Joint Publications Research Service, No. 32790, 1965. (Originally published in Russian, 1962.)

Easton, T. A. On the normal use of reflexes. *American Scientist*, 1972, *60*, 591–599.

Fant, G. *Speech sounds and features.* Cambridge, Mass.: MIT Press, 1973.

Fowler, C. Coarticulation and theories of extrinsic timing. *Journal of Phonetics*, 1980, *8*, 113–133.

Fowler, C. A., Rubin, P., Remez, R. E., & Turvey, M. T. Implications for speech production of a general theory of action. In B. Butterworth (Ed.), *Speech production.* New York: Academic Press, 1980.

Fujimura, O., & Lovins, J. B. Syllables as concatenative phonetic units. In A. Bell & J. B. Hooper (Eds.), *Syllables and segments.* Amsterdam: Elsevier/North-Holland, 1978, pp. 107–120.

Geschwind, N. The apraxias: Neural mechanisms of disorders of learned movement. *American Scientist,* 1975, *63,* 188–195.

Gibbon, D. *Perspectives of intonation analysis (Forum Linguisticum,* Band 9). Bern: Herbert Lang, 1976.

Glencross, D. J. The effect of changes in task conditions on temporal organization of a repetitive speed skill. *Ergonomics,* 1975, *18,* 17–28.

Halwes, T., & Jenkins, J. J. Problem of serial order in behavior is not resolved by context-sensitive associative memory models. *Psychological Review,* 1971, *78,* 122–129.

Henke, W. L. *Dynamic articulatory model of speech production using computer simulation.* Unpublished doctoral dissertation, Massachusetts Institute of Technology, 1966.

Itoh, M., Sasanuma, S., Tatsumi, I., & Kobayashi, Y. Voice onset time characteristics of apraxia of speech. *Annual Bulletin, Research Institute of Logopedics and Phoniatrics, (University of Tokyo),* 1979, *13,* 123–132.

Johns, D. F., & LaPointe, L. L. Neurogenic disorders of output processing: Apraxia of speech. In H. Avakian-Whitaker & H. A. Whitaker (Eds.), *Current trends in neurolinguistics,* vol. 1. New York: Academic Press, 1976.

Kent, R. D. A cinefluorographic–spectrographic investigation of the component gestures in lingual articulation. Unpublished doctoral dissertation, University of Iowa, 1970.

Kent, R. D. Models of speech production. In N. J. Lass (Ed.), *Contemporary issues in experimental phonetics.* New York: Academic Press, 1976.

Kent, R. D. Sensorimotor aspects of speech development. In R. N. Aslin, J. R. Alberts, & M. R. Peterson (Eds.), *The development of perception: Psychobiological perspectives.* New York: Academic Press, 1982.

Kent, R. D. & Forner, L. L. Speech segment durations in sentence recitations by children and adults. *Journal of Phonetics,* 1980, *8,* 157–168.

Kent, R. D., & Minifie, F. D. Coarticulation in recent speech production models. *Journal of Phonetics,* 1977, *5,* 115–133.

Kent, R. D., & Moll, K. L. Vocal tract characteristics of the stop consonants. *Journal of the Acoustical Society of America,* 1969, *46,* 1549–1555.

Kent, R. D. & Moll, K. L. Tongue body articulation during vocal and diphthong gestures. *Folia Phoniatrica,* 1972, *24,* 286–300.

Kent, R. D., & Rosenbek, J. C. Prosodic disturbance and neurologic lesion. *Brain and Language,* 1982, *15,* 259–291.

Kent, R. D., & Rosenbek, J. C. Acoustic patterns of apraxia of speech. *Journal of Speech and Hearing Research,* 1982, in press.

Kent, R. D., Carney, P. J., & Severeid, L. Velar movement and timing: Evaluation of a model for binary control. *Journal of Speech and Hearing Research,* 1974, *17,* 470–488.

Klapp, S., Abbott, J., Coffman, K., Greim, D., Snider, R., & Young, F. Simple and choice reaction time methods in the study of motor programming. *Journal of Motor Behavior,* 1979, *11,* 91–101.

Klich, R. J., Ireland, J. V, & Weidner, W. E. Articulatory and phonological aspects of consonant substitutions in apraxia of speech. *Cortex*, 1979, *15*, 451–470.

Kozhevnikov, V. A., & Chistovich, L. A. *Speech: Articulation and perception.* Washington, D.C.: Joint Publications Research Service, No. 30, 1965. (Originally published in Russian, 1965.)

Kuehn, D. P., & Tomblin, J. B. The use of cineradiographic techniques for the study of articulation disorders. Paper presented at the Annual Convention of the American Speech and Hearing Association, Las Vegas, Nev., 1974.

Künzel, H. J. Some observations on velar movements in plosives. *Phonetica*, 1979, *36*, 384–404.

LaPointe, L. L. Neurologic abnormalities affecting speech. In D. B. Tower (Ed.), *The nervous system* (Vol. 3): *Human communication and its disorders.* New York: Raven Press, 1975.

LaPointe, L. L., & Johns, D. F. Some phonemic characteristics in apraxia of speech. *Journal of Communication Disorders*, 1975, *8*, 259–269.

Lebrun, Y., Buyssens, E., & Henneaux, J. Phonetic aspects of anarthria. *Cortex*, 1973, *9*, 126–135.

Lindblom, B. E. F. Spectographic study of vowel reduction. *Journal of the Acoustical Society of America*, 1963, *35*, 1773–1781.

MacKay, D. G. Aspects of the syntax of behavior: syllable structure and speech rate. *Quarterly Journal of Experimental Psychology*, 1974, *26*, 642–657.

Macken, M. A., & Barton, D. The acquisition of the voicing contrast in English: A study of voice onset time in word-initial stop consonants. *Journal of Child Language*, 1980, *7*, 41–74.

MacNeilage, P. F. Motor control of serial ordering of speech. *Psychological Review*, 1970, 77, 182–196,

MacNeilage, P. F., & DeClerk, J. L. On the motor control of coarticulation in CVC monosyllables. *Journal of the Acoustical Society of America*, 1969, *45*, 1217–1233.

Martin, A. D. Some objections to the term apraxia of speech. *Journal of Speech and Hearing Disorders*, 1974, *39*, 53–64.

Moll, K. L., & Daniloff, R. G. Investigation of the timing of velar movements during speech. *Journal of the Acoustical Society of America*, 1971, *50*, 678–684.

Newell, K. M., Hoshizaki, L. E. F., & Carlton, M. J. Movement time and velocity as determinants of movement timing accuracy. *Journal of Motor Behavior*, 1979, *11*, 49–58.

Norman, D. A. Copycat science or does the mind really work by table look-up? In R. A. Cole (Ed.), *Perception and production of fluent speech.* Hillsdale, N. J.: Lawrence Erlbaum Associates, 1980.

Öhman, S. E. G. Coarticulation in VCV utterances: Spectrographic measurements. *Journal of the Acoustical Society of America*, 1966, *39*, 151–168.

Öhman, S. E. G. Numerical model of coarticulation. *Journal of the Acoustical Society of America*, 1976, *41*, 310–320.

Paillard, J. The patterning of skilled movements. In J. Field, H. W. Magoun, & V. E. Hall (Eds.), *Handbook of physiology*, Section I: *Neurophysiology* (Vol. 3.). Washington, D.C.: American Physiological Society, 1960.

Perkell, J. S. *Physiology of speech production: Results and implications of a quantitative cineradiographic study* (Research Monograph No. 53). Cambridge, Mass.: MIT Press, 1969.

Pike, K. L. *The intonation of American English*. Ann Arbor: University of Michigan Press, 1945.

Pilch, H. *Phonemtheorie 1. Teil.*, 2nd rev. ed. Basel, 1968 (cited by Gibbon (1976)).

Rosenbek, J. C., & Wertz, R. T. Veterans Administration Workshop on Motor Speech Disorders, Madison, Wis. (unpublished), 1976.

Rosenbek, J., Wertz, R. T., & Darley, F. L. Oral sensation and perception in apraxia of speech and aphasia. *Journal of Speech and Hearing Disorders*, 1973, *38*, 462–472.

Schmidt, R. A. A schema theory of discrete motor learning. *Psychological Review*, 1975, *82*, 225–260.

Semjen, A. From motor learning to sensorimotor skill acquisition. *Journal of Human Movement Studies*, 1977, *3*, 182–191.

Shewan, C. M. Phonological processing in Broca's aphasics. *Brain and Language*, 1980, *10*, 71–88.

Sternberg, S., Monsell, S., Knoll, R., & Wright, C. The latency and duration of rapid movement sequences: Comparison of speech and typewriting. In G. Stelmach (Ed.), *Information processing in motor control and learning*. New York: Academic Press, 1978.

Sussman, H. M. What the tongue tells the brain. *Psychological Bulletin*, 1972, *77*, 262–272.

Sussman, H. M., & Westbury, J. R. The effects of antagonistic gestures on temporal and amplitude parameters of anticipatory labial coarticulation. *Journal of Speech and Hearing Research*, 1981, *46*, 16–24.

Tatham, M. A. A. A speech production model for synthesis-by-rule. *Ohio State University Working Papers in Linguistics*, 1970, *6*.

Thompson, A. E., & Hixon, T. J. Nasal air flow during normal speech production. *Cleft Palate Journal*, 1979, *16*, 412–420.

Wickelgren, W. A. Context-sensitive coding, associative memory, and serial order in (speech) behavior. *Psychological Review*, 1969, *76*, 1–15.

Chapter 5

Development of Speech Production: Perspectives from Natural and Perturbed Speech

D. KIMBROUGH OLLER and PETER F. MACNEILAGE

I. Introduction

By five years of age normal children produce speech that sounds much like that of adults. Before this time, their approximations include a number of well-documented systematic errors. Children from 20 to 30 months of age commonly:

1. reduce[1] consonant clusters;
2. delete[1] final consonants;
3. assimilate[1] the phonetic features of one syllable to other syllables in the attempted string; and
4. collapse[1] certain phonemic categories systematically—for example,
    (a) initial fricatives, affricates, and stops collapse to stops,
    (b) initial and final stops of all voicing types collapse to voiceless un-aspirated stops,
    (c) liquids and glides become glides, and
    (d) dorsal and apical consonants collapse to apical ones.

Explanation of these commonly observed patterns is a primary (if not *the* primary) goal of research in child phonology. Explanations for these patterns have posited important roles for (1) perceptual, (2) cognitive, or (3) motor factors.

---

[1]These terms (reduce, delete, etc.) are traditional descriptors of the pattern of relationship of child and adult pronunciations; they should not be taken to indicate the authors' views on the mechanism of production.

II. Perceptual Factors

A common contention is that a child's failure to pronounce certain element types is due to inability to discriminate among certain types (Carrell, 1968; Berry, 1969; Peizer & Olmsted, 1969; Waterson, 1971; Salus & Salus, 1974). This claim has been contested by others who have asserted that children have all the necessary discrimination skills relevant to speech (Stampe, 1972). The latter view has several kinds of apparent (and we emphasize "apparent") empirical support. One point is that many minimal speech sound contrasts have been demonstrated to be discriminable in infancy: for example, voiced and voiceless stop and fricative consonants in various positions (Eimas, Siqueland, Juszyck, & Vigorito, 1971; Eilers & Minifie, 1975), stop consonants differing in place of articulation (Morse, 1972), and stops and glides (Hillenbrand, Minifie, & Edwards, 1977).

However, to show that a minimal pair *can be* discriminated is not necessarily to show that the discrimination will be easy enough to be used practically in real speech settings. Recent evidence (Eilers, Gavin, & Oller, in press; Oller & Eilers, 1982) suggests that sounds discriminable in 6- to 9-month-old infants may not uniformly be *used* discriminably in real speech settings by young children (24–36 months). Furthermore, it should be noted that very few infant studies have been directed toward assessing discrimination of multiple tokens of speech sound types (see Kuhl, 1979) and none have addressed open sets of representatives of sound types to be studied. Instead, a single tape-recorded token of, say, /ba/ is generally contrasted repetitively with a single token of, say, /pa/. Results showing discrimination in such studies may have limited generalizability to the extremely varied sounds of real speech, where no two /ba/'s are identical, and where /b/'s and /p/'s may have quite different acoustic character depending on phonetic context, speaker, ambient noise level, and so on. It appears important, then, to maintain a healthy skepticism about how generally applicable the infant's speech discrimination abilities are, in spite of some positive scientific evidence of skills.

Another kind of evidence apparently favoring the notion that children *can* discriminate sounds they do not produce has been called the *"fish–fis* phenomenon"* (Moskowitz, 1970). Consider this interchange:

Mommy: What's this?
Two-year-old child: A fis.
Mommy: A fis?
Child: No, a fis!
Mommy: A fis?
Child (perturbed): No, a fis!
Mommy: Oh, a fish?
Child: Yes, a fis.

It has been asserted that the commonness of such interactions (and they are widely reported) shows that children auditorily discriminate what they do not produce discriminably. In the case presented the child certainly does auditorily discriminate the mother's *fish* and *fis*, but what is not at all clear is that such discrimination had been available throughout the child's learning experience. At an earlier stage the productive collapse of *fish* and *fis* may indeed have been influenced by auditory discrimination difficulty. To show, as this example does, that *at some stage* there is an ability to recognize distinctions without an ability (or willingness) to pronounce them, is not to show that the pronunciation is uninfluenced by possible perceptual problems from an earlier stage. Furthermore, it is emphatically not true that *fish-fis*-type interchanges occur whenever one imitates a child's systematic phonetic errors. Often the child accepts such renderings without apparent notice. The *fish–fis* phenomenon does not, then, prove that discrimination difficulties are irrelevant to speech sound errors in general.

Yet another claim that presumably indicated that perception could not account for production errors was made by Stampe (1972). His contention was that when children overcome a pronunciation error (e.g., collapse of liquids and glides), they overcome it with precipitous thoroughness, applying the correction in all phonetic environments immediately. This, he asserted, indicated that the problem could not be perceptual (apparently assuming that perceptual changes would have to be gradual). However, the facts do not support Stampe's claim. Actually, child pronunciation changes appear to occur with many fits and starts, a new and more correct pronunciation often appearing first in very limited contexts and then spreading, across weeks or months, to a variety of additional ones (Warren, 1975).

It is not, then, possible to rule out perceptual influences on childhood phonological errors. In fact, some positive evidence supports the idea that certain sound errors may at least in part be perceptual at root. For example, the English contrast of /f/ and /θ/ has been shown to be relatively difficult (compared to other contrasts) in a variety of studies with adults (Miller & Nicely, 1955), 2-year-old children (Eilers & Oller, 1976; Johnson, Hardee, & Long, 1981), and infants (Eilers, Wilson, & Moore, 1977). The very common collapse of /f/ and /θ/ in child speech (in, e.g., *baftub*) is amenable to an explanation emphasizing perceptual difficulties.

While it is not possible to rule out perceptual influences on pronunciation errors, it *is* possible to show that at least one characteristic of these errors is *not* perceptual in nature. This characteristic is unidirectionality. Note that /θ/ → /f/, but not /f/ → /θ/ (except in hypercorrections occurring at later developmental stages). Similarly, /r/ → /w/ but not /w/ → /r/, and so on. Also, in cases of assimilation, the choice of "assimilator" and "assimilatee" (e.g., in velar assimilation of an alveolar: /dɔgi/ → /gɔgi/) does not appear to be explicable on perceptual grounds. Neither does the choice of a particular form of consonant cluster simplification. Perception might offer an explanation as to why sounds are undifferentiated in production, but it cannot explain why the child consistently chooses a particular alternative for pronunciation (Compton, 1970).

III. Cognitive Factors

It has been suggested that child sound errors may be attributable to difficulties with the phonological storage of lexical items. There are reported instances of children pronouncing a contrast correctly in immediate imitation but failing to produce the same contrast discriminably in a naming situation. A common case of this is seen in progressive pronunciations (Leonard, Schwartz, Folger, & Wilcox, 1978). For example, a child is asked to imitate a new word (e.g., *pretty*) involving some element (/r/) generally deleted in the child's system. The child's first imitation attempt (or first several attempts) *includes* the normally avoided element (/r/) but later that element is dropped and the pronunciation is made consistent with the rest of the system in spontaneous use of the word. Such a pattern cannot be reconciled with the notion that avoidance of /r/ is motivated by either strict perception or strict production constraints. It has been reasoned that the avoidance is most appropriately viewed as more central. Ingram (1976) has referred to such avoidance as "organizational."

Further indications of an organizational explanation for some speech sound errors come from a perception and production study of eight children from 18 to 30 months of age (Johnson et al., 1981). The investigators tested the production of 11 pairs of nonsense syllables in a pure imitation task. The same syllables were then taught to the children as names for dolls. In the last phase of the experiment, the 11 pairs of syllables were tested in a meaningful speech perception study. For example, one pair of syllables employed was [sa] versus [ʃa]. In the imitation study each child was asked to imitate [sa] and [ʃa] several times, and adult judgments were made as to whether the productions were collapsed or distinct. Then the children were taught to identify dolls named [sa] and [ʃa]. Finally the child was asked to "pull [sa] (or [ʃa]) in the wagon."

The results of the study showed that of contrastive syllable pairs that were treated correctly in the meaningful speech perception (pull-the-doll) task, 81% had been produced contrastively in imitation. Since it is common for some perceived contrasts to be productively collapsed (as in the *fish–fis* phenomenon), a pattern showing better perception than production might be expected. However, it is logically impossible for a child to produce a systematic imitative distinction between sounds that the child cannot discriminate perceptually. Johnson et al.'s results showed that 55% of pairs that were "perceptually confused" in the meaningful speech discrimination task were distinctly articulated in the imitation task. Since the imitative success of the children clearly shows a perceptual (and productive) discrimination capacity, we must look for an explanation of the confusions in the meaningful speech perception task in a realm beyond peripheral perception or production. An explanation involving cognitive organization of phonetic units seems necessary. Apparently the child can sometimes hear a distinction and pronounce it, as long as the task is cognitively simple and does not require involvement of his full linguistic (including lexical) and action control systems. Initial imitation of nonsense words would not necessarily involve lexical search. The subsequent learning of the syllables as names for dolls *would* involve establishment of lexical categories, although the precise composition of the sound-related aspects of lexical representation may not yet be optimal. It may then be that under the demanding conditions of comprehending an entire sentence and designing an action accordingly, the lexical representation may not be adequate to consistently support a correct response.

On the basis of evidence from the Johnson et al. study, it appears reasonable to conclude that organizational factors do play a role in some speech production errors of childhood. It should be stressed, however, that evidence has not ruled out the possibility that storage or organizational constraints may be instituted in response to *relative* perception or production difficulty.

IV. Motor Factors

Perhaps the factor most widely assumed to account for common childhood speech sound errors is production (motor) difficulty, or an "ease of articulation" principle. However, a major barrier to universal acceptance of the importance of this factor has been the view of Jakobson (1941). He argued that although all possible speech sounds are (according to his understanding) produced with equal ease in the prelinguistic babbling stage, sounds used in the child's first words develop in a fixed order, determined by an innate linguistic mechanism for maximizing perceptible phonological distinctions. Since Jakobson assumed that babbling productions showed all sounds to be easy, he concluded that ease of articulation could not explain the later errors. This view has problems on all counts. In the first place, babbling data do *not* show an ability of infants to produce all sounds with ease. Contrary to Jakobson's claim, some types (e.g., ejectives) occur rarely, if ever, in babbling as judged by adult listeners, and the ones that occur frequently are largely the ones that are also judged to occur in early meaningful speech (see Lewis, 1936; Menyuk, 1968; Cruttenden, 1970; Oller, Wieman, Doyle, & Ross, 1975). Thus, in fact, the data on babbling show a high similarity with patterns observed in early meaningful speech, and leave open the possibility that avoidance of certain element types or sequences (e.g., consonant clusters, fricatives, liquids, dorsal consonants) may be motivated in both cases by relative difficulty of production.

Sounds in the child's first words develop in a *relatively* fixed order, but not in the *absolutely* fixed order required by Jakobson's theory. The sounds most frequent in the child's babbling tend to be the ones first used in words. There are some differences from child to child, so that the hierarchy of preferences is a statistical one. But even the statistical picture is not the one to be expected from a theory based on maximization of perceptual differentiation. Ohala (1979) has pointed out that if consonant preferences in the world's languages (which are very similar to the consonant preferences in children's first words) were chosen to maximize perceptual differentiation, they would be very different from what they are.

V. Speech Motor Development: Theoretical Issues

Of the three factors that appear to be involved in the development of speech patterns of children—perceptual, cognitive, and motor factors—motor factors may, in spite of Jakobson's objections, be the dominant ones. There seem to be productive preferences for certain sounds over others regardless of context and an extremely pervasive hierarchy of contextual preference effects. One thing that is obviously needed is an objective definition of the possible explanatory concept—ease of articulation. Some steps have been taken in that direction. For example, the obvious difficulty of maintaining the transglottal air flow necessary for voicing during vocal-tract obstruction is a plausible explanation for the preference of children (and languages) for voiceless rather than voiced obstruents (Ohala, 1981; MacNeilage, 1982). However, we seem a long way from explanatory principles that would cover the wide range of context-dependent effects.

There is a temptation to speculate that a child gradually learns specific rules for correct production of sounds in each context. This would imply that by the time he no longer makes the errors described above (usually by 5 years), he is essentially performing at adult levels. However, recent work on adult speech production encourages a somewhat different view. A salient feature of this work has been the demonstration that adults show a remarkable versatility in producing acceptable speech by means of compensatory maneuvers in the presence of unusual and sometimes unexpected perturbations of their articulations (e.g., placement of bite blocks between the teeth—Lindblom, Lubker, & Gay, 1979). These remarkable adaptations suggest that rather than learning a subset of fixed motor patterns for particular contexts, the adult speaker has learned general-purpose algorithms for goal attainment. Furthermore, it becomes possible to understand the purpose of such algorithms when one views speech in an ecological perspective, and notes the extremely wide variety of postural perturbations (e.g., lying down, turning one's head, eating) under which speech is normally successfully produced (MacNeilage, 1981).

It is not at all obvious that children have such extensive compensatory speech abilities. Indeed, the learning of pronunciation systems for languages may require extraordinary efforts in the realm of adapting to a wide variety of postural and situational perturbations. The requirements of developing adaptation algorithms might be a primary source of the motor difficulty of speech from the earliest stages, and thus might be a major factor in the systematic sound errors described earlier. Children might be thought to use simple, restricted sound inventories precisely because only a small number of elements can be adapted at early stages to a sufficiently wide variety of settings and postures. In this context it is of interest to determine the compensatory ability of children developing speech. We report here an initial study of this question.

VI. A Preliminary Bite Block Study with Two Normal Children

A. Goal

The goal of this pilot study was to determine whether or not two normal children could pronounce acoustically and auditorily acceptable vowels with their teeth clenched and with bite blocks clenched between their teeth. In addition, we planned to compare pronunciations of the vowels at the beginning and end of sessions and look for change (possibly attributable to experience) in resonance patterns in the bite block and teeth clenched conditions. It was hoped that the results of the study would provide a preliminary view of childhood compensatory speech abilities and encourage additional research. Because the children were relatively old with respect to those studied in child phonology research in general, the results of this first study would, in any case, represent only a beginning.

B. Methods

1. Subjects Two English-speaking children, a boy of 4 and a girl of 8, were used as subjects. Both children are clear speakers and neither had had any experience in any previous study examining compensatory speech abilities. In both cases the children's hearing and general intelligence were verified as normal.

2. Apparatus The two bite blocks employed were made of white Teflon. They were 100 mm long, 6 mm wide (horizontal dimension in use), and either 15 or 20 mm wide (vertical dimension) at the point of tooth contact. The point of contact was a groove at one end of the block into which the teeth of these subjects fitted securely. At the end distal from the groove, the blocks had a hole through which a thick leather thong was threaded. The experimenter held the thong while the child had the block clenched between his or her teeth.

The recordings both for model stimuli and for child's pronunciations were made in a single-wall IAC sound-insulated chamber. The recordings were made and stimuli were played on a TEAC tape recorder (3300-2T) using Scotch 250 tape. Stimuli were played to the children through a high-fidelity amplification system and a Pioneer HPM100 speaker in the sound chamber. The recording microphones were battery powered.

The acoustic analyses were obtained with a Kay Sonagraph (6061B).

Narrow-band Type A spectra were obtained for each relevant vowel produced. Type B spectra were used to supplement interpretations and to determine locations for placement of sectioner pins.

3. Stimuli A native speaker of American English pronounced three [i]'s and three [æ]'s, which were recorded as stimuli on a master tape. Each vowel was approximately 500 msec in duration with approximately 300 msec inter-stimulus interval (ISI). These were judged by independent listeners as being unambiguous as to vowel quality.

A stimulus tape was made by dubbing the master pronunciations repeatedly. The two vowels /i/ and /æ/ always occurred in groups of three (e.g., /i/, /i/, /i/ then /æ/, /æ/, /æ/) but the relative order of occurrence of /i/'s and /æ/'s on the tape was quasi-random and counterbalanced with regard to experimental conditions.

4. Recording Procedure The subjects were individually seated in the sound-treated booth. They were informed that they would hear a voice from the loudspeaker in the booth pronouncing vowels like /i/, /i/, /i/ or /æ/, /æ/, /æ/. They were asked to imitate the sounds and "say just what the voice says." A practice trial with three pronunciations of a vowel not involved in the study was given to verify that the subjects understood the imitation task.

The subjects were further informed before the recordings began that there would be three ways they would be asked to imitate the sounds. In one case they would be biting on a block while they spoke. The 15-mm bite block was then shown to the children. They were told they would be asked to bite firmly and not to let the block slip around as they spoke. In another case, they were told, they would be asked to speak with their teeth clenched. Finally, they would on some occasions be asked to speak normally. These explanations were given before the subjects had any practice with the blocks because the experimenters wished to record the very first attempts at articulation in the fixed-jaw conditions.

The three experimental conditions (jaw free, bite block, teeth clenched) were presented for recording in a quasi-random order. For the 4-year-old child, 15 pronunciations of each vowel were elicited in each condition. Thus his data represent 45 productions of each vowel. The 8-year-old pronounced 30 exemplars in each condition for a total of 90 productions per vowel. Only the /i/ pronunciations have been analyzed for the 8-year-old. At the end of the basic session, the 4-year-old pronounced an additional 5 and the 8-year-old an additional 10 /i/ vowels with the 20-mm bite block. During the entire recording procedure, elicited productions were always in three trial blocks of the same vowel (either /i/, /i/, /i/, or /æ/, /æ/, /æ/).

5. Spectrographic Analysis Difficulties of analyzing resonances of child vowels are discussed by Fant (1966), taking particular account of fundamental frequency. Because childhood F_0 is high, harmonics are widely spaced and error of formant estimation is high. As in any study of resonances in child speech, the present study was required to deal with the relatively high error of formant estimation. One indication of such error is that the average remeasurement error for resonance peaks in this study was approximately 100 Hz.

Another difficulty in the present study is that the first formants of childhood vowel productions were often difficult to assess because first harmonics represented peaks in the spectra, indicating that the first formant frequency may have been near or below the fundamental. For this reason, we resolved to ignore first formants in the data analysis.

Type A Sonagrams (frequency by amplitude spectra) were made for each child vowel. The second major resonance peak was determined by assuming a half-power bandwidth of -3 dB. In the case of /i/ vowels this resonance ($R2$ in the figures) was often a combination of second, third, and even fourth formants, since clustering of the formants produced a very wide-band resonance in the spectrographic displays, and $F2$ could not be isolated by using the chosen bandwidth criterion. Because $R2$ is influenced by $F3$ and $F4$, the values for $R2$ are clearly higher than the $F2$ data reported for other children of the age of the present subjects (see Kent, 1979).

The spectrographic displays were made for the central portion (in time) of each vowel. It is thus reasonable to expect that auditory feedback could be involved in determining the accuracy of the resonances of the vowels pronounced by the children.

6. Listener Judgments In addition to the spectrographic analysis of the produced vowels, two experimentally blind listeners, both phonetically trained, were asked to judge independently the vowel quality of each child's pronunciation. Listeners were seated in a quiet room and were told that they would hear the voices of two children pronouncing vowel sounds. Their task was to transcribe each vowel as one of eight possibilities: [i], [I], [ɑ], [E], [æ], [ə], or [a]. They were informed that there were no "wrong" answers and that not all the seven vowels would necessarily occur. If the pronunciation seemed ambiguous as to vowel quality, listeners were given the option of recording two alternatives.

The tape was then played to the listeners, with only the voices of the children being audible. The order of playback was the same as that produced by the children.

C. Results

1. Spectographic Data The data show wide discrepancies between the two children. The 8-year-old produced relatively stable $R2$ values of /i/ for the three conditions across 30 pronunciations (displayed as 10 blocks of three trials each in Figure 5-1), while the 4-year-old produced changing $R2$'s for /i/ across 15

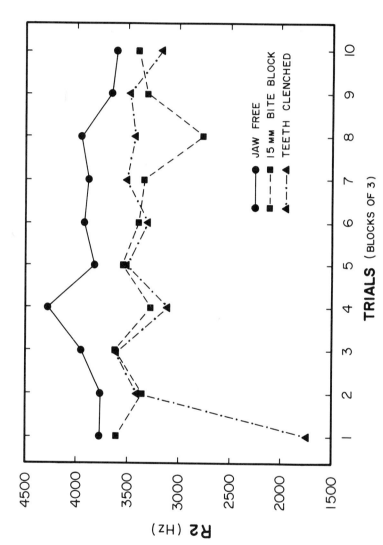

Figure 5-1. Resonance complex $R2$ in the production of the vowel /i/ by the 8-year-old child.

trials (displayed as five blocks of three trials in Figure 5-2). Excluding the first block of three trials in the teeth clenched condition (which we take to indicate lack of attention), $R2$'s of the 8-year-old child had trial-to-trial standard deviations of only 259, 288, and 190 Hz for the jaw free, bite block (15 mm), and the teeth clenched conditions, respectively. These standard deviations represent only 7% of the mean $R2$ values. In the 4-year-old's case, the inconsistency is much greater. His standard deviations of 553, 796, and 891 Hz for $R2$'s in the three conditions represented 15% of the mean $R2$ values.

The data from the 8-year-old also show a consistent relationship of $R2$'s for the three conditions. The $R2$ for the jaw free condition ($\bar{X} = 3861$ Hz) is uniformly higher than the other two conditions for all 30 trials. Values for the bite block and teeth clenched conditions are quite similar to each other (3357 and 3392 Hz, respectively), again ignoring the first three trials in the teeth clenched condition. The difference between the jaw free and other conditions is not only consistent but large, and it is about five times the estimated measurement error. No obvious tendency toward "improvement" of the $R2$ values in the fixed-jaw conditions is seen.

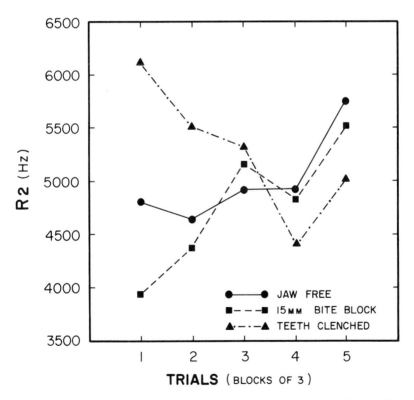

Figure 5-2. Resonance complex $R2$ in the production of the vowel /i/ by the 4-year-old child.

Another indication of the effect of fixed-jaw conditions on the 8-year-old subject's resonance patterns for /i/ is that a larger bite block (20 mm) produced a greater discrepancy of values. In Figure 5-3, the first six jaw free *trials* (not *blocks*) are compared with the first and last six trials with the 15-mm block and the six trials with the 20-mm block (administered at the end of the session). The mean $R2$ with the 20-mm block is 3024 Hz ($SD= 94$ Hz), more than 300 Hz down from the 15-mm condition. Note also that the last six 15-mm trials do not appear closer to the jaw free condition than the first six trials.

The 4-year-old's data, on the other hand, suggest an extensive adaptation to the fixed-jaw conditions across 15 trials. The $R2$ value for the teeth clenched condition begins highest (over 6000 Hz), while the value with the bite block (15-mm) begins lowest. After nine trials, the values for the three conditions are quite similar. Surprisingly, even the jaw free condition shows considerable variability, especially in the last three trial blocks.

In Figure 5-4, the 4-year-old's data on the 20-mm and 15-mm blocks are compared. The abscissa here represents trial-by-trial data, and indicates that in the first five trials the 15-mm block yielded a considerable decrement in $R2$

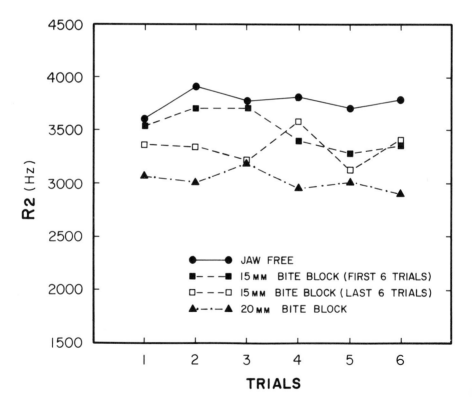

Figure 5-3. Resonance complex $R2$ in the production of the vowel /i/ by the 8-year-old child showing serial effects and effects of different-sized bite blocks.

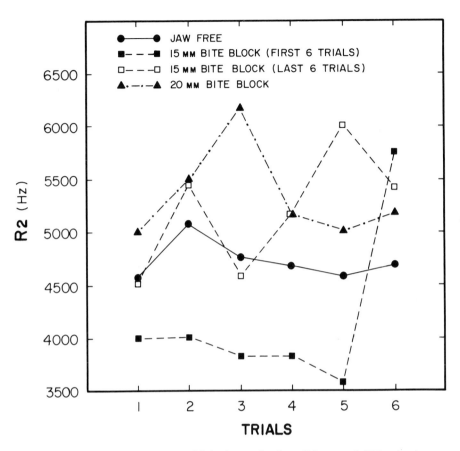

Figure 5-4. Resonance complex R2 in the production of the vowel /i/ by the 4-year-old child showing serial effects and effects of different-sized bite blocks.

from the jaw free condition (first six) but that on the sixth bite block trial the child began producing a much higher R2. The last six trials with the 15-mm block as well as the six trials with the 20-mm block (occurring at the end of the session) both show higher R2's than the jaw free condition's first six trials. Thus, the data on the vowel /i/ for the 4-year-old suggest variable performance and a substantial change in pronunciation strategy across the session, resulting in an apparent overcompensation. Even the jaw free condition seems to have been affected by the strategy change (see Figure 5-2, fifth trial block), and the relative ordering of R2's for the three conditions is scrambled with respect to the beginning of the session.

An additional indication of adaptation by the 4-year-old across the session is seen in Figure 5-5, where data on 15 trials of imitation of /æ/ are displayed. The resonance focused on, referred to as R1A, has a −3-dB bandwidth and represents the second peak in the Type A Sonagram. Note that this resonance

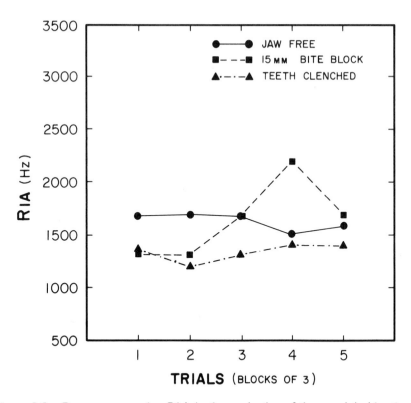

Figure 5-5. Resonance complex $R1A$ in the production of the vowel /æ/ by the 4-year-old child.

was fairly stable across 15 trials for the jaw free condition (8% variability, SD = 132 Hz) as well as for the teeth clenched condition (9% variability, SD = 129 Hz). In the latter condition it was consistently depressed. In the 15-mm bite block condition, however, the child began with a depressed $R1A$ but by the third trial block adjusted the pronunciation, overshooting on the fourth block and realigning on the fifth. The variability of $R1A$ in the bite block condition is considerable (28% variability, SD = 463 Hz) indicating extensive adjustment.

2. Listener Judgment Data The listener judgments of the pronunciations described in the section on spectrographic data indicate that in spite of substantial differences in pronunciations from condition to condition most of the vowels were heard appropriately as /i/ or /æ/. Even the extremely variable /i/ vowels of the 4-year-old were normally heard as /i/. On the other hand, some differences between the jaw free and jaw fixed conditions could be discerned, especially if pronunciations judged to be ambiguous as to vowel quality were considered. All of the 30 jaw free /i/'s of the 8-year-old were heard as /i/ by the listeners but 6 of 30 with teeth clenched were heard by at least one listener as either not /i/ at all or as ambiguous (either /i/, /I/, or /E/). In the 15-mm bite block condition 9 of 30 were heard by at least one listener as ambiguous or mistaken, and with the 20-mm block all six pronunciations were heard as ambiguous. It can thus be concluded that, while compensation for the jaw fixed conditions must have occurred, it did not, from an auditory perspective, completely overcome the limitations imposed by the physical restrictions for the 8-year-old child.

The listener judgment data for the 4-year-old child are more difficult to interpret. All his /i/ vowels pronounced in the jaw free condition were heard unambiguously as /i/. Surprisingly, given the wide shifts in $R2$, the jaw fixed conditions also produced near uniform perceptions of /i/ (14 of 15 for both the teeth clenched and 15-mm bite block conditions and 5 of 6 for the 20-mm bite blocks). For the vowel /æ/, the listeners did not generally hear unambiguous correct imitation even in the jaw free condition (9 of 15 attempted /æ/'s were heard as other vowels). The teeth clenched and bite block conditions produced even more perceived errors (14 and 13, respectively). Thus, although the data for the 4-year-old show some complications, there is a trend toward a larger number of perceived errors in the jaw fixed conditions.

VII. Conclusion

This chapter has been intended not only to provide a rationale for studies of compensatory speech abilities in childhood, but also to begin addressing the study empirically. What has been determined is that in the case of two normal children, some degree of adjustment for fixed-jaw conditions does occur, but that, unlike normal adults, adjustment is not always sufficient to eliminate auditorily identifiable anomalies in the vowel qualities produced. For the younger child, acoustic analysis suggested rather radical adjustments in the jaw fixed conditions until by the end of the brief session he appeared to be overcompensating for the limitations of a fixed jaw and even introducing acoustically extended jaw free pronunciations of the vowel /i/. For the older child, the jaw fixed conditions produced relatively stable acoustic patterns with resonances identifiably different from those produced in jaw free conditions. These differences did not, however, always yield differences in perceived vowel quality.

Such results offer reason to pursue further the study of compensatory speech in childhood. The results of such studies will surely be of interest to those who wish to gain perspective on the manner in which compensatory abilities develop. Further, if relative inabilities of children (especially younger ones) to compensate consistently and effectively can be verified in additional work, it will provide support for the contention that systematic childhood sound errors may represent an adaptation to the difficulties of pronouncing various phonetic elements in a wide variety of physical settings.

VIII. Discussion of Results

The discussion of the present work at the conference on speech programming from which this volume arose was informative and useful in suggesting a variety of possible additional steps in such research and in offering notes of caution on the interpretation of this preliminary study. Several discussants addressed the methodology for resonance estimation and offered suggestions about how to improve it. By using a buzzer simulating a low F_0 introduced in the middle of vowel productions, formant resolution might be improved (Dr. Lindblom). Similarly, having the children whisper their pronunciations could considerably improve resonance estimation (Dr. Kent). Also, by tracking resonance changes in diphthong productions, resolution of individual formants might be made possible (Dr. Fujimura). These sorts of options were presented in part as means of clarifying what the children's particular formant patterns were, since it is some conjunct of formants that yields the $R2$ complex and that may produce the primary perceptual cue for /i/ vowels. Further, by resolving formant patterns it might be possible to understand better the articulatory gestures used to achieve acoustic adjustments. Other discussants further encouraged direct monitoring of articulation patterns, for example, with strain gauge systems and the like.

A basic question in interpretation (raised by Dr. Diehl) concerned the possibility that the 8-year-old's data may have represented a literal anatomical inability to acoustically adjust sufficiently (in jaw fixed conditions). In response we pointed out that at least in the case of the 15-mm bite block, some individual pronunciations yielded $R2$'s of 3800 Hz or more. It thus seems reasonable to conclude that the subject had the anatomical capacity to match the $R2$ of the jaw free condition. The same reasoning does not, of course, unambiguously indicate that relative anatomical limitations did not encourage the depression of $R2$'s. Furthermore, the six pronunciations of /i/ with the 20-mm block by the 8-year-old subject were all substantially depressed (see Figure 5-3), leaving open the possibility of an absolute anatomical limitation in this case.

Beyond the issue of the child's capacity to produce similar resonance patterns with and without jaw fixing, discussants questioned what precisely the child might be attempting to do in fixed-jaw conditions. Dr. Porter suggested that the child might readjust his acoustic targets in the fixed-jaw conditions and might be satisfied with less than "perfect" approximations, recognizing that normal speech allows some variations from norms without loss of phonetic information. Dr. Abbs pointed out that the listener judgment data suggest that the children may have made adjustments for the jaw fixings in realms other than resonance patterns, for example, in F_0 and in vowel duration. These suggestions have merit, and the possibility that the children did cope with jaw fixings in unexpected ways simply cannot be ruled out given the present data.

The discussion of the chapter has offered several important suggestions for further work. A concerted effort to unravel patterns of the development of compensatory speech abilities may produce benefits both for child phonological theory and for the general understanding of the manner in which speakers adjust to a wide variety of physical contexts in speech communication.

Acknowledgments. This research has been supported by the Mailman Foundation. The authors thank Rebecca Eilers, Robert Rosov, and Livia Gomez for assistance in the experiment.

References

Berry, M. *Language disorders of children.* New York: Appleton-Century-Crofts, 1969.

Carrell, J. *Disorders of articulation.* Englewood Cliffs, N. J.: Prentice-Hall, 1968.

Compton, A. J. Generative studies of children's phonological disorders, *Journal of Speech and Hearing Disorders,* 1970, *35* (4), 315–339.

Cruttenden, A. A phonetic study of babbling, *British Journal of Disorders of Communication,* 1970, 5 (2), 110–118.

Eilers, R. E., Gavin, W. J., & Oller, D. K. Cross-linguistic perception in infancy: The role of the linguistic experience, *Journal of Child Language,* in press.

Eilers, R. E., & Minifie, F. D. Fricative discrimination in early infancy, *Journal of Speech and Hearing Research,* 1975, *18*, 158–167.

Eilers, R. E., & Oller, D. K. The role of speech discrimination in developmental sound substitutions, *Journal of Child Language,* 1976, *3*, 319–329.

Eilers, R. E., Wilson, W. R., & Moore, J. M. Developmental change in infant speech perception, *Journal of Speech Hearing Research,* 1977, *20*, 766–780.

Eimas, P., Sigueland, E., Juszyck, P., & Vigorito, J. Speech perception in infants, *Science,* 1971, *4*, 303–306.

Fant, C. A note on vocal tract size factors and non-uniform *F*-pattern scalings, *STL-QPR,* 1966, *4*, 22–30.

Hillenbrand, J., Minifie, F. D., & Edwards, T. Tempo of frequency change as a cue in speech sound discrimination by infants. Paper presented at the biennial meeting of the Society for Research in Child Development, 1977.

Ingram, D. *Phonological disability in children.* New York: Elsevier, 1976.

Jakobson, R. *Kindersprache, Aphasie, und allgemeine Lautgesetze.* Uppsala: Almqvist & Wiksell, 1941.

Johnson, C. J., Hardee, W. P., & Long, S. W. Perceptual basis for phonological simplification of the fricative class. Paper presented for the American Speech, Language and Hearing Association, 1981.

Kent, R. D. Imitation of synthesized vowels by preschool children. *Journal of the Acoustical Society of America,* 1978, *63*, 1193–1198.

Kuhl, P. K. Speech perception in infancy: Perceptual constancy for spectrally dissimilar vowel categories, *Journal of the Acoustical Society of America,* 1979, *66* (6), 1668–1679.

Leonard, L., Schwartz, R. G., Folger, M. K., & Wilcox, M. J. Some aspects of child phonology in imitative and spontaneous speech, *Journal of Child Language,* 1978, *5*, 403–415.

Lewis, M. M. *Infant Speech: A study of the beginnings of language.* New York: Harcourt, Brace & World, 1936.

Lindblom, B., Lubker, J. F., & Gay, T. Formant frequencies of some fixed-mandible vowels and a model of speech motor programming by predictive simulation. *Journal of Phonetics, 1979, 7,* 147–161.

MacNeilage, P. F. Feedback in speech production: An ecological perspective. In T. Myers, J. Laver, & J. Anderson (Eds.), *The cognitive representation of speech.* Amsterdam: Elsevier/North-Holland, 1981, 39–44.

MacNeilage, P. F. Speech production mechanisms in aphasia. In S. Grillner, B. Lindblom, J. Lubker, & A. Persson (Eds.), *Speech Motor Control.* Wenner-Gren International Symposium series, Vol. 36. New York: Pergamon Press, 1982, 43–60.

Menyuk, P. The role of distinctive features in children's acquisition of phonology, *Journal of Speech and Hearing Research,* 1968, *11,* 138–146.

Miller, G. A., & Nicely, P. E. An analysis of perceptual confusions among some English consonants, *Journal of the Acoustical Society of America,* 1955, *27,* 338–352.

Morse, P. A. The discrimination of speech and non-speech stimuli in early infancy, *Journal of Experimental Child Psychology,* 1972, *14,* 447–492.

Moskowitz, A. The two-year-old stage in the acquisition of English phonology, *Language,* 1970, *46,* 426–441.

Ohala, J. Discussion of Symposium No. 1. Phonetic universals in phonological systems and their explanation. *Proceedings of the 9th International Congress of Phonetic Sciences,* 1979, *2,* 5–8.

Ohala, J. Chapter 9, this volume.

Oller, D. K., & Eilers, R. E. Speech identification in Spanish- and English-learning two-year-olds, *Journal of Speech and Hearing Research,* 1982, in press.

Oller, D. K., Wieman, L., Doyle, W., & Ross, C. Infant babbling and speech, *Journal of Child Language,* 1975, *3,* 1–11.

Peizer, D., & Olmsted, D. Modules of grammar acquisition, *Language,* 1969, *45,* 68–96.

Salus, P. R., & Salus, M. W. Developmental neurophysiology and phonological acquisition order, *Language,* 1974, *50,* 151–160.

Stampe, D. *A dissertation on natural phonology.* Unpublished doctoral dissertation, University of Chicago, 1972.

Warren, I. *The development of phonological processes in the young child.* Unpublished doctoral dissertation, University of Washington, 1975.

Waterson, N. Child phonology: A prosodic view, *Journal of Linguistics,* 1971, *7,* 170–221.

Chapter 6

Sublexical Units and Suprasegmental Structure in Speech Production Planning

STEFANIE SHATTUCK-HUFNAGEL

I. Introduction

A number of elements have been suggested as units of sublexical processing during planning for speech production, some derived from grammatical theory and some from observed variations and constancies in the acoustic and articulatory patterns of speech. Candidates range from muscle-group control mechanisms to distinctive features, individual phonemic segments, diphones, demisyllables, syllable onsets and rhymes, and even syllables themselves. Proposals vary widely, partly because different levels of processing are being modeled, but also because the production planning process is highly complex, and our understanding of its many aspects is still quite rudimentary. To cite just a few areas where our models are particularly primitive, little is known about the planning mechanisms that might impose serial order on abstractly represented units, those that integrate adjacent elements with each other, those that coordinate all of the factors influencing segment duration, and those that compute motor commands; even less is known about the relationships among such possible processing components.

This chapter deals with a type of evidence from spontaneous language behavior, and with the light this evidence sheds on one particular aspect of production. The evidence comes from speech errors and it bears on the question of the sublexical units that undergo serial ordering. The discussion will leave aside the possible relation of serial ordering processes to lexical retrieval on the one hand, and questions about coarticulatory integration and articulatory motor control on the other, and focus instead on one surprising fact: Fragments of

Table 6-1.   Submorphemic Error Units

---

1. . . . ponato . . . (tomato)
2. . . . tar cowed . . . (car towed)
3. Doing neep dee bends . . . (deep knee)
4. *Journal of Vernal Lerbing* . . . (*Verbal Learning*)
5. There's this /baiθ pæk/ . . . (bike path)
6. . . . theep droat . . . (deep throat)
7. . . . dretter swying . . . (sweater drying)
8. . . . shu flots . . . (flu shots)
9. . . . journicle article . . . (journal article)
10. Matatchie, Washington: the appital capital of the world. (apple capital)
11. Is it a blue building with stained glass wildings? (stained glass windows)
12. . . . rabbit habbits on the arm . . . (rabbit hops)
13. Roy and Joy . . . (Roy and Josh)
14. he said "Have you studied a lot?" and I sot—and I said "No, not very much."
15. . . . and the -anguage of lacquisition . . . (acquisition of language)

---

lexical elements can become misordered in speech production errors. In particular, such fragments can change places, resulting in exchange errors like those shown in Table 6-1. The set of sublexical units that can participate in exchange errors seems to range from distinctive features to base morphemes, and includes the segment, the syllable, and other sublexical strings of segments.

The first question this observation raises is, Why should sublexical elements participate in exchange errors at all? It is much less surprising that we find errors which involve the misordering of word and morpheme units, since we expect the generation of normal spontaneous utterances to invoke mechanisms for the retrieval and appropriate serial ordering of whole lexical items. We expect this because we presume that conversational speech is not cobbled together out of stored sequences of words. Instead, retrieved lexical entries are arranged in order afresh during the processing of each new utterance. Since there must be a mechanism to accomplish this task, it is not surprising to find that it may occasionally misfire, causing exhanges like "take up and sit notice" for "sit up and take notice," and "thinking down and sitting" for "sitting down and thinking." The question is, Why should smaller sublexical elements, like features, segments, and sequences of segments, participate in exchange errors as well? Is there also a mechanism in the production planning apparatus that imposes serial order on fragments of lexical items?

The ubiquitous occurrence of exchange errors that involve these elements suggests that there is such a mechanism, although its operation is not yet clearly understood. The argument goes like this: We know from observation that when the production planning process malfunctions, it sometimes results in a misordering of sublexical fragments (for our purposes, these are units smaller than the morpheme). We assume that in most cases a speech error results from what is essentially a normal sequence of planning events, marred only by a minor malfunction, rather than from a grossly atypical series of events that occurs only during the planning of utterances that contain errors. On this assumption, the occurrence of misorderings (i.e., exchanges) between sublexical elements strongly suggests that these elements normally undergo a serial ordering process during production planning; in other words, errors in ordering imply a normal ordering process that sometimes malfunctions.

The major question addressed in this chapter concerns the nature of the processing units over which this mechanism operates. Any constraints that can be observed on which of the sublexical elements of an utterance can interact with each other in errors will provide information about this normal ordering process, the units it operates over, and the form of their representation.

Evidence for Sublexical Error Units

Evidence that sublexical error units do indeed arise comes from a growing number of error corpora. For example, in 1971 Fromkin published observations on her University of California at Los Angeles (UCLA) corpus of spontaneous speech errors, reporting several types of exchange errors in which sublexical units changed places. The subsequent finding that close to half of the several thousand entries in the Massachusetts Institute of Technology (MIT) corpus of spontaneous speech errors also involved sublexical error units confirmed the widespread occurrence of this kind of error (Garrett, 1975; Shattuck, 1975). Fromkin was particularly interested in error units that correspond to the descriptive elements of linguistic theory: features, segments, syllables, and morphemes. The MIT survey focused on a wider variety of error unit types, adding syllable onset, syllable rhyme, and other "string-of-segment" units to the list. The error unit called *string of segments* consists of at least one consonant and one adjacent vowel which together form only part of a morpheme; for example, strings like "-anguage" (as in the error "the -anguage of lacquisition" for "the acquisition of language"). Error units like this raise the question whether we can identify any constraints at all on sublexical error units. Can any two strings of segments in an utterance exchange with each other in an error? The evidence that will be reviewed here suggests not, and supports instead the following hypothesis: The primary sublexical exchange error unit is neither the distinctive feature nor the syllable, but a structural unit very close to the single phonemic segment. There is some evidence that the syllabic subcomponents of onset, nucleus, and coda may provide a slightly better description of the data, but this possibility awaits experimental confirmation. Other error units, including the feature, the syllabic rhyme, and the syllable itself, as well as longer sublexical strings, arise comparatively rarely. Although the occurrence of errors that involve these units will have to be accounted for in an adequate model of the production planning process, the preponderance of single-segment (or possibly onset, nucleus, and coda) error units strongly suggests that these are the units over which sublexical serial order is normally computed.

To sum up the organization of the chapter: It will be argued that, although other sublexical units may play important roles in some aspects of representation and processing for production, it is individual phonemic segments (or possibly the syllable onset, nucleus, and coda) that normally undergo serial ordering. Evidence to support this view comes from (1) distribution patterns in a corpus of spontaneous speech errors, and (2) results of a series of error elicitation experiments using tongue-twister-like sequences of CVC syllables. Suprasegmental structures and patterns, on the other hand, constrain the ways in which these sublexical fragments can interact; again, both observational and experimental evidence supports this view. Finally, a preliminary model embodying these claims will be briefly described.

II. Error Evidence on the Nature of Sublexical Computational Units

A. Evidence from Spontaneous Speech Errors

The set of sublexical exchange errors in the MIT corpus that can be unambiguously classified as to the number of segments in the error unit involved are divided for our purposes into two groups: those that involve a single segment and those that do not. In addition, a large number of errors are ambiguous as to the unit involved. For example, does the error "cat fat" for "fat cat" involve a segment, a syllable onset, a syllable, or an entire morpheme? Is the error unit in "canpake" for "pancake" a feature, a segment, or a syllable onset? Although ambiguities of this type make precise enumeration difficult, the weight of the evidence supports a unit smaller than the syllable and larger than the feature as the most commonly exchanged sublexical unit. In addition, three further observations are supported by the data:

1. Exchanges of whole syllables are rare, as are exchanges of the rhyme component of syllables.
2. Single distinctive features rarely appear as exchange error units, even though many pairs of exchanged segments differ by only one feature.
3. The existence of a small number of sublexical errors that involve either (a) a single feature, or (b) strings of segments containing both a consonant and a vowel does not obviate the claim that the single segment predominates among exchanged sublexical elements. However, these nonsegmental errors will have to be accounted for in an adequate model of production and its possible malfunctions.

The arguments that support each of these statements will be examined in turn, under "Further Observations," below.

1. Distribution in the Spontaneous Corpus A brief word is in order here about the MIT error corpus, which has been described in more detail elsewhere (Garrett, 1975, 1976, 1980; Shattuck, 1975; Shattuck-Hufnagel, 1979). As of this date, more than 6000 errors have been collected, by the above authors and others, who monitor ongoing speech and write down mistakes as they are heard. Transcription includes as much of the sentential context as can be recalled and uses normal English orthography except where a broad phonetic transcription is necessary (e.g., to avoid the ambiguity of English vowel spelling.) The criteria for inclusion are (1) that the error is a clear departure from the speaker's intended output, normally with some indication that the speaker judges it to be different from his or her intention (a correction, a chuckle, a twitch, positive response to a direct interrogation by the listener, or, in a few cases, the strong intuition of the listener), and (2) that it is written down immediately, because errors are hard to remember for more than a few tens of seconds.

The corpus collected in this way at MIT contains at least a few examples of exchange error units for every descriptive unit on Fromkin's list, including the feature (e.g., "tik of the tum" for "tip of the tongue"), the segment (e.g., "gudget bap" for "budget gap"), the syllable (e.g., "How about Al Lucindor?" for "...Lou Alcindor"), and the base morpheme (e.g., "I've been reading this book about woodpecker-eating houses" for "house-eating woodpeckers"). In addition, there are exchanges that involve syllable onsets, rhymes, nuclei, and codas as well as apparently unmotivated sublexical strings of segments. For the present analysis we have removed the errors that clearly involve the exchange of entire base morphemes, like "I hate raining on a hitchy day" for "I hate hitching on a rainy day," because these error units may correspond to lexical entries rather than sublexical fragments. In addition, we have deleted the following categories of sublexical exchanges:

1. Within-word exchanges, like "tykipal" for "typical," which seem to behave differently from between-word exchanges with regard to stress and syllable-position constraints, and thus may arise by a different mechanism.
2. Incomplete errors, like "invate's—inmate's visitation rights," which are corrected in midstream. These interrupted errors may be incipient exchanges (e.g., "invate's misitation rights") but may also be the first parts of anticipatory substitution errors (e.g., "invate's visitation rights"), a type not discussed further in this chapter. Traditionally these errors have been classed as anticipatory substitutions; since we can neither accept nor rule out the possibility that they are incipient exchanges, they are omitted from our analysis here.
3. Errors that occur in function words, like "shince see" for "since she," which again appear to show different patterns from those found in exchanges between fragments of content words.
4. Exchanges in which the two target words have segments in common adjacent to the error, so that it cannot be determined how many segments are included

in the error unit. For example, in an error like "a mike meeld professor" for "a meek mild professor," the error unit could have been either V (i.e., /i/ exchanged for /ai/) or the initial CV (i.e., /mi/ exchanged for /mai/). With this subset removed, we can compare the frequency of unambiguous single-segment errors with that of unambiguous multisegment exchanges, presuming that the exchanges in which the error units share common segments are distributed in the same proportion. As an alternative to this approach, it could be argued that exchanges like "neep dee bends" for "deep knee bends," where the error unit could be either the initial C or the initial CV, should be included as syllable errors, or at least as CV errors. However, since it is impossible to determine the error unit in these cases, it seems safest to count them in neither class.

Moreover, any claim that syllables tend to serve as error units more readily when they have at least one identical segment would be impossible to distinguish from the claim that two phonemic segments exchange more readily when they are followed or preceded by an identical segment in their respective syllables. To avoid such problems, we have removed these unit-ambiguous errors from this analysis.

Of the 210 remaining exchange errors in the 1981 count of the MIT corpus (i.e., those that are complete, unambiguous as to the number of segments in the error unit, occur in content words, and are clearly sublexical), the majority—66% of the total, as shown in Table 6-2,—involve single segments. This subset includes only the single-segment exchanges: those between single consonants, between single vowels, and between single consonants located in clusters, as in "sprit blain" for "split brain." It does not include exchanges between a single consonant and a cluster, as in "shu flots" for "flue shots."

The remaining 34% of the sublexical exchange errors is divided among other error units, of which the next most frequent is the consonant cluster (16% of the total). This subset includes exchanges between single consonants and clusters (like "show snoveling" for "snow shoveling," and "lightly britt" for "brightly lit"), and a few exchanges of whole clusters (like "blink it drack" for "drink it black"). Another 4% are syllabic nuclei that include a vowel and a liquid, as in

Table 6-2.   Distribution of Sublexical Error Units

Unit	Number of errors	Percentage of total
Feature	2	1
Segment	138	66
CC or VV (includes V + liquid)	43	20
CV or VC (less than a syllable)	16	8
Syllable	6	3
String of Segments (more than a syllable)	5	2

"Sarmon and Gifunkel" for "Simon and Garfunkel," or "Is the merk bilning?" for "Is the milk burning?" Together, the C, V, syllable onset, and syllable nucleus exchanges make up 86% of the sublexical exchanges. This observation suggests that, at the level where sublexical exchange errors occur, the elements being processed are represented as individual phonemic segments and clusters, rather than as syllables or other subunits containing both C's and V's.

What of the remaining 14% of the unambiguous, complete, between-content-word sublexical exchange errors? What is the composition of this subset? In particular, what is the frequency with which the syllable and the distinctive feature participate in exchange errors? In the next section we turn to an analysis of these remaining errors.

2. Further Observations: Syllable and Syllable–Rhyme Exchanges, Feature Exchanges, and Other Error Units

Syllable and syllable-rhyme exchange errors are rare. Despite the overall predominance of the segment among sublexical exchange error units, it is possible that the syllable might make up a significant proportion of the nonsegmental errors. To test this possibility, we examined the distribution of nonsegmental sublexical exchange units in the 1981 count of the MIT corpus. Nonsegmental exchange units were classified as

1. single feature,
2. syllable onset cluster,
3. complex vowel nucleus (e.g., vowel plus liquid in the context, VCC),
4. syllable rhyme,
5. CV, when this sequence forms only part of a syllable (as in "the cutting widge of his et" for "the cutting edge of his wit"),
6. entire syllable, and
7. longer strings of C's and V's within a morpheme.

Recall that cases like "where did you get those sues, shoe?" for "where did you get those shoes, Sue?", where the exchanged segments are followed or preceded by identical phonemic contexts, were omitted from the analysis because the number of segments in the error unit could not be unambiguously determined.

The results of this classification, shown in Table 6-3, clearly indicate that the syllable does not predominate among nonsegmental exchange error units. Less than 3% of the complete and unambiguous between-content-word exchange errors involve the exchange of two syllables. Of course, many monosyllabic word and morpheme errors are equivalent to single-syllable units, but we assume here that these errors involve units that are best defined at the higher level.

While the rarity of whole-syllable exchanges is clear, it is more difficult to evaluate the status of the syllabic components of onset and rhyme, as well as of nucleus and coda, as exchange error units. This is because so many of the errors

Table 6-3. Nonsegmental Error Units

Unit	Number of errors	Percentage of total
Feature	2	1
CC	34	16
VV (includes V + liquid)	9	4
CV (less than a syllable)	4	2
VC (less than a syllable)	12	6
Syllable	6	3
String of Segments (more than a syllable)	5	2

involve single-segment units that are equivalent to a syllable onset ("bate of dirth" for "date of birth"), nucleus ("sedden duth" for "sudden death"), or coda ("stick neff" for "stiff neck"). To illustrate this problem, Table 6-4 shows the percentage of errors that can be accounted for under three separate assumptions about the units of sublexical serial ordering: that they are (a) single phonemic segments, (b) the syllabic subcomponents of onset and rhyme (prefigured in MacKay, 1972), and (c) the syllabic subcomponents of onset, nucleus, and coda. About half the errors are accounted for by all three assumptions, since they occur between single-consonant onsets (as in "marsing Pontague" for "parsing Montague"). Each of the assumptions is violated by some of the errors, but the assumption of representational units equivalent to onset, nucleus, and coda is the most successful. This is because there are more errors that preserve polysegmental onsets than break them up, and more errors that preserve (vowel plus liquid) nuclei than break them up.

It must be noted that 12 errors or 6% of the total are best described as syllable rhymes, as in "you bind while I grone" for "you bone while I grind," and "my sole has a hock" for "my sock has a hole." With the 138 errors that can be described as syllable onsets, the assumption of the onset and rhyme as processing units accounts for 71% of the errors. This is worse than the 81% that results from the assumption of onset, nucleus, and coda, and better than the 66% from the assumption of the single phonemic segment. Thus, the issue of which sublexical units best account for the units of exchange errors awaits experimental resolution.

Table 6-4. Proportion of Exchange Errors Accounted for under Three Different Assumptions about the Processing Units

Assumed units	Percentage	
	Accounted for	Unaccounted for
Single segments	66	34
Syllable onset, syllable rhyme	71	29
Syllable onset, nucleus, and coda	81	19

Although some of the errors break up these syllabic subcomponents, there are two kinds of dissolution that do not appear in the corpus: (1) CV units in the context CCV, as in the /lai/ of "glide" or the /rei/ in "straight," and (2) (liquid) + C units in the context of V(liquid)C, as the /lt/ of "belt" or the /rt/ of "cart." Instead, the consonants of an onset cluster tend to function as a unit, as in "stover cory" for "cover story." The sequence of vowel-plus-liquid in a syllabic nucleus follows a similar pattern, serving as a unit in such errors as "basketbore callt" for "basketball court."

In general, the hypothesis that the syllable onset, nucleus, and coda are the primary units of sublexical serial misordering accounts for a higher proportion of sublexical exchange errors than does the single-segment hypothesis or the onset and rhyme hypothesis, but all three hypotheses run into difficulties in accounting for some of the observed errors, and each can account for some errors that the others cannot. The question which sublexical sequences *can* serve as exchange error units, and which units most often *do*, is presently being pursued with error elicitation experiments; see Section II.B for some discussion of these methods and preliminary results.

The second further observation to be made about sublexical errors in the spontaneous corpus is that *single-feature* exchange errors are rare, despite the large proportion of errors in which the exchanged segments differ by only one feature.

Evidence showing that exchanged segments undergo readjustment to fit their new context (Fromkin, 1971, 1973; Garrett, 1975, 1976) suggests that, at the point where serial ordering occurs, the segments are at least somewhat abstractly represented. In view of these observations, a reasonable working hypothesis about the nature of the sublexical serial ordering process might be that it involves some operation on the distinctive features, since they define the abstract phonological elements in the grammar. What do sublexical exchange errors reveal about this hypothesis?

The question is a significant one because it has been shown, for a number of speaker populations, that when one segment (the intrusion) substitutes for another segment (the target), target and intrusion tend to have a high degree of similarity (Blumstein, 1973, English-speaking aphasics; Goldstein, 1977, normal English speakers, UCLA and MIT corpora; Johns, 1972, Portuguese speakers; MacKay, 1970, German speakers, Merringer's corpus; Nooteboom, 1969, Dutch speakers; Shattuck-Hufnagel & Klatt, 1979a, 1979b, English speakers, MIT corpus). This target–intrusion similarity can be described in a number of different ways: in terms of shared distinctive features, articulatory characteristics, or even acoustic similarities. Unfortunately, our present methods of analysis do not allow us to determine which of these possible frameworks best captures the relationship between target and intrusion segments (although see Goldstein, 1977, and van den Broecke & Goldstein, 1980, for an evaluation of distinctive feature constraints on error matrices). However, the fact that the similarity patterns are compatible with a feature interpretation makes it important to determine whether apparent whole-segment exchanges can be as well or better described as the misordering of single-feature-like elements. For example, is the error "pits and beeses" for "bits and pieces" best described as the exchange of two segments (/b/ and /p/) or as an exchange of the feature values plus and minus voiced? (The arguments presented below are discussed in greater detail in Shattuck-Hufnagel & Klatt, 1979a.)

To what extent, then, can sublexical exchange errors be described in feature terms? First, although indisputable feature exchanges are rare in the MIT corpus, they do occur. For example, in "tik of the tum" for "tip of the tongue," the exchange of nasal for oral stop results in two new segments (/p/ and /ŋ/ become /k/ and /m/), so the error cannot be described as the exchange of two entire segments. The UCLA corpus contains a larger number of single-feature exchanges: the list of examples of single-feature errors (Fromkin, 1973) includes nine unambiguous feature exchanges, and more have been added since. It is unlikely that these errors can be accounted for as two independent segmental substitutions occurring in the same utterance which happen by chance to look like feature exchanges. If this were the case, they should form a small subset in a much larger group of pairs of concurrent errors within a single utterance that do not display this fortuitous feature symmetry. A constructed example of the kind of error that would be expected is "the mod was diven" for "the nod was given," where the substitutions of /m/ for /n/ and of /d/ for /g/ occur independently. But this larger set of double substitution errors is not found in the MIT corpus. Unrelated double substitutions within a single utterance are extremely rare if they occur at all; the MIT corpus contains no examples for nonadjacent segments. We conclude that these symmetric single-feature errors that create two new segments do in fact involve the transposition of individual feature values.

In contrast to errors that clearly involve interactions between single features, exchanges like "red-fud worests" for "red-wood forests," which would require several feature changes to describe, are more appropriately classified as whole-segment exchanges. Finally, there are a number of exchange errors in which the unit could be equally well described as a single feature or as a single segment, because the exchanged segments differ by only one feature (e.g., the exchange of /m/ and /b/, or of /d/ and /t/). What is the critical evidence that will distinguish between the feature description and the segment description?

We need a subset of errors that permits unambiguous determination of the kind of error unit involved. If we can isolate such a subset, and we find that whole-segment errors rather than individual-feature errors predominate there, it will strongly suggest that the set of ambiguous exchange errors (like /m,b/ exchanges) follows the same pattern, that is, that most of them are in fact exchanges of whole-segment planning units.

To qualify as candidates for unambiguous assignment to single-feature error unit rather than whole-segment error unit status, a pair of interacting segments must satisfy two criteria. First, the two segments must differ by more than one feature, so that single-feature and whole-segment exchange errors will produce distinct results. Segment pairs that differ by only one feature do not satisfy this requirement; for example, using the three-way classification of place, manner, and voice, the pairs /m,b/ or /p,k/. Segment pairs like /p,n/ and /f,k/ do satisfy this requirement. Second, the single-feature errors that could ocur between the segments of the pair must result in segments that are phonemically admissible in American English. The pair /s,k/ satisfies the first criterion, because the segments differ in both manner and place, but if place or frication features exchange, the result will include a velar fricative, a segment that is not part of the phonemic inventory of English. Since this circumstance may make a feature error less likely, such pairs have been removed from the set under analysis.

In the 1979 count of the MIT corpus, there were at least 70 unambiguous exchange errors whose target segment pairs met the two criteria just presented. Of these, only 3 interactions resulted in single-feature errors. The remaining 67 interactions changed more than one feature in each half of the error, and so are more parsimoniously described as whole-segment exchanges. This observation makes it highly unlikely that features or featurelike dimensions are the primary units of normal sublexical serial ordering.

The last of the further observations about sublexical error units is that although the single segment predominates as the error unit among exchanges that are unambiguous as to unit, there remains a small proportion that involves either single features or longer strings of segments (Table 6-3). Their numbers are relatively small compared to single-segment exchanges, but they raise some interesting questions. It is unlikely that they can be accounted for as the result of several independently occurring exchanges that happen to involve adjacent segments, because multiple exchanges almost never occur even for nonadjacent segments. The most likely explanation is probably either that they occur at some other point in production planning, or that once a misselection has occurred, there is some tendency for the processor to keep misselecting segments until it reaches the end of a larger sublexical constituent. In any case, the exchange of sequence-of-segment units will have to be accounted for separately in an adequate model of the production process, just as single-feature exchanges must be.

One step toward this end would be to specify constraints on polysegmental error units. There is some evidence that these constraints are quite powerful. For example, exchanged sequences that break up morphemes are almost always fragments of single morphemes; they do not span word or morpheme boundaries. That is, sequences like "-ome ba–" in "come back" do not function as error units (Shattuck, 1975). Further, certain patterns of breakdown in syllabic components are not observed; as noted earlier, we do not find the /ri/ of "treat" and other similar sequences appearing as error units. Very roughly, the constraint seems to be that larger units can break apart into their constituents in errors, but the resulting error units are almost never made up of fragments of one subcomponent plus fragments of another. This formulation is obviously unsatisfactory, and points out the need for a model that will account for the occasional occurrence of longer sequences of consonants and vowels as error units.

In the MIT corpus, there are a few cases where the error unit that might be called the "rest of the word" arises for polysyllabic target words, as in "Haire and Cloward" for "Howard and Claire." These data hint at a level of representation in terms of (1) initial segments of the word, and (2) the rest of the word. Hockett (1967) has proposed this analysis for monosyllabic mono-morphemes, but it is possible that it might be appropriate for all words at some level of processing. The large number of word-onset error units among sub-lexical exchanges, discussed earlier as evidence for syllabic subcomponents, is equally compatible with this alternative description in terms of components of words. This description would be particularly appropriate for a process of lexical access or retrieval, where word onsets are presumed to play a critical role (Shattuck-Hufnagel, 1981b). Analysis of larger numbers of sublexical errors, and experimental confirmation of observed patterns, will no doubt reveal further constraints on the sequences of segments that can serve as error units, and provide information that will be useful in evaluating claims about the units of sublexical production planning.

3. Summary: Spontaneous Error Evidence The observation that the segment or something close to it is the predominant error unit for sublexical exchange errors in the MIT corpus suggests the existence of a serial ordering mechanism that operates over elements that are represented in terms of these segments. In contrast, it does not support a model in which either whole syllables or distinctive features normally undergo such ordering. However, the distribution of error unit types in a spontaneous corpus is sure to be affected by any existing listener bias against certain kinds of error units. A stronger test of the segmental representation hypothesis would be provided by a similar analysis of errors elicited in the laboratory and tape-recorded to permit repeated listening and perhaps more objective transcription. In this way we could determine whether substantial numbers of syllable-sized or other errors have been systematically omitted from the corpus. In addition, since elicitation permits the use of stimuli that are prescribed by the experimenter, it allows greater control over the phonemic structure of utterances. In Section II.B we describe the results of an elicitation experiment that tests the notion that utterances are more likely to come apart into individual segments than into longer sublexical strings containing both C's and V's.

B. Evidence from Elicited Speech Errors

The error elicitation experiments are part of a general investigation of phonemic patterns that are particularly likely to be associated with errors involving sublexical units. The stimuli used in these experiments are designed to test specific predictions about the contextual factors that influence error rates and types. The stimuli used to elicit spoken errors contain four nonsense CVC syllables (e.g., /pof bis baf pis/) with initial and final consonants alternating in pairs. In this example, the initial pair /p,b/ alternates in the pattern ABBA and the final pair /f,s/ in the pattern ABAB. This "alternating alternation," much like the pattern in the tongue twister "She sells sea shells," is very effective in eliciting errors.

Our predictions about elicited error units were based on the preponderance of single-segment errors in the spontaneous corpus. If this predominance accurately reflects the underlying units of sublexical planning, then single-segment errors should similarly outnumber other types in a corpus of tape-recorded elicited errors that can be monitored more carefully than unrecorded spontaneous speech. On the other hand, if the spontaneous error data have been distorted by a listener bias (in either perception or memory) against multi-segment error units, and if, instead, syllables, onsets, and rhymes, or other sequences, are the primary units of sublexical serial ordering, then under the improved observation conditions of a taped elicitation experiment the most common elements should include #CV-, -VC#, and/or #CVC# units.

1. Stimuli Ten consonant pairs that often interacted in errors in the MIT corpus were selected: /t,k/, /m,n/, /č,t/, /p,f/, /m,b/, /g,d/, /k,p/, /r,l/, /f,s/, /b,p/. Each stimulus string of four syllables used two consonant pairs, one pair alternating in syllable-initial and another in syllable-final position. Ten such four-syllable strings were generated, balanced for which type of alternation (ABBA vs. ABAB) occurred in initial and which in final position. Each of the four syllables in a string contained a different vowel, so that any misordered units could be unambiguously identified. (If all of the vowels had been the same, then a #CV-error unit would be indistinguishable from a #C-, and a -VC# unit indistinguishable from a -C#.) The vowels /a,i,o,u/ were rotated through the four syllable positions as needed, to generate the 10 strings.

A second set of 10 strings was constructed using the same consonant pairs, but reversing their positions in initial and final syllable slots, so that /pof bis baf pus/ became /fop sib fab sup/. Thus, each pair was tested in both initial and final syllable position.

2. Stimulus Presentation The stimulus strings, typed on 3 × 5″ cards, were presented visually, one at a time, to 14 adult normal native speakers of English, half male and half female. The speaker was instructed to read the string aloud three times, and then to turn the card over and attempt to repeat it twice from memory, for a total of five consecutive renditions of each utterance by each speaker. Seven speakers produced the first set of 10 and seven more the second set, for a total of 700 renditions. Since this speech task is somewhat demanding, the stimulus cards were interspersed with others instructing the speaker to generate a normal English sentence and speak it aloud; this interpolation was designed to reduce the possibility that elements from one stimulus string might influence errors in the subsequent string. No attempt was made to control the rate of speech. Utterances were tape-recorded for later transcription, and exchange errors were tabulated by error unit size as before.

3. Results Like the spontaneous error corpora, the results of this elicitation experiment reveal a strong asymmetry in favor of single-segment errors. Of the 84 exchange errors observed, 83, or 99%, involved single segments (left half of Table 6-5). The structure of the stimuli does not permit a distinction to be drawn between single-segment units and the syllabic subcomponents of onset, nucleus, and coda; since all of these components are made up of single segments, but the error units CV and VC are clearly not functional here. No unambiguous single-feature errors occurred, although this may be because few of the pairs of alternating consonants differed by more than one feature.

It is interesting to note that almost all of the exchange errors occurred during the recitation rather than the reading condition. Does this mean that the predominance of single-segment error units can be accounted for as a memory constraint on the speaker, unrelated to the demands of speech production processing? Several lines of evidence argue against this interpretation.

First, the elicited error results parallel the asymmetry between single-segment and string-of-segment error units in spontaneous speech, suggesting that the two speaking conditions tap similar underlying planning processes. Although it is possible that the similar results arise in two separate ways, the hypothesis that the two kinds of processing overlap is more parsimonious.

A second argument comes from the distribution of nonexchange error units in the reading condition, that is, from substitutions (e.g., /pof bis/ becomes /pof pis/ or /bof bis/) and incomplete or interrupted errors (e.g., /pof bis/ is rendered as /bof—pof bis/). In the analysis of spontaneous errors earlier we ignored nonexchange errors, because the evidence they provide for the interaction of segment-sized units is more difficult to interpret than that provided by exchanges. For example, in the anticipatory substitution error "light letter" for "night letter," is the substitution /l/ for /n/ necessarily related to the occurrence of /l/ in "letter"? Perhaps the error unit is the word "light." In an exchange error

Table 6-5. Error Unit Distribution, by Elicitation Condition, for Tongue Twister Experiment

	Exchange errors		Other error types	
Condition	Single segment	CV, VC, CVC	Single segment	CV, VC, CVC
Reading	4	0	49	0
Recitation	79	1	81	6
	83	1	130	6

of the form "light netter," the symmetry of the two error events provides more compelling evidence for the claim that the units involved were single segments.

Because exchange errors allow us to triangulate in on the error unit, they have been heavily relied on as evidence for the nature of the sublexical processing unit. In this experiment, however, nonexchange errors like substitutions give a clear picture of the unit involved, because the targets are nonsense syllables (so that word substitution is a less likely alternative account) and because the vowels in the four syllables are all different (so that CV or VC error units can be distinguished from those involving single C's or V's, at least for interactions among elements in the utterance). Thus the distribution of nonexchange errors like anticipatory and perseveratory substitutions and incomplete errors is of considerable interest.

The distribution for all nonexchange elicited errors that involved an interaction between two portions of the target utterance is shown in the right half of Table 6-5. Although the number of errors remains smaller in the reading condition than in the recitation condition, it is large enough to reveal an asymmetry in favor of single-segment errors. This suggests that if the pool of exchange errors in the reading condition were large enough, it would show the same asymmetry, indicating that the asymmetry in favor of single-segment error units arises in production planning rather than short-term memory.

One further question arises about the accuracy with which these results reflect the units of submorphemic planning in normal speech production. Since the pattern of alternating alternations that contributed to the difficulty of articulating the elicitation stimuli is defined in terms of single consonants, the stimuli might be biased toward the elicitation of single-segment errors and against the movement of longer strings. Does this mean that the overwhelming predominance of single-segment error units is specific to the structure of these elicitation stimuli? We think not; if the syllable were the primary ordering unit in submorphemic processing, it is unlikely that a bias in stimulus structure could reduce it to less than 10% of the total error units (and 1% of the exchange error units) in tongue twisters. However, further experiments are clearly needed in order to contrast the hypothesis of single-segment units with that of syllable onset, nucleus, and coda, and to determine whether the size of the alternating units in a tongue twister determines or influences the size of the error unit.

C. Summary: The Segment as Computational Unit

Observations from both spontaneous and elicited speech errors support the hypothesis that sublexical serial ordering errors are likely to involve individual phonemic segments. This finding is compatible with a model in which a serial ordering process occurs at a point in production planning when the constituents of an utterance are represented in terms of their phonemic segments, or possibly in terms of the syllable components of onset, nucleus, and coda. In contrast, neither the syllable nor the distinctive feature appears to be the independent representational element operated on by the process that gives rise to sublexical serial order errors. If, as has been argued here, suprasegmental elements like the syllable do not serve as discrete, independently represented elements to be processed by a serial ordering mechanism, what *is* the role of suprasegmental facts in production planning? More specifically, what can we discover about the answer to this question from speech error patterns? We turn now to a discussion of two suprasegmental phenomena, word stress and syllable structure, and to an examination of what error evidence suggests about their influence on the serial ordering process for sublexical elements.

III. Role of Suprasegmental Structure in Sublexical Serial Order Processing

One constraint on sublexical exchange errors that emerges from the foregoing discussion is that no one multisegmental structural unit with at least one C and one V (such as the syllable) appears as an error unit as often as does the single phonemic segment. It is clear that neither the syllable nor the distinctive feature is the major unit of sublexical serial order processing. What then *is* the role of these elements in constraining exchange errors, and (by implication) in constraining the normal serial ordering process? In the remainder of this chapter, we will have little to say about the role of the distinctive feature. The data are compatible with the view that sublexical representational elements are represented in terms of their distinctive feature values (e.g., occasional single-segment exchanges, the shared features of target and intrusion segments, and perhaps even the tendency for consonant clusters to interact with single consonants with many of their feature values, as in /f/ for /sp/). It is possible, however, that some set of auditory or articulatory dimensions can be formulated that will provide an even better account of these aspects of the data.

We will explore the effects on sublexical exchange errors of two kinds of suprasegmental facts: word stress patterns and syllable structure. In general terms, the influence of these two factors reveals itself as a set of similarity constraints on the segments in an utterance that can interact in an error. That is, two exchanged segments generally have in common

1. the word stress value of their syllables, and
2. their structurally defined positions in larger units (although the precise nature of the larger units over which this positional constraint should be stated is not yet clear).

We will examine error evidence that supports a role for these factors in the representations operated on by the sublexical serial ordering process, and then briefly summarize a model of serial ordering, proposed in an earlier paper, that incorporates them.

A. The Influence of Word Stress Patterns and Position on Segmental Exchanges

For each error that involves an exchange between two segments of an utterance, we can ask the question, Along what dimensions are the two interacting elements similar? The assumption behind this question is that the answer will reveal something about the representation of the utterance in the speaker's head at the time when the error occurred. One kind of similarity, *intrinsic* similarity between the two interacting segments of an exchange error, has been demonstrated for both consonant and vowel exchanges (Shattuck-Hufnagel & Klatt, 1975, 1979a; Goldstein, 1977; Nooteboom, 1969; and others). The intrinsic similarity between two segments is determined by their relationship in the sound system of the language, independent of their function in a particular utterance.

A second kind of similarity involves the phonemic, morphological, and syntactic environments in which the two interacting segments appear. This might be called *extrinsic* similarity, defined by the contexts of the segments in the particular utterance in which the error occurred. Two aspects of extrinsic similarity that will concern us here are the word stress value of the syllables in which the two segments appear, and the positions of the two segments in their respective syllables.

1. Stress and Positional Similarity The majority of single-consonant exchanges in the 1981 count of the MIT corpus appear to follow a stress-similarity constraint. That is, for the 210 complete exchanges that occur between content words and are unambiguous as to the number of segments involved because the error units share no segments, 86% occur before the primary stressed vowel of the word (as in "gudget bap" for "budget gap"), and 9% occur either (1) after the primary stressed vowel in syllable-final position, or (2) syllable initially before an unstressed vowel. Thus, 95% of the single-consonant exchanges occur between segments whose syllables have similar word stress values (using the simple distinction between syllables with primary word stress vs. those without). Only 5% of the single-consonant exchange errors in this set violate word-stress similarity, as in "rath meview" for "math review," or "pult of cursonality" for "cult of personality."

On its face, this observation indicates that the word stress value of the syllable in which a segment occurs in a given utterance strongly influences the selection of segments in the utterance that it can interact with in an error. One might say that shared word stress value makes it possible for the processor to confuse the segments from two syllables. Yet, the interpretation of this seemingly straightforward pattern is complicated by the fact that the position of segments in their respective words and syllables can account for the observations about equally well. This is true because all but one of the prestressed vowel errors occurs in word-initial position. That is, most of the errors occur in initial position in words that have their primary stress on the first syllable. Fromkin (1977) has pointed out a similar pattern in her UCLA corpus: Of the stressed syllables involved in a corpus of 612 segmental errors, 88% are word-initial syllables. Thus, either or both of the two factors, stress similarity or positional similarity, could be the source of the constraint.

A further source of obscurity for the precise nature of this constraint is the high proportion of exchange errors that occur in one syllable words, as in "gerd of hoats" for "herd of goats," and "greep grain" for "green grape." For these errors, word stress and word position constraints are also confounded with syllable position constraints.

Although these data are compatible with the claim that stress similarity defines the pool of segments in an utterance that can be misselected for each other, they might also be produced by a proclivity for errors in initial position, combined with the large proportion of words in conversational English with primary stress on the first or only syllable. An interaction between these two factors could not, however, account for the whole of the position constraint. It leaves unaccounted for at least two sets of errors that are subject to the constraint: syllable-final exchanges and exchanges between segments in syllables in different word positions (like "no bout adoubt it" for "no doubt about it").

Moreover, the phonotactic or morpheme structure constraints of English are not adequate to account for the position constraint. If we assume that the phonotactic constraints are stated over abstract segments rather than over positional allophones, they would permit errors such as "sly faft" for "fly fast," where the exchanging /s/ and /f/ appear in opposite syllable positions and where both are permissible phonotactically. But these errors occur extremely rarely in the MIT corpus (fewer than 1%), suggesting that some other mechanism must be postulated to impose the positional constraint. In the model to be described here, this mechanism is the scan-and-copy component of a sublexical serial ordering process, which scans sets of segments defined by their syllabic positions.

2. Stress and Positional Asymmetries In addition to the suprasegmental *similarity* constraints observed on single-element exchange errors in the MIT corpus, there are powerful stress and positional *asymmetries*. There are two forms that these asymmetries could take: (a) within-error asymmetries, in which one type of segment tends to replace another type within an error, and (b) across-error asymmetries, in which similar segment types interact with each other but comparison across a number of errors shows that certain types are more likely to be involved in an error. An example of the first, or within-error, type of asymmetry would be a pattern of systematic replacement of, say, stop consonants with fricatives. An example of the second, or across-error, type would be the finding that stops interact with stops, and fricatives with fricatives, but that stops as a class are more subject to error than fricatives as a class. In other words, across-error asymmetries arise not when there is a tendency for one class of segment to replace another but when interacting segments come from similar classes and certain classes are more subject to error than others. Across-error asymmetries are consistent with a model in which similarity is an important constraint on the possibility that two segments can interact in an error. Within-error asymmetries are not consistent with such a model.

In general, I have argued that speech errors show across-error asymmetries rather than within-error asymmetries. For example, it is not the case that one subset of the segments of English systematically displaces the other subset; rather, each segment is about equally likely to appear as a target or as an intrusion (with the exception of the palatal segments /šžčj/; Shattuck-Hufnagel, 1979; Shattuck-Hufnagel & Klatt, 1980). This shows the lack of a within-error asymmetry in favor of, for example, unmarked segments. At the same time, the rate of participation in errors by the segments of English is proportional to their frequency of occurrence (Shattuck-Hufnagel & Klatt, 1979a). This indicates an across-error asymmetry in favor of frequently occurring segments.

With respect to word stress and position, speech errors are again characterized by asymmetries of the across-error type. That is, we find that most interactions occur between segments defined by some value A on a dimension fewer interactions occur between segments with the value $-A$, and almost no interaction occurs between members of the two classes $+A$ and $-A$. For example, pairs of word-initial segments often interact with each other in exchange errors, noninitial segments interact with each other less frequently, and initial and final segments almost never interact, at least for the set of exchange errors defined as above.

Similarly, pairs of segments from primary word stress syllables interact with each other freely, whereas pairs of segments from nonprimary stress syllables and segments drawn from one stressed syllable and one unstressed syllable interact only rarely. The findings of Boomer and Laver (1968) for a corpus of errors of all types in English might be described in similar terms. They report that "where target and origin are located in different (usually adjacent) tone groups, each will be in the tonic word of its own tone group." That is, for interactions that cross tone-group boundaries, pairs of segments from tonic words interact more often than either pairs from nontonic words or pairs from one tonic and one nontonic word.

The most notable exception to this recurring pattern of across-error asymmetries (accompanied by within-error similarities) has been reported by MacKay (1971). He surveyed a corpus of segmental exchanges collected from German speech by Merringer (1908) and Merringer and Meyer (1895). These errors differed from the English errors described above in that they occurred within words rather than between words. An example is the error *"justizifierte"* for *"justifizierte"* (Merringer, 1908, p. 19). For this subset of exchange errors, MacKay found an interesting within-error asymmetry, which he describes as "stress pre-entry." That is, a segment from a stressed syllable late in the word tends to "preenter," replacing a segment in an unstressed syllable in the word, in the first half of the exchange. Of course, the segment displaced from the early unstressed syllable then "postenters" in the later stressed syllable to complete the error, but the important point is the asymmetry in the first portions of the errors. An illustrative example of this phenomenon in English is the within-word error "pretipisation" for "precipitation." An English example of the reverse pattern, preentry of the unstressed-syllable segment and postentry of a stressed-syllable segment, is the error "narimating" for "marinating"; these errors occur much less frequently in the within-word corpus in German.

Noting a slight tendency toward a similar asymmetry in several small corpora in English, MacKay ascribes it to a kind of special early processing, suggesting that stressed syllables undergo "a higher level of subthreshold activation . . . than unstressed ones," and thus that their segments might tend to reach the threshold for activation earlier than they should.

Leaving aside a number of questions about these data (Do stress patterns and average word length combine in German to form a large pool of late-stress words with room to move the stress forward? Why does the early activation not lead the stress to move with the moved segments, at least for vowels?), we can examine the distribution of within-word exchange errors in the MIT corpus. In contrast to the German corpus, complete single-consonant exchanges within content words in the MIT corpus show no tendency toward stress preentry. Of the 56 examples, 21 involve preentry from an *un*stressed syllable, 14 involve preentry from a stressed syllable, and 21 are neutral, since they do not involve any segments from the primary stress syllable of the word (as in "ajeribonie" for "aborigine").

For the small number of complete within-content-word vowel exchanges, the pattern is similar. There are seven cases of preentry from unstressed syllables (as in "cartyourd" for "courtyard"), and four of stress preentry (e.g., "zicchuni" for "zucchini"). In sum, 26% of the complete, unambiguous single-segment exchanges within content words support the stress preentry hypothesis, 42% are not compatible with it, and 32% are neutral. This pattern of errors in English offers little support for the necessity of positing a stress preentry mechanism.

B. Further Observations on Suprasegmental Constraints

Three further facts about suprasegmental constraints on sublexical errors can be noted here.

1. The first concerns the question whether stress values can exchange in the way that segments and other planning units apparently can. For example, the error "lin*guist*" for "*lin*guist" could be described either as an exchange of two stress values or as the misassignment of primary stress by some other mechanism. Cutler (1980) has noted that stress misplacements occur primarily in polymorphemic (often derived) words like "photo*gra*pher." She observes that for each of these words there is a related word bearing stress on

the syllable that receives it in the error (in this case, "photo*gra*phic"). Cutler argues that this constraint on main-stress misplacement indicates that various allomorphs of a given morpheme are stored near each other in the lexicon, along with their separately represented stress patterns. In her model, the lexical selection mechanism occasionally malfunctions, selecting the phonemic representation for the target allomorph but the stress pattern for a different one stored nearby.

Most of Fromkin's (1977) examples can be similarly described: "*or*igin," "*progress*" (for "pro*gress*"), "eco*no*mists," "diffe*re*nces," and "*pho*netic" (although not "mobi*li*ty"). She argues that these and more complex errors involving both stress and segmental disarray, as in "pro*fes*soral" for "profes*so*rial" and "descri*ba*tion" for "des*crip*tion," show that stress placement rules are actively applied during the generation of an utterance. Thus although conflicting interpretations of the data are possible, it is clear that stress errors fall into definable patterns that can be described as the misassignment or misselection of stress patterns, rather than as the exchange of stress values. This is compatible with the notion that stress value is not an independently represented element that must undergo serial ordering separate from its syllable or nucleus.

2. A second observation about suprasegmental constraints concerns the precise nature of the position similarity constraint proposed above. As noted, the unit over which the constraint should be stated cannot be specified with any certainty on the basis of distributions in the presently available corpora, because the number of errors in which we can distinguish the position in the foot, word, morph, and syllable is very small. The syllable position constraint describes all but two of the consonantal exchanges in our corpus, but the limited context recorded for each error does not always permit evaluation of the foot; experimental test of the hypothesis that this rhythmic unit is the basis of the position constraint is under way.

It should be noted, however, that whatever the basic unit of the positional constraint, the constraint itself cannot be stated in an absolute left-to-right manner. Instead, it must take into account the structure of the syllables involved. For example, in the error "sprit blain" for "split brain," the /l/ was the third target segment in "split" and the /r/ was the second target segment in "brain." The description misses the fact that the /l/ and /r/ are targets for similar slots in their respective syllables; that is, the last slot before the nucleus.

One way of capturing the position constraint on such error interactions is to state it over a canonical template some of whose slots will be empty for most words of English. For example, the template might have three slots in the onset, two in the nucleus, and three or four in the coda. The position constraint would specify that when an exchange error breaks up an onset cluster, only segments destined for structurally similar slots in their respective syllables could interact with each other because only such sets of segments are subject to the search performed by the scan-and-copy mechanism for any given slot (see the discussion of the model, section IV). Such a template would account for constraints on errors between onset segments (permitting errors like "skop tarving" for "stop carving"), as well as for the failure of syllable-onset segments to interact with those in syllable-final clusters. When the onset functions as a unit, of course, the question of position constraints within it does not arise.

Beyond the position constraint on interacting segments, one further observation suggests a role for the template. Many errors move segments into locations that would otherwise be empty. For example, exchange errors move the segment that was displaced by the intrusion in the first part of the error into the downstream slot from which that intrusion came; apparently, there is some mechanism that preserves that downstream slot even when it is not occupied by its target segment. Similarly, segment shifts (like "play a f-at fee" for "pay a flat fee") move segments into slots that would be empty in a correct production of the utterance. Finally, additions that appear to be a kind of duplication from context (like "striped brass" for "striped bass") also insert a segment into a location that would otherwise remain empty. The occurrence of errors that move segments into an empty location (rather than simply substituting one segment for another) seems to suggest a representation in terms of a canonical syllable or foot framework with appropriate empty slots available. That the error slot is structurally similar to that of the presumed source is, of course, further evidence for the position constraint.

3. The final observation concerns the predictions that this model might make about the possible violation of phonotactic constraints in errors. Absolute phonotactic constraints, like that against engma /ŋ/ in initial position, may be less likely to be violated in errors than combinatorial constraints like that against initial /tl/. This is because engma will never be available in the set of segments destined for syllable-onset slots in an English utterance, and so it will never be misselected for insertion in an onset by mistake. In contrast, since both /t/ and /l/ can appear in syllable onsets, they may be simultaneously available in the pool of segments destined for onset slots in a given utterance, and by error they may be misselected to fill slots in the same syllable. If the slot specifications are stated so that /t/ is only available for the middle of the three onset slots, and /l/ only for the third, we might expect an occasional /tl/ error (but no /lt/ errors) to occur.

The number of errors in the MIT corpus that violate phonotactic constraints is small, as we might expect if perceptual processes are influenced by expectations based on the structure of the listener's language. The few that have been recorded, however, are of anecdotal interest. There are no errors that move engma into an onset slot, but there are several that result in onsets that violate the combinatorial constraints of English morpheme structure: one initial /tl/, two /vr/, two /zw/, and a number of šm/ and /šn/ (although the latter, as Fromkin, 1973, has pointed out, may be slowly slipping into the language for other reasons).

Clearly, rigorous experimentation will be necessary to determine how these two factors might play a role in sentence production planning: (1) phonotactic constraints, (2) the notion of a template the size of the syllable or other large rhythmic unit. One aspect of the tongue twister experiments described earlier offers some preliminary support for the observation that segments do not exchange across syllable position, and thus indirectly for the template hypothesis. Many of the four-syllable stimuli had confusable pairs not only in initial position and in final position but also across initial and final position. For example, the twister /fut pon pait fin/ has the initial pair /f,p/ and final pair /t,n/, but also the cross-position pair /p,t/. Yet, no cross-syllable-position interactions occurred between these two segments or between similarly arranged pairs in other sets of stimuli. Apparently, in this highly artificial speaking situation (just as in normal spontaneous speech), structural position in the syllable helps to determine the set of segments within an utterance that can interact with each other in an exchange error.

C. Summary of Suprasegmental Constraints on Sublexical Errors

From analysis of the MIT corpus of spontaneous errors involving sublexical units, we have established the likelihood of positional and stress constraints that imply a significant role for syllable (or foot) structure and for stress patterns in the normal serial ordering process of spontaneous speech planning. We do not know precisely what unit the position constraint should be stated over, nor can we specify either the details of its representation of hierarchical structure within syllables or other units, or the theoretical framework that will best capture stress similarity constraints. We do not know exactly what is implied by the across-error asymmetries that favor errors involving word-initial segments from stressed syllables, nor by the apparent rarity of within-error asymmetries. But as we have begun to formulate questions about these matters with greater precision, to pursue their implications for models of production processing, and to test the predictions made by these models with a variety of experimental methods, we have come closer to making full use of the rich data provided by malfunctions in the speech production planning process to understand its normal workings. In the meantime, the incompleteness of our understanding should not prevent us from formulating a model, however crude, that embodies those aspects of error constraints about which we can be reasonably confident. The remainder of this chapter summarizes such a data-based model, one that is described more comprehensively in Shattuck (1975) and Shattuck-Hufnagel (1979). Recent findings (Shattuck-Hufnagel, 1981, 1982) suggest that a number of extensions and additions to the model will be necessary, but it remains basically a slot-plus-filler mechanism, in which sets of sublexical components undergo serial ordering by transfer from a short-term store into a framework of slots provided by a canonical representation in terms of larger units, perhaps syllables or feet. Other models can be found in Baars, Motley, and MacKay (1975), Dell and Reich (1981), Ellis (1979), Fromkin (1973), Jarrett (1980), Laver (1980), MacKay (1970), and MacNeilage and MacNeilage (1973).

IV. A Serial Ordering Component in the Production Planning Model

The model for the process that accomplishes the serial ordering of sublexical fragments, proposed in Shattuck (1975) and Shattuck-Hufnagel (1979) on the basis of constraints on error patterns, has three components: (1) two independent representations of the utterance, consisting of (a) the segments to be ordered, and (b) the suprasegmental framework (perhaps defined by rhythmic units) into which they will be copied; (2) a scan-copier, which serially selects segments from the set to be ordered, under the descriptions provided by the framework; and (3) several monitors, which will (a) prevent multiple copying of a given target segment into more than one slot (by deleting it or marking it as used after copying), (b) detect suspiciously similar sequences that might have arisen by error (and perhaps edit them), and so on.

This serial ordering component operates over a candidate set of lexical entries selected for possible inclusion in the utterance on the basis of a surface structure generated by a separate component (Garrett, 1975, 1976, 1980.) Normally, after the generation of a framework of slots, the scan-copier examines the set of candidate segments to find the target segment appropriate for the first slot, selects the target, and copies it into the slot. The monitor then deletes that segment from the set of target segments or marks it in some way as "used." As this process is repeated for successive slots, a separate monitor examines the stretch of filled slots for suspicious-looking strings that are likely to have arisen by error, sometimes "correcting" sequences like "top total taste" to "top total saste," and so on.

When one or another of the three aspects of the serial order processor malfunctions, the different types of errors that have been observed will arise: substitutions, shifts, exchanges, additions, omissions, and incomplete (or interrupted) errors. Imagine for a moment that the scan-copier errs and selects the wrong candidate segment for a particular slot. For example, in the utterance "shop talk," suppose that the /t/ destined for the initial slot in "talk" is misselected to fill the initial slot in "shop." The stage is now set for a number of possible error types to occur when the scan-copier reaches the slot in which that misselected /t/ *should* have appeared: the initial slot in "talk." What will happen? If the scan-copier finds no segment that satisfies its instructions for this slot, it may abort the utterance and start again, resulting in the interrupted error "top—shop talk." If it settles for the next-best still-available target segment, the displaced /š/, the speaker will produce the exchange "top shalk." Finally, if there is a second malfunction, this time in the deletion monitor, so that the copied /t/ is not removed from the set of candidate items but remains available to be selected for its correct target slot, the anticipatory substitution "top talk" will be produced. All other observed error types that involve an interaction within the utterance can be similarly produced by one or more failures in one or more of the mechanisms in the serial ordering process.

This model forms the basis for a number of predictions about other aspects of speech error patterns. For example, errors that do not involve an interaction within the utterance, and thus do not arise by this mechanism, may have different characteristics. This prediction has been confirmed by the finding that substitution errors with no apparent source in the utterances (e.g., "the fourt decided" for "the court decided") show a different pattern of feature similarity between target and intrusion segments (Shattuck-Hufnagel & Klatt, 1979b).

The model also makes some predictions about the relative frequency with which various types of errors should occur. Errors that involve a single malfunction (like interrupted errors) should occur more frequently than errors that involve several concomitant malfunctions (like anticipatory substitutions). This prediction is confirmed in the MIT corpus, where incomplete sublexical errors outnumber complete anticipatory substitutions by more than three to one.

A third prediction is that certain kinds of sequences of similar segments may be edited out of the utterance. This process is sometimes observed in sequences like "be behaving" and "to tomorrow's party." Finally, the model predicts that when a completed error is detected and corrected, "leftover" or unused segments from the candidate set may show up in the correction. Corrections of word blends, as in "patch—back of cigarettes," (for "pack" or "batch") occasionally show this pattern.

Suprasegmental structure plays two closely related roles in this model of the serial ordering process. First, it provides a framework of serially ordered slots represented separately from the segments that will fill them. This ensures that slots can be maintained even when they are empty of their target segments, a requirement if we are to account for the fact that a displaced segment, if it appears at all, appears in the target location of the segment that did the displacing. It also provides empty slots into which segments can be shifted or added.

The second influence of suprasegmental structure follows directly from its provision of a serially ordered framework: It imposes constraints on which of the candidate segments in an utterance will be scanned for the target segment destined for a particular slot. In this way, it largely determines which segments in the utterance can interact with each other in an error. For example, if the scanning of candidate segments is restricted to those destined for structurally similar slots, this model can account for the tendency of errors to move a displaced or added segment into a slot that is structurally similar to its target slot. In its first pass through the set of segments it might scan only those destined for onset slots, ensuring that onset segments are more likely to interact than onset and coda segments. Similarly, the scanner might search the set of stressed syllable segments separately from those without stress, making it more likely that segments from stressed syllables will interact with each other than with segments from unstressed syllables. In these ways, the proposed serial ordering mechanism could account for some of the extrinsic or contextual similarity constraints on interacting error segments. It also accounts for the intrinsic similarity of interacting segments, since misselections will be more likely to occur between segments that are similarly represented.

V. Conclusion

Two lines of investigation look especially promising for further research. First, there is a need for more error corpora, both from normal adult speakers and from other speech communities; and second, we need to pursue the experimental testing of hypotheses generated from observed corpora.

The expansion of error corpora would be most useful if it included (a) tape-recorded corpora, to ensure that distribution figures are accurate and to permit the transcription of stress and intonation; (b) corpora from children, the aged, and speakers with language pathologies; and (c) corpora in languages other than English. There are several substantial corpora in American English (collected by Fromkin at UCLA, Garrett and Shattuck-Hufnagel at MIT, Dell and Reich at Toronto and the University of New Hampshire, and Stemberger at the University of California at San Diego), but none of them contain appreciable numbers of taped errors. The published corpora in German, Portuguese, and Dutch are limited in scope. As far as I know, no corpus exists in a non-Indo-European language. It would be particularly interesting to test, in a highly inflected language, Garrett's (1975, 1980) proposal that the syntactic framework that provides the ordering principle for the lexical items in an utterance is formed by closed-class items (including the syntactic affixes). This test requires a corpus of base-morpheme exchanges, so that one can see whether the case markers remain behind, as Garrett's model predicts and as pronoun exchanges in English suggest (e.g., "he called her" for "she called him").

Experimental tests of hypotheses generated from analysis of spontaneous-error corpora have been few (Baars, Motley, & MacKay, 1975; Dell and Reich, 1981; Kupin, 1979; MacKay, 1978; Shattuck-Hufnagel, 1980). One problem with experimental elicitation methods is the difficulty of being sure that they tap the normal processes of spontaneous speech planning. We presume that the planning of elicited speech must share a final common pathway with spontaneous speech, but we cannot be sure how far up into the process this pathway extends. Yet, elicitation methods provide an opportunity to focus attention on particular structures and relations, and on their effects on error rates and error types. They also provide some insurance against perceptual and memory biases in the collection of spontaneous errors. Recent attempts at eliciting spontaneous utterances with certain prescribed phonemic characteristics look promising (Shattuck-Hufnagel, 1981a, 1981b). With careful interpretation of results, and with converging evidence from a number of different experimental methods, we may well find that speech error patterns paradoxically provide us with one of the clearest available views of the processes of normal speech production planning.

References

Baars, B. J., Motley, M. T., & MacKay, D. G. Output editing for lexical status from artificially-elicited slips of the tongue. *Journal of Verbal Learning and Verbal Behavior*, 1975, *14*, 382–391.

Blumstein, S. E. *A phonological investigation of aphasic speech*. The Hague: Mouton, 1973.

Boomer, D. S., & Laver, J. D. M. Slips of the tongue. *British Journal of Disorders of Communication*, 1968, *3*, 2–12.

Cutler, A. Queering the pitch: errors of stress and intonation. In V. A. Fromkin (Ed.). *Errors in linguistic performance: Slips of the tongue, ear, pen and hand. New York:* Academic Press, 1980.

Dell, G. S., & Reich, P. A. Toward a unified theory of slips of the tongue. In V. A. Fromkin (Ed.), *Errors in linguistic performance*. New York: Academic Press, 1980.

Dell, G. S., & Reich, P. A. Stages in sentence production: An analysis of speech error data. Unpublished manuscript, Dartmouth College, Hanover, N. H., 1981.

Ellis, A. W. Speech production and short-term memory. In J. Morton and J. C. Marshall (Eds.), *Psycholinguistics* (Vol. 2: *Structures and processes*). Cambridge, Mass., and London, England: MIT Press, 1979.

Fromkin, V. A. The non-anomalous nature of anomalous utterances. *Language*, 1971, *47*, 27–52.

Fromkin, V. A. Introduction. In V. A. Fromkin (Ed.), *Speech errors as linguistic evidence*. The Hague: Mouton, 1973.

Fromkin, V. A. Putting the emPHAsis on the wrong sylLAble. In L. M. Hyman (Ed.), *Studies in stress and accent* (Southern California Occasional Papers in Linguistics No. 4). Los Angeles: UCLA Department of Linguistics, 1977.

Garrett, M. F. The analysis of sentence production. In G. Bower (Ed.), *The psychology of learning and motivation* (Vol. 9). New York: Academic Press, 1975.

Garrett, M. F. Syntactic processes in sentence production. In E. C. T. Walker and R. Wales (Eds.), *New approaches to language mechanisms*. Amsterdam: North-Holland, 1976.

Garrett, M. F. Levels of processing in sentence production. In B. Butterworth (Ed.), *Language Production* (Vol. 1). New York: Academic Press, 1980.

Goldstein, L. Features, salience and bias. UCLA Working Papers in Phonetics 39, 1977.

Hockett, C. F. Where the tongue slips, there slip I. In *To Honor Roman Jakobson* (Janua Linquarum Series Major No. 32). The Hague: Mouton, 1967.

Johns, C. *Speech errors in Portuguese*. Unpublished master's thesis, University of Edinburgh, 1972.

Kupin, J. Tongue twisters as a source of information about speech production. Unpublished doctoral dissertation, University of Connecticut at Storrs, 1979.

Laver, J. A model of the speech production process. In V. A. Fromkin (Ed.), *Errors in linguistic performance.* New York: Academic Press, 1980.

MacKay, D. G. Spoonerisms: The structure of errors in the serial order of speech. *Neuropsychologia,* 1970, *8,* 323–350.

MacKay, D. G. Stress pre-entry in motor systems. *American Journal of Psychology,* 1971, *1,* 35–51.

MacKay, D. G. The structure of words and syllables. *Cognitive Psychology,* 1972, *3,* 210–227.

MacKay, D. G. Speech errors inside the syllable. In A. Bell and J. B. Hooper (Eds.), *Syllables and Segments.* Amsterdam: North-Holland, 1978.

MacNeilage, P. F., & MacNeilage, L. A. Central processes controlling speech production during sleep and waking. In F. J. McGuigan & R. A. Schoonover (Eds.), *The psychophysiology of thinking.* New York: Academic Press, 1973.

Merringer, R. *Aus dem Leben der Sprache.* Berlin: Behr Verlag, 1908.

Merringer, R., & Meyer, C. *Versprechen und Verlesen.* Berlin: Verlag, 1895.

Nooteboom, S. G. The tongue slips into patterns. In A. G. Sciarone et al. (Eds.), *Nomen: Leyden studies in linguistics and phonetics.* The Hague: Mouton, 1969.

Shattuck, S. R. *Speech errors and sentence production.* Unpublished doctoral dissertation, Massachusetts Institute of Technology, 1975.

Shattuck-Hufnagel, S. Speech errors as evidence for a serial order mechanism in sentence production. In W. E. Cooper & E. C. T. Walker (Eds.), *Sentence processing.* Hillsdale, N. J.: Lawrence Erlbaum Associates, 1979.

Shattuck-Hufnagel, S. Speech error units smaller than the syllable. *Journal of the Acoustical Society of America,* 1980, *68* (Suppl. 1).

Shattuck-Hufnagel, S. Position constraints on segment exchange errors in production and memory. *Journal of the Acoustical Society of America,* 1981, *70* (Suppl. 1).

Shattuck-Hufnagel, S. Word position *vs* stressed-syllable-position constraints on elicited speech errors: implications for a processing model. *Journal of the Acoustical Society of America,* 1982, *72* (Suppl. 1).

Shattuck-Hufnagel, S., & Klatt, D. H. An analysis of 1500 phonetic errors in spontaneous speech. *Journal of the Acoustical Society of America,* 1975, *58* (Suppl. 1)

Shattuck-Hufnagel, S., & Klatt, D. H. The limited use of distinctive features and markedness in speech production: Evidence from speech error data. *Journal of Verbal Learning and Verbal Behavior,* 1979, *18,* 41–55. (a)

Shattuck-Hufnagel, S., & Klatt, D. H. Similarity constraints on phoneme errors of different types. *Proceedings of the 9th International Congress of Phonetic Sciences,* 1979, *1,* 317. (b)

Shattuck-Hufnagel, S., & Klatt, D. H. How single phoneme error data rule out two models of error generation. In V. A. Fromkin (Ed.), *Errors in linguistic performance.* New York: Academic Press, 1980.

Stemberger, J. P. Lexical entries: Evidence from speech errors. Unpublished manuscript, University of California at San Diego, La Jolla, 1980.

van den Broecke, M. P. R., & Goldstein, L. Consonant features in speech errors. In V. A. Fromkin (Ed.), *Errors in linguistic performance.* New York: Academic Press, 1980.

Chapter 7

A "Dynamic Pattern" Perspective on the Control and Coordination of Movement

J. A. Scott Kelso, Betty Tuller, and Katherine S. Harris

I. Introduction

That speech is the most highly developed motor skill possessed by all of us is a truism; but how is this truism to be understood? Although the investigation of speech production and that of motor behavior have proceeded largely independently of each other, they share certain conceptions of how skilled movements are organized. Thus, regardless of whether one refers to movement in general or to speech as a particular instance, it is assumed that for coordination to occur, appropriate sets of muscles must be activated in proper relationships to others, and correct amounts of facilitation and inhibition have to be delivered to specified muscles. That the production of even the simplest movement involves a multiplicity of neuromuscular events overlapping in time has suggested the need for some type of organizing principle. By far the most favored candidates have been the closed-loop servomechanism accounts provided by cybernetics and its allied disciplines, and the formal machine metaphor of central programs. The evidence for these rival views seems to undergo continuous updating (e.g., Adams, 1977; Keele, 1981) and so will not be of major concern to us here. It is sufficient to point out the current consensus on the issue, namely, that complex sequences of movement may be carried out in the absence of peripheral feedback, but that feedback can be used for monitoring small errors as well as to facilitate corrections in the program itself (e.g., Keele, 1981; Miles & Evarts, 1979).

But at a deeper level, none of these models offers a principled account of the coordination and control of movement. The arguments for this position have been laid out in detail elsewhere (Fowler, Rubin, Remez, & Turvey, 1980; Kelso, Holt, Kugler, & Turvey, 1980; Kugler, Kelso, & Turvey, 1980; Turvey, Shaw, & Mace, 1978) and will be elaborated here only inasmuch as they allow us to promote an alternative. To start, let us note that programs and the like— though intuitively appealing—are only semantic *descriptions* of systemic behavior. They are, in Emmett's (1980) terms, "externalist" in nature and are quite neutral to the structure or design characteristics of that which is being controlled. By assuming, a priori, the reality of a program account, we impose from the outside a descriptive explanation that allows us to interpret motor behavior as rational and coherent. But it would be a categorical error to attribute to the concept *program* causal status. Nevertheless, it is commonplace in the analysis of movement for investigators to observe some characteristic of an animal's performance, such as the extent of limb movement, and conclude that the same characteristic is represented in the motor program (e.g., Taub, 1976). In like vein, the observation that lip rounding precedes the acoustic onset of a rounded vowel and therefore coarticulates with preceding consonants is explained by the presence of the feature [+ rounding] in the plan for a speech gesture (cf. Fowler, 1977). Such an interpretative strategy is akin to that of the observer of bee behavior who attributes the product of a behavior—honey arranged in hexagonal form—to a hexagon program possessed by all bees. A more careful analysis would reveal that hexagonal tessellation, or "close packing," occurs whenever spherical bodies of uniform size and flexible walls are packed together. That is to say, close packing is a consequence of dynamic principles that allow for the minimization of potential energy (least surface contact), and it is dynamics that determines the emergence of hexagonal patterns such as honeycombs (for further examples of complex form arising from dynamic principles, see Thompson, 1942; Kugler et al., 1980; Stevens, 1974).

The gist of the message here is that if we adopt a formal machine account of systemic behavior, we take out, in Dennett's (1978, p. 15) words, a "loan on intelligence" that must ultimately be paid back. Rather than focusing our level of explanation at an *order* grain of analysis in which all the details of movement must be prescribed (see Shaw & Turvey, 1981), a more patient approach may be to seek an understanding of the relations among systemic states as necessary a posteriori facts of coordinated activity (see Rashevsky, 1960; Shaw, Turvey, & Mace, 1981). In essence we would argue, as Greene (Note 1) does, that in order to learn about the functions of the motor system we should first seek to identify the informational units of coordination.

Although the latter topic—coordination—has received some lip service in the motor control literature, a rigorous analysis of muscle collectives has (with few exceptions) not been undertaken as a serious scientific enterprise. We venture to guess that one of the reasons for such a state of affairs is that extant models of movement control (and skill learning) assume that the system is already coordinated. Thus, servomechanism accounts speak to the positioning of limbs or articulators in terms of, for example, some reference level or spatial target, but are mute as to how a set of muscles might attain the desired reference or target. Similarly, program descriptions of motor behavior assume that the program represents a coordinated movement sequence and that muscles simply carry out a set of commands (e.g., Keele, 1981; Schmidt, 1975). Any systemic organization of the muscles themselves is owing to the program—a *fait accompli* that explains nothing.

But what does an adequate theory of movement coordination (and skilled behavior as well) have to account for? Fundamentally, the problem confronting any theorist of systemic behavior in living organisms is how a system regulates its internal degrees of freedom (Bernstein, 1967; Boylls, 1975; Greene, 1972; Iberall & McCulloch, 1969; Tsetlin, 1973; Turvey, 1977; Weiss, 1941). A first step toward resolving this issue in motor systems is to claim—following the insights of the Soviet school (e.g., Bernstein, 1967; Gelfand, Gurfinkel, Tsetlin, & Shik, 1971; Tsetlin, 1973)—that individual variables, say muscles, are partitioned into collectives or synergies where the variables within a collective change relatedly and autonomously. Combinations of movements are produced by changes in the mode of interaction of lower centers; higher centers of the nervous system do not command; rather they tune or adjust the interactions at lower levels (Fowler, 1977; Greene, 1972, Note 1; Kelso & Tuller, 1981; Tsetlin, 1973; Turvey, 1977). As Gelfand et al. (1971) suggest, learning a new skill (within the foregoing style of organization) consists of acquiring a convenient synergy, thus lowering the number of parameters requiring independent control (see Fowler & Turvey, 1978, for a skill learning perspective and Kugler, Kelso, & Turvey, 1982, for a developmental analysis). Before going any further, we should note that the term *synergy* is used here in a way that is different from Western usage: A synergy (or coordinative structure as we prefer to call it) is not limited to a set of muscles having similar actions at a joint, nor is it restricted to inborn reflex-based neurophysiological mechanisms (Easton, 1972). Rather, synergies and coordinative structures connote the use of muscle groups in a behavioral situtation: They are functional groupings of muscles, often spanning several joints that are constrained to act as a single unit. To paraphrase Boylls (1975), they are collections of muscles, all of which share a common pool of afferent and/or efferent information, that are deployed as a unit in a motor task.

In this chapter we do not propose to continue the polemic for a coordinative structure style of organization. The evidence for coordinative structures in a large variety of activities is well documented (e.g., for speech, see Fowler, 1980; for locomotion, see Boylls, 1975; for postural balance, see Nashner, 1977; for human interlimb coordination, see Kelso, Southard, & Goodman, 1979a, 1979b) and the rationale for such an organizational style is compelling, though perhaps not accepted by all. Instead we want to focus first on the following question: When groups of muscles function as a single unit, what properties (kinematic and electromyographic) do they exhibit? We intend to show that there are certain features of neuromuscular organization that are common to many, if not all, modes of coordination, including human speech. Second, and more important, we shall attempt to provide a principled rationale for why coordinative structures have the properties that they have. Such an account will not be in the algorithmic language of formal machines, where each aspect of the movement plan is explicitly represented. Rather we shall develop the argument—based on dynamic principles that have their groundings in homeokinetic physics (Iberall, 1977; Kugler et al., 1980; Yates & Iberall, 1973) and dissipative structure (dynamic pattern) theory (Katchalsky, Rowland, & Blumenthal, 1974; Prigogine & Nicolis, 1971)—that real systems (as opposed to formal machines) consist of ensembles of coupled and mutually entrained oscillators and that coordination is a natural consequence of this organization.

Although in previous work coordinative structures have been linked to dissipative structures (Kelso, Holt, Kugler, & Turvey, 1980; Kugler et al., 1980; see also Kugler et al., 1982), here we shall prefer Katchalsky's term *dynamic pattern* (cf. Katchalsky et al., 1974). Traditionally, the word *structure* has referred only to static *spatial* patterns that are at or near thermodynamic equilibrium. In contrast, the term *dissipative structure* applies also to the temporal domain and refers to open nonequilibrium systems that require energy to maintain spatiotemporal patterns. Thus the term *dynamic pattern* is preferred not only because it removes the ambiguity between classical notions of the term *structure* and Prigogine's dissipative structures, but also because it captures the flavor of what is, in effect, a functional or dynamic organization. We are persuaded of the importance of dynamic patterns because they provide an accurate description of the appearance of qualitative change, or emergent properties, that cannot be understood with reference to quantitatively known component processes.

According to Katchalsky et al. (1974; see also Yates, 1980; Yates & Iberall, 1973) there are three essential ingredients for a system to display dynamic patterns. First, there should be a sufficiently large density of interacting elements or degrees of freedom. Second, the interactions should be nonlinear in nature; and finally, free energy should be dissipated. As we shall see, the "stuff" of the motor system—synergies or coordinative structures—consists of precisely these ingredients.

The continuous dissipation and transformation of energy results in a fundamental property of living systems—cyclicity—and motivates the physical theory that complex systems are ensembles of nonlinear, limit cycle oscillators (homeokinetics; e.g., Iberall & McCulloch, 1969; Soodak & Iberall, 1978). This claim necessarily suggests that coordinated movement will be subject to particular kinds of constraints whose form we will attempt to elucidate shortly. But it is to the general issue of constraints that we turn first.

II. Coordinative Structures as Constraints

As Mattingly (1980) points out in his review of *Gödel, Escher, Bach: An Eternal Golden Braid* (Hofstadter, 1979), it has long been recognized by linguistic theoreticians that a formal theory of grammar that allows an un-restricted use of recursive devices would be simply too powerful. Such a theory would permit the grammars that occur in natural languages, as well as an infinite number of grammars that bear no relation whatsoever to natural languages. Thus the claim that programs can be developed to model the human mind is vacuous: Without the incorporation of constraints, one program may be as good as any other, and none may have anything to do with how real biological systems work.

In a similar vein, current theories of motor control fail to embody the concept of constraint: They do not capture the distinction between those acts that occur and those that are physically possible but never will occur. The motor program notion, for example, is a description of an act—specified in terms of the contractions of muscles—that is too powerful because it can describe acts that could never be performed by an actor. Theoretically, the motor program is as viable for unorganized convulsions as it is for coordinated movement (cf. Fowler, 1977). Boylls (1975) expresses an identical view of servomechanistic models. The concept of coordinative structure (in his terms, muscle linkages)

> by no means represents a conventional engineering approach to the control of motor performance, because the brain is not viewed as having the capacity to transfer an existing state of the musculature into any other arbitrary state, however bio-mechanically sound. Most such unconstrained states would have no behavioral utility. Hence the linkage paradigm . . . naturally assumes that evolution has econ-omized the motor system's task through constraints restricting its operation to the domain of behaviorally useful muscle deployments. (p. 168)

If the proper unit of analysis for the motor system is indeed the coordinative structure, then the difference between coordinated and uncoordinated move-ment—between control and dyscontrol—is defined by what acts are actually performed, since the coordinative structure by definition is functional in nature.

We should clarify what we mean by *functional* here, for some may view it as a buzzword that glosses over underlying mechanisms. This would be a mis-understanding, for as Fentress (1976) has taken pains to point out, mechanism itself is a functional concept and can only be considered in relative terms. Thus what constitutes a mechanism at one level of analysis becomes a system of interrelated subcomponents at a more refined level of analysis.[1] Questions pertaining to mechanisms (e.g., are coordinative structures mechanisms?) are applicable only when the context for the existence of a particular mechanism is precisely defined (Kelso & Tuller, 1981). This brings us to an important point: Coordinative structures are functional units in the sense that the individual degrees of freedom constituting them are constrained by particular behavioral goals or effectivities (Turvey & Shaw, 1979). Sharing the same degrees of

---

[1]For example, the structure DNA can be taken as a mechanism at one level of analysis, but at another level DNA is more appropriately described as a set of interacting components such as proteins and enzymes.

freedom without reference to the effectivity engaged in by an actor would not constitute a functional unit.

Nowhere is this claim (insight?) more apparent than in modern ethological research, where there is growing recognition that nervous systems are organized with respect to the relations among components rather than to the individual components themselves (cf. Bateson & Hinde, 1976; Rashevsky, 1960). Thus, in seeking to understand the nature of behavior, some ethologists consider it more appropriate to look for generalities across dimensions that are physically distinct but normally occur together (e.g., pecking and kicking during fights) rather than across dimensions that share the same physical form (e.g., pecking for food and pecking in fights; cf. Fentress, Note 2). In our attempts to relate divergent levels of organization in biological systems we do well to keep the "functional unit" perspective to the forefront, for such units may well have been the focus of natural selection. Moreover, the implications for the acquisition of skill and motor learning are apparent. For example, if one were to ask whether speaking is a complex act, one answer would be that it is complex for the child who is learning to speak but simple for the adult who has already acquired the necessary coordination to produce the sounds of the language. In the sense that the degrees of freedom of the speech apparatus are subject to particular constraints in the adult speaker (which it is our role to discover), then there is reason to believe that his or her neuromuscular organization is actually *simpler* than that of the child *for the same act* (see Yates, 1978, on complexity). Similarly, it is quite possible that so-called complex tasks that fit existing constraints may be much more easily acquired than the "simple" tasks we ask subjects to perform in a laboratory. We turn now to consider exactly what form such constraints appear to take.

III. Properties of Coordinative Structures

A. Local Relations

If, as Gurfinkel, Kots, Paltsev, and Fel'dman (1971) argue, there are many different synergies or coordinative structures, then the key problem for a science of movement is to detect them and to define the context in which they are naturally realized. What should we be looking for and how should we be looking? If the constraint perspective is correct, then we may well expect to see—in any given activity—a constancy in the relations among components of a coordinative structure even though the metrical values of individual components may vary widely. For example, the temporal patterning of muscle activities may be fixed independent of changes in the absolute magnitude of activity in each muscle. Similarly, the temporal patterning of kinematic events may be fixed independent of changes in the absolute magnitude or velocity of individual movements.

One obvious strategy for uncovering relations among components is to change the metrical value of an activity (e.g., by increasing the speed of the action). In this fashion, we can observe which variables are modified and which variables, or relations among variables, remain unchanged. Notice that if one searches for canonical forms of an activity, then changing metrical properties obscures the basic form by altering properties of individual components that would otherwise remain stable. For example, in the study of speech, changes in speaking rate and syllable stress pose major problems for researchers looking for invariant acoustic definitions of phonemes. Alternatively, these changes may provide the major ways that invariance can be observed; some aspects of phonemes must change and other aspects must remain the same in order to preserve phonemic identity over changes in speaking rate and stress.

The properties of coordinative structures have been more fully articulated in a number of recent papers (Fowler, 1977; Kelso, Holt, Kugler, & Turvey, 1980; Kugler et al., 1980; Turvey et al., 1978). Here we shall present only a small inventory of activities that reveal those properties. We shall try to show—at macroscopic and microscopic levels of behavior—that certain relations among variables are maintained over changes in others. In addition, a primary goal will be to extend this analysis, in a modest way, to the production of speech and beyond that to the intrinsic relations that hold across the systems for speaking, moving, and seeing.

Electromyographic (EMG) investigations of locomotion illustrate the properties of coordinative structures discussed briefly above. For example, in freely locomoting cats (Engberg & Lundberg, 1969), cockroaches (Pearson, 1976), and humans (Herman, Wirta, Bampton, & Finley, 1976), increases in the speed of locomotion result from increases in the absolute magnitude of activity during a specific phase of the step cycle (see Grillner, 1975; Shik & Orlovskii, 1976), but the timing of periods of muscle activity remains fixed relative to the step cycle. In keeping with the notion of coordinative structures, the temporal patterning of muscle activities among linked muscles remains fixed over changes in the absolute magnitude of activity in individual muscles.

The literature on motor control of mastication offers an abundance of data understandable within a constraint perspective. For example, Luschei and Goodwin (1974) recorded unilaterally from four muscles that raise the mandible in the monkey. The cessation of activity in all four muscles was relatively synchronous whether the monkey was chewing on the side ipsilateral or contralateral to the recorded side. In contrast, the amplitude of activity in each muscle was very sensitive to the side of chewing. In other words, the timing of activity periods of the four muscles remained fixed over large changes in amplitude of the individual muscle activities.

Similar timing relations have been reported in human jaw-raising muscles. Møller (1974) observed that the timing of activity in the medial pterygoid and anterior temporalis muscles relative to each other remains unchanged during natural chewing of an apple, although the individual chews are of varying durations and amplitudes; the muscles acting synergistically to raise the jaw generally show fixed temporal patterns of activity over substantial changes in the magnitude of activity. Thexton's (1976) work suggests that this constancy of temporal relations holds for antagonistic muscle groups as well. Specifically, the timing of activity in the muscles that lower and raise the jaw is not sensitive to changes in consistency of the chewed food, although the amplitudes of activity in the muscles that raise the jaw decrease markedly as the food bolus softens.

The two activities discussed, locomotion and mastication, are easily described as fundamental patterns of events that recur over time. The observed pattern is not strictly stereotypic because it is modifiable in response to environmental changes, such as bumps in the terrain or changes in consistency of the food. This style of coordination, in which temporal relationships are preserved over metrical changes, may also hold for activities that are less obviously rhythmic and whose fundamental pattern is not immediately apparent. Examinations of kinematic aspects of two such activities, handwriting and typewriting, reveal these properties of coordinative structures.

At first blush, the control of handwriting does not appear to be in terms of a fundamental motor pattern that recurs over time. The linguistic constraints are considered primary, precluding the possibility of regularly occurring motor events. However, when individuals are asked to vary writing speed without varying movement amplitude, the relative timing of certain movements does not change with speed (Viviani & Terzuolo, 1980). Specifically, the tangential velocity records resulting from different writing speeds reveal that overall duration changed markedly across speeds. But when the individual velocity records are adjusted to approximate the average duration, the resulting pattern is invariant. In other words, major features of writing a given word occur at a fixed time relative to the total duration taken to write the word. The same timing relationships are preserved over changes in magnitude of movements, over different muscle groups, and over different environmental (frictional) conditions (Denier van der Gon & Thuring, 1965; Hollerbach, 1980; Wing, 1978).

The control of typewriting, like handwriting, does not appear to be in terms of a fundamental motor pattern that recurs over time. But Terzuolo and Viviani (1979) looked for possible timing patterns in the motor output of professional typists and found that for any given word, the set of ratios between the times of occurrence of successive key-presses remained invariant over changes in the absolute time taken to type the word. When weights were attached to the fingers, the temporal pattern of key-presses (the set of time ratios) was unaffected, although the time necessary to type the words often increased. Thus, temporal relationships among kinematic aspects of typewriting appear to be tightly constrained, although the time necessary to accomplish individual keystrokes may change.

A synergistic or coordinative structure style of organization appears to hold over diverse motor acts. The question remains whether this view can be applied to the production of speech. Specifically, do temporal relationships among some aspects of articulation remain fixed over metrical changes in the individual variables? Two obvious sources of metrical change in speech that have been extensively investigated are variations in syllable stress and speaking rate. If the view of systemic organization that we have elaborated here holds for speech production, we would expect to see a constancy in the temporal relationships among articulatory components (muscle activities or kinematic properties) over stress and rate variations. Allow us first to step back and examine briefly a general conception of how changes in stress and rate are accomplished.

Many current theories of speech motor control share the assumption that changes in speaking rate and syllable stress are independent of the motor commands for segmental (phonetic) units. Articulatory control over changes in speaking rate and syllable stress is considered as "the consequence of a timing pattern imposed on a group of (invariant) phoneme commands" (Shaffer, 1976, p. 387). Lindblom (1963), for example, suggests that each phoneme has an invariant "program" that is unaffected by changes in syllable stress or speaking rate (tempo). Coarticulation results from the temporal overlap of execution of successive programs.[2] Thus, when a vowel coarticulates with a following consonant, it is because the consonant program begins before the vowel program is finished (see also Kozhevnikov & Chistovich, 1965; Stevens & House, 1963). According to these views, when speaking rate increases or stress decreases, the command for a new segment arrives at the articulators before the preceding segment is fully realized. The articulation of the first segment is interrupted, resulting in the articulatory undershoot and temporal shortening characteristic of both unstressed syllables and fast speaking rates. This scheme predicts that the relative temporal alignment of control signals for successive segments, and their kinematic realizations, will change as stress and speaking rate vary, a prediction contrary to the constancy in temporal relationships observed in locomotion, mastication, handwriting, and typewriting.

There exists EMG evidence, albeit quite limited, that the coordinative structure style of organization may hold for speech production, that is, that temporal relationships among aspects of intersegmental articulation remain constant over changes in stress and speaking rate. Experiments by Tuller, Harris, and Kelso (1982) and Tuller, Kelso, and Harris (1982) explored this question directly by examining possible temporal constraints over muscle activities when stress and speaking rate vary. The five muscles sampled are known to be associated with lip, tongue, and jaw movements during speech.

When speakers were asked to increase their rate of speech or to decrease syllable stress the acoustic duration of their utterances decreased as expected. The magnitude and duration of activity in individual muscles also changed markedly. However, the relative timing of muscle activity was preserved over changes in both speaking rate and syllable stress. Specifically, the relative

---

[2]Although Lindblom's later work does not adhere to the originally described model (e.g., Lindblom, 1974), it has strongly influenced recent experimental work (e.g., Fant, Stålhammar, & Karlsson, 1974; Gay, 1978; Gay, Ushijima, Hirose, & Cooper, 1974; Harris, 1978) and, we believe, is representative of a class of theories of speech motor control.

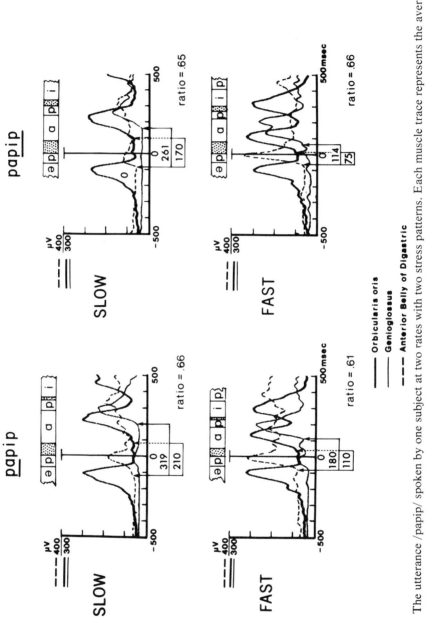

Figure 7-1. The utterance /papip/ spoken by one subject at two rates with two stress patterns. Each muscle trace represents the average of 12 repetitions of the utterance. Arrows indicate onsets of activity for anterior belly of digastric (jaw lowering for /a/; broken line), orbicularis oris (lip movement for /p/; thick line), and genioglossus (tongue fronting for /i/; thin line). The ratio of the latency of consonant-related activity relative to the vowel-to-vowel period is indicated for each stress and rate condition. (From Tuller, Kelso & Harris, 1982.)

timing of consonant activity and activity for the flanking vowels remained fixed over suprasegmental change.

The preservation of relative timing of muscle activities is illustrated in Figure 7-1, which is essentially a 2 × 2 matrix of stress and rate conditions for the utterance /papip/. Each muscle trace represents the average of 12 tokens produced by one subject. Arrows indicate the onsets of activity for /a/ (anterior belly of digastric), /p/ (orbicularis oris inferior), and /i/ (genioglossus). Onset values, defined as the time when the relevant muscle activity increased to 10% of its range of activity, were determined from a numerical listing of the mean amplitude of each EMG signal, in microvolts, during successive 5-msec intervals.

As is apparent from the figure, the onset of consonant-related activity was strongly linked to the timing of activity for the flanking vowels. In this case, the ratio of latency to period was unaffected by suprasegmental changes, although variations in duration and peak amplitude of activity in individual muscles were evident. In all cases, the relationship maintained was highly linear, though not necessarily ratiomorphic. This preservation of relative timing of consonant- and vowel-related muscle activity was observed for all utterances and muscle combinations sampled, and was independent of the large variations in magnitude and duration of individual muscle activity (for details see Tuller, Kelso, & Harris, 1982). These data fit the primary characteristic of coordinative structures outlined above; namely, there is a constancy in the relative temporal patterning of components, in this case muscle activities, independent of metrical changes in the duration or absolute magnitude of activity in each muscle.

In the brief review of locomotion, mastication, handwriting, and typewriting, we noted that these activities show temporal constraints at either an EMG or a kinematic level, constraints that fit a coordinative structure style of organization. Activities such as speech, handwriting, and typewriting, usually described as less stereotypic or repetitive than locomotion or mastication, can also be described within a synergistic or coordinative structure style of control (see also Kelso, Southard, & Goodman, 1979a, 1979b). In the next section we will attempt to extend this type of analysis to the relations that hold across different structural subsystems, such as the systems for speaking, moving, and seeing.

B. Global Relations

The inventory presented above offers a view of motor systems that Gelfand and Tsetlin (1971) refer to as *well organized*. Thus the working parameters of the system appear to fall into two distinct groups: essential parameters that determine the form of the function (also called the structural prescription, cf. Boylls, 1975; Kelso et al., 1979a, 1979b; Grimm & Nashner, 1978; Turvey et al., 1978), and nonessential parameters that lead to marked changes in the values of the function but leave its topology essentially unchanged. It is possible that a subdivision of this nature does not exist for every function; nevertheless, the distinction between essential and nonessential variables (between coordination and control—see Kugler et al., 1980) is apparent in a wide variety of activities.

As a historical note, we remark that the distinction between variables of coordination and control is not entirely new (although there is little doubt of our failure to appreciate it). Over 40 years ago von Holst (1937/1973), following his extensive studies of fish swimming behavior, hypothesized the presence of a duality between frequency and amplitude of undulatory movement (see also Webb, 1971). Invariantly, amplitude of fin movement could be modulated (sometimes by as much as a factor of 4) by, for example, the application of a brief pricking stimulus to the tail, without affecting frequency in any way. Von Holst (1937/1973) concluded that this behavior may be explained as follows: "The automatic process (a central rhythm) determines the frequency, whilst the number of motor cells excited by the process at any one time defines—other things being equal—the amplitude of the oscillation" (pp. 88–89). There seems little doubt that neurophysiological research of the last decade has borne out von Holst's thesis—in general, if not in detail—with its discovery of numerous central rhythm generators (see Davis, 1976; Dellow & Lund, 1971; Grillner, 1975; Stein, 1978). We shall have much more to say about the nature of rhythmical activity in the next section; for the moment let us consider the possibility that the partitioning of variables into essential and nonessential is a basic design strategy for motor systems.

In Section III.A we presented a brief inventory of activities that highlighted the nature of constraints on large numbers of muscles. Yet these activities illustrate the partitioning of variables within local collectives of muscles— muscles acting at single or homologous limbs or within a single structural subsystem. The arguments that a synergistic style of organization constitutes a design for the motor system would surely be strengthened if it could be shown that the same classification of variables into essential and nonessential holds for more than one structural subsystem. We turn then to examine a potential relationship that has intrigued numerous investigators, namely, that between speaking and manual performance.

There is reason to believe that the two activities may be linked by virtue of their privileged status as unique functions of the left hemisphere. This fact has been used to suggest that language lateralization arises as a result of the requirement for unilateral motor control of a bilaterally innervated vocal apparatus (Liberman, 1974).

Relatedly, in their well-known "functional cerebral space" model, Kinsbourne and Hicks (1978a, 1978b) suggest that because the human operator has access to a limited amount of functional cerebral space, excitation from putative cortical control centers that are close together (e.g., for speaking and controlling the right hand) is likely to overflow and cause intrahemispheric interference. Conversely, the greater the functional distance between control centers, the less likely is contamination from one center to the other and the better is performance on simultaneous tasks. Experiments showing that right-hand superiority in balancing a dowel on the index finger is lost when subjects are required to speak while doing the task (e.g., Kinsbourne & Cook, 1971; Hicks, 1975; Hicks, Provenzano, & Rybstein, 1975) all seem to support some type of functional space or intrahemispheric competition model.

These experiments also motivate a view of cerebral function in which speaking is considered dominant over the manual task. Unfortunately, the dependent measures employed—dowel balancing or number of taps on a key—do not allow us to examine possible interactions with speaking (e.g., whether pauses in tapping and pauses in speaking co-occur). This design deficiency is in part to blame for the focus on manual performance as it reflects intrahemispheric interference with little or no emphasis on possible complementary effects on speech dynamics. Indeed, the failure to find effects on global measures of vocal performance (e.g., number of words generated in response to a target letter in 30 sec) has led some investigators to conclude that interference is a "one-way street," with "cognitive tasks having priority over motor systems" (Bowers, Heilman, Satz, & Altman, 1978, p. 555).

From our perspective it makes little sense to talk of interference, competition, and rigid dominance relations in a coordinated system. If speech and movement control systems are governed by the same organizational principles, the issue for lateralization concerns the tightness of fit between these systems when control is effected by one limb or the other. Although we shall not speak to the laterality issue directly at this point, we do want to illustrate that apparent competition and interference between the subsystems for speaking and manual performance may be more correctly viewed as an effect of their mutual collaboration.

Consider the following experiment, in which subjects[3] are asked to produce cyclical movements of a comfortable frequency and amplitude with their right index finger while simultaneously uttering a homogeneous string of syllables ("stock," "stock," etc.).[4] Obviously, subjects have no problem whatsoever in following these instructions. Now imagine that the subject is told to vary the stress of alternate syllables in a strong–weak manner (phonetically, /'stak, stak, 'stak, stak ... /) while maintaining amplitude and frequency of finger movement constant. The waveform data for one such subject are shown in Figure 7-2. It is quite obvious that finger movements are modulated—in spite of instructions not to do so—such that they conform to the speech stress pattern;

---

[3]We have tested a total of seven subjects in a number of different experimental situations. Although we shall not present averaged data here, the figures shown are representative of the performance of all of our subjects. In fact, some subjects show greater effects than those illustrated here.

[4]The apparatus for recording finger movements has been described in detail elsewhere (Kelso & Holt, 1980). Basically, the finger slips into a sleeve whose axis of rotation is coupled to a potentiometer, thus enabling us to obtain a full complement of kinematic characteristics. Both finger and speech waveforms were recorded on FM tape for later off-line analysis on a PDP 11/45 computer.

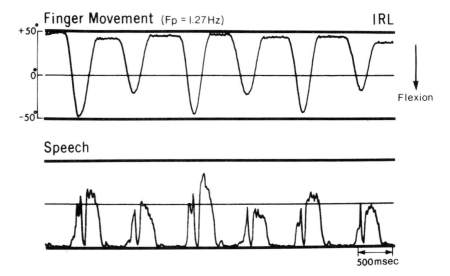

Figure 7-2. Alternate stress of speaking: Simultaneous finger movement (top) and integrated speech waveform (bottom) produced by a subject when told to vary the stress of alternate syllables but maintain the amplitude and frequency of finger movements constant.

that is, longer finger movements accompany stressed syllables, and shorter finger movements accompany unstressed syllables. Is this the outcome of the speech system "driving," as it were, the motor system? A parallel experiment in which subjects were asked to keep stress of speaking constant but to vary the extent of finger movement (i.e., alternating long and short excursions) suggests not. Often the result was that the change in amplitude of finger movement was accompanied by a change in the pattern of syllable production such that there was increased stress[5] with the longer finger movement. The waveform data for one such subject are shown in Figure 7-3.

These data speak to several issues. Of primary importance is the demonstration of *mutual interactions* among the subsystems for speaking and manual performance. Interestingly, this theme is also borne out in recent work on aphasic patients by Cicone, Wapner, Foldi, Zurif, and Gardner (1979). Speech and gesture seem to follow an identical pattern in aphasia: Anterior (Broca's) aphasics seem to gesture no more fluently than they speak, and posterior (Wernicke's) aphasics (who generate much empty speech) gesture far more than normals.

But the broader impact of these data on speaking and manual activity is not

---

[5]We use the word *stress* here guardedly because we have not yet performed listener tests on subjects' productions. It is clear, however, that the amplitude of the audio waveform is modulated according to what the finger is doing.

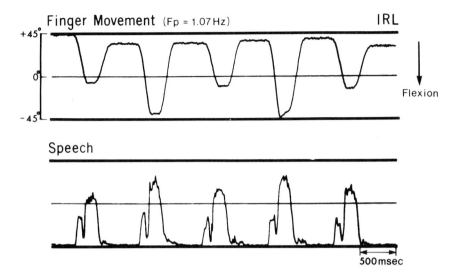

Figure 7-3. Alternate extent of finger movements: Simultaneous finger movement (top) and integrated speech waveform (bottom) produced by a subject when told to vary the extent of alternate finger movements but produce all syllables exactly like all other syllables.

only their indication that the two activities share a common organizational basis (see also Studdert-Kennedy & Lane, 1980, for additional commonalities between spoken and signed language); rather it is that the same design theme emerges in "coupled" systems as in "single" systems (such as those for walking, chewing, handwriting, typewriting, and speaking, reviewed in the preceding section). When an individual speaks and moves at the same time, the degrees of freedom are constrained such that the system is parameterized as a total unit. The parameterization in this case, as in the case of single systems, takes the form of a distribution of force (as reflected in the mutual amplitude relations) among all the muscle groups involved.

An important property of collectives of muscles is their ability to establish and maintain an organization in the face of changes in contextual conditions. Thus Kelso and Holt (1980) show that human subjects can achieve invariant end positions of a limb despite changes in initial conditions, unexpected perturbations applied during the movement trajectory, and both of these in the absence of awareness of limb position. The organization of limb muscles in this case appears to be qualitatively similar to a nonlinear vibratory system (for more details and further evidence see Bizzi, Dev, Morasso, & Polit, 1978; Cooke, 1980; Fel'dman, 1966; Kelso, 1977; Kelso, Holt, & Flatt, 1980; Polit & Bizzi, 1978; Schmidt, 1980; see also below). Similarly, in the well-known speech experiment of Folkins and Abbs (1975), loads applied to the jaw yielded "compensatory responses" in the lips to preserve ongoing articulation. In fact, the movement of the jaw and lower lip covaried in such a way that the sum of their displacements tended to remain constant (but see Sussman, 1980, for possible methodological problems with compensation studies).

Is the preservation of such "equations of constraint" in the face of unexpected changes in environmental context also characteristic of coupled systems? In short, the answer appears to be yes, at least if the following experiment is representative. Imagine that as an individual is synchronizing speech and cyclical finger movements (in the manner referred to earlier), a sudden and unexpected perturbation is applied to part of the system. In this case a torque load (approximately 60 ounce-inch of 100-msec duration) is added to the finger in such a way as to drive it off its preferred trajectory (see Kelso & Holt, 1980, for details of this technique). In order for the finger to return to its stable cycle, additional force must be supplied to the muscles. Qualitatively speaking, an examination of the movement waveform of Figure 7-4 reveals that the finger is back on track in the *cycle following the perturbation*. Of interest, however, is the speech pattern (again, the individual audio envelopes in Figure 7-4 correspond to the syllable /stak/ spoken at preferred stress and frequency). We see that the audio waveform is unaffected in the cycle in which the finger is perturbed: It is in the following cycle that a dramatic amplification of the waveform occurs. This result is compatible with the present thesis that systems, when coupled, share a mutual organization and that this organization may be preserved over efference (as in the stress–amplitude experiments) or afference (as in the present experiment). Thus a peripheral disturbance to one part of the

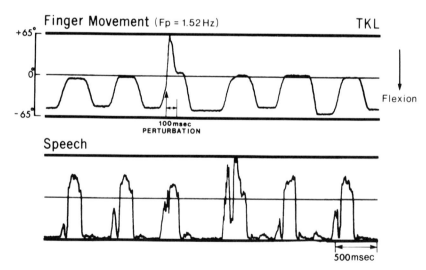

Figure 7-4. Unexpected finger perturbation: Simultaneous finger movement (top) and integrated speech waveform (bottom) produced during a sudden, unexpected finger perturbation. Notice the increase in amplitude of the syllable in the cycle following the perturbation.

system (requiring an additional output of force to overcome it) will have a correlated effect on other parts of the system to which it is functionally linked. Note that as in the previous experiments on speaking and moving, there is no support whatsoever for a one-way dominance of speech over manual performance. Were that the case, there is little reason to expect speaking to be modified in any way by finger perturbations.

Why then does the adjustment (maladjustment may be a more appropriate word) to speaking occur on the cycle *after* the perturbation? Some insight into this issue may be gleaned from a clever experiment on locomotion by Orlovskii and Shik (1965). Dogs were fitted with a force brake at the elbow joint and then were allowed to locomote freely on a treadmill. A brief application of the brake during the transfer-flexion phase not only retarded the movement of the elbow but also that of the shoulder, suggesting that both joints are constrained to act as a unit within the act of locomotion. Spinal mechanisms were implicated because the joints returned to their original velocities within 30 msec of the brake application. But of even greater interest was the *next* locomotory cycle, some 800–900 msec following the original perturbation. Here the transfer-flexion phase was delayed again, as if the perturbation (along with an appropriate response) had reoccurred. Note that had the brake actually been applied, this "phantom braking response" (Boylls, 1975) would have constituted an *adaptation*; indeed, this phenomenon of modifying current acts based on perturbations occurring in antecedent ones is called *next-cycle adaptation*.

Although our understanding of such phenomena is still rather primitive (see Boylls, 1975, pp. 77–79, for one speculation of a neural type), the present equations-of-constraint perspective on coupled systems offers at least a descriptive account (see also Saltzman, 1979). From the mutual relations observed in the stress and finger amplitude experiments, we can generate the following simple constraint equation:

$$f(x,y) = k$$

where the variables x and y represent the set of muscles (subsystems) for speaking and manual activity, respectively, such that a specific change in x will be accompanied by a corresponding change in y to preserve the function, f, constant. Now imagine that at time t_1 the variable y is altered via a peripheral perturbation such that a change in its value (in the form of an increase in muscular force) is necessary to overcome the disturbance. As a consequence of "mechanical" constraints (e.g., neural conduction times, mechanical properties of muscles) the variable x cannot immediately adopt an appropriate value *on the perturbed cycle*. On the next cycle, however, the variable x takes on a complementary value as a necessary consequence of the fact that force is distributed among both systems.

Let us clarify one important aspect of this simple formulation. The interrelations observed here are not meaningfully described as "compensatory." That is, x is not incremented because it has to compensate for changes in y. The synergistic relations observed between speaking and manual activity are not based on a causal logic (because y, then x). Rather, the coherency between systems is captured by an *adjunctive* proposition (since y is incremented, then x must also be incremented).[6] In the stress–finger amplitude experiment, x and y were simultaneously adjusted; in the perturbation experiment, as a consequence of inherent neuromechanical factors, x was not adjusted until the next cycle, even though y had returned to its preferred state. In both cases the basic notion is the same. That is, the *complementary* relations observed are a consequence of the total system functioning as a single, coherent unit.

The global relations between speaking and manual activity that we have identified above are, it seems, far from exotic, if we look for them through the right spectacles. Other systems with quite different structural designs appear to share the same style of coordination. Consider, as a final example, coordination between the eye and the hand. Imagine a situation in which the oculomotor system is partially paralyzed with curare and the subject asked to point ballistically at a target N degrees from visual center (Stevens, 1978). The typical result is that the limb overshoots the designated target—a phenomenon called *past pointing*. A common explanation of this finding is that the subject estimates the movement as farther than N degrees because the *intended* eye movement (registered by an internal copy of the command or corollary discharge of N degrees) and the actual eye movement ($N-k$ degrees) are discrepant. If the subject uses the mismatch information to adjust the limb movement, he will overshoot the target. But an alternative to this hypothesis is offered on the basis of a set of experiments on past pointing in patients with partial extraocular paralysis[7] (see Perenin, Jeannerod, & Prablanc, 1977).

While Perenin et al. argue that the mechanism leading to spatial mis-localization involves "the monitoring of the oculomotor output itself" rather than corollary discharge, we believe that their results can be explained within the present framework. We contend that the *actual* amount of force required to move the partially paralyzed eye to a visual target accounts for past pointing. Thus in a task involving the coupling of oculomotor and limb subsystems, parameterization occurs over the total coupled system, so that the increase in force required to localize a partially paralyzed or mechanically loaded eyeball (cf. Skavenski, Haddad, & Steinman, 1972) is necessarily distributed to the system controlling the hand in a task that requires their coupled activity. There is no need to invoke a corollary discharge (Brindley, Goodwin, Kulikowski, &

---

[6]The idea that adjunctive logic rather than conditional or causal logic is necessary in order to capture the mutual compatibilities among system components is owing to Shaw and Turvey (e.g., Shaw & Turvey, 1981; Turvey & Shaw, 1979). There is growing acceptance of this view in ecological science (cf. Patten, Note 3; Patten & Auble, in press).

[7]We are indebted to Edward Reed for bringing these data to our notice. Reed properly argues that the integration of experiments on extraocular paralysis favoring corollary discharge theory (cf. Teuber, 1966) is based on an argument from exclusion: All other possible accounts are excluded, therefore corollary discharge theory is correct. We concur with Reed, and offer a simpler account of the data.

Leighton, 1976; Stevens, 1978) or an efference monitoring mechanism (Perenin et al., 1977); the eye–hand system is simply utilizing the design strategy that seems to work for many other activities that involve large numbers of degrees of freedom. In short, the fascinating aspect of the data linking the eye, the speech apparatus, and the hand is that the relations observed apply to systems whose structural features are vastly different, just as these same coordinative structure properties apply to more "local" collectives of muscles that share common structural elements.

IV. Rationalizing Coordinative Structures as "Dynamic Patterns"[8]

We have seen in the previous sections that a ubiquitous feature of collectives of muscles is the independence of the force or power distributed into the collective and the relative timing of activities (electromyographic and kinematic) within the collective. In fact, we have presented evidence suggesting that the motor system has a preferred mode of coordination: Where possible, scale up on power but keep relative timing as constant as possible. The flexibility of the system is attained by adjusting the parametric values of inessential variables without altering the basic form of the function as defined by its essential variables. It remains for us now to rationalize why nature has adopted this strategy. In particular let us consider why timing constraints are a principal characteristic of coordinated movement. In fact, this question could take a more general form: Why are humans inherently rhythmic animals?[9] A short excursion into dynamics offers an answer to these questions in terms of physical principles. As we shall see, the physics of systems in flux defines living creatures as rhythmic; no new mechanisms need be introduced to account for the inherent rhythmicity (Morowitz, 1979).

Dynamics—the physics of motion and change—has not been considered particularly appropriate for an analysis of biological systems because until quite recently it has dealt almost exclusively with linear conservative systems. In simple mechanical systems such as a mass–spring, the equation of motion describes a trajectory toward an equilibrium state. Thus a linear system represented by the second-order differential equation

$$m\ddot{x} + c\dot{x} + kx = 0 \qquad (1)$$

will decay in proportion to the magnitude of its viscous (frictional) term (c), and

---

[8]Parts of this section also appear, with minor modifications, in Kelso (1981).

[9]We do not believe this to be a trivial question. Even "at rest" man is operating periodically (see Desmedt, 1978, for review on normal "resting" tremor). At more macroscopic levels we are subject to circadian phenomena (e.g., Aschoff, 1979). Even the structure of language—if recent generative theories are a yardstick (e.g., Liberman & Prince, 1977)—is inherently rhythmic.

oscillatory motion will cease. All this is predicated on the second law of thermodynamics—time flows in the direction of entropy. Yet living systems are characterized by sustained motion and persistence; as Schrödinger (1945) first remarked, they "accumulate negentropy." Living systems are not statically stable; they maintain their form and function by virtue of their *dynamic stability*.

How might we arrive at a physical description of biological systems that does not violate thermodynamic law? Consider again the familiar mass–spring equation, but this time with a forcing function, $F(\theta)$:

$$m\ddot{x} + c\dot{x} + kx = F(\theta). \tag{2}$$

Obviously it is not enough to supply force to the system; to guarantee persistence (and to satisfy thermodynamic principles) the forcing function must exactly offset the energy lost in each cycle. Real systems meet this requirement by including a function—called an escapement—to overcome dissipative losses. The escapement constitutes a nonlinear element that taps some source of potential energy (as long as it lasts) to compensate for local thermodynamic losses. Thus, a pulse or "squirt" of energy is released via the escapement such that, averaged over cycles, the left-hand side of Equation 2 equals the right-hand side and sustained motion is thereby assured.

The foregoing description is of course the elementary theory of the clock (see Andranov & Chaiken, 1949; Iberall, 1975; Kugler et al., 1980; Yates & Iberall, 1973, for many more details), but it draws our attention to some fundamentally important concepts: First, stability can only be established and maintained if a system performs work; second, work is accomplished by the flow of energy from a high source of potential energy to a lower potential energy "sink;" third, stated as Morowitz's theorem, the flow of energy from a source to a sink will lead to at least one cycle in the system (Morowitz, 1979).

That cyclical phenomena abound in biological systems is hardly at issue here (see Footnote 9, the chronobiology literature [Aschoff, 1979], and reviews by Oatley & Goodwin, 1971; Wilke, 1977). Nor is the notion—favored by investigators of movement over the years —that "clocks," "metronomes," or rhythm generators may exist for purposes of timing (e.g., Keele, 1980, for recent discussion; Kozhevnikov & Chistovich, 1965; Lashley, 1951). However, we might emphasize that the many extrinsic "clock" mechanisms are not motivated by thermodynamic physical theory. The view expressed here—which can only mirror the emphatic remarks of Yates (1980)—is that cyclicity in complex systems is ubiquitous because it is an *obligatory manifestation of a universal design principle for autonomous systems*.

Such a foundation for complex systems leads us, therefore, away from more traditional concepts. The Bernard–Cannon principle of homeostasis, for example, which provides the framework on which modern control theory—with its reference levels, comparators, error correction mechanisms, and so on—is built, is obviated by a dynamic regulation scheme in which internal states are a consequence of the interaction of thermodynamic engines (Soodak & Iberall, 1978). The latter scheme, appropriately termed *homeokinetic*, conceives of systemic behavior as established by an ensemble of nonlinear oscillators that are entrained into a coherent harmonic configuration. For homeokinetics, many degrees of freedom and the presence of active, interacting components is hardly a "curse" in Bellman's (1961) terms; rather it is a necessary attribute of complex systems.

That the constraints imposed on coordinated activity—whether of speech or limbs (or both)—should take the form of a dissociation between power and timing is now less mysterious within this framework than before. Coordinative structures *are* nonlinear oscillators (of the limit cycle type, see below) whose design necessarily guarantees that the timing and duration of "squirts" of energy will be independent of their magnitude within a fixed time frame (a period of oscillation; see Kugler et al., 1980). Referring back to Equation 2, we see that the magnitude of the forcing function will be some proportion of the potential energy available, but the forcing function itself is not dependent on time (Iberall, 1975; Yates & Iberall, 1973). Nonconservative, nonlinear oscillators are truly *autonomous* devices in a formal mathematical sense; time is nowhere represented in such systems (Andranov & Chaiken, 1949) and energy is provided in a "timeless" manner.

An example may be helpful at this point. It comes from a fascinating experiment by Orlovskii (1972) on mesencephalic locomotion in the cat. If one selectively stimulates the hindlimb areas of Red and Dieters nuclei in a stationary cat, the flexor and extensor synergies (corresponding to swing and stance phases, respectively) can be energized. During induced locomotion, however, continuous stimulation of one site or the other has an effect *only when the respective synergies were actually involved in the step cycle.* Supraspinal influences (the energy supply) are tapped only in accordance with the basic design of the spinal circuitry. It is the latter—as in real clocks—that determines *when* the system receives its pulse of energy as well as the duration of the pulse (see also Boylls, 1975, for a discussion of spinal "slots," and Kots's 1977 analysis of the cyclic "quantized" character of supraspinal control, pp. 225–229).

The organization realized by coordinative structures—as we have noted—is not obtained without cost; nonlinear dynamic patterns emerge from the dissipation of more free energy than is degraded in the drift toward equilibrium. Thus the stability of a collective is attained by the physical action of an ensemble of "squirt" systems in a manner akin to limit cycle behavior (cf. Katchalsky et al., 1974; Prigogine & Nicolis, 1971; Soodak & Iberall, 1978). It remains for us now to illustrate—albeit briefly and in a very preliminary way— some of the behavioral predictions of the dynamic perspective on coordinated movement. These necessarily fall out of the properties of nonlinear limit cycles—a topic that we can address here only in a rather terse way.

Homeokinetic theory characterizes biological systems as ensembles of nonlinear oscillators coupled and mutually entrained at all levels of organization. It predicts the discovery of numerous cyclicities and evidence of their mutual interaction. As noted above, the only cycles that meet the nonlinear, self-sustaining, dynamic stability criteria that homeokinetics demands are called *limit cycles* (Goodwin, 1970; Soodak & Iberall, 1978; Yates & Iberall, 1973), and it is from their properties that insights into behavior might emerge. Here we give a sampling of work in progress (Kelso, Holt, Rubin, & Kugler, 1981). By and large, the research involves cyclical movements of the hand alone or in combination with speech (see Section III.B).

A. Response to Perturbations and Changes in Initial Conditions

As Katchalsky et al. (1974) note, the essential difference between linear or nonlinear conservative oscillators and limit cycle oscillators (which obey nonlinear dissipative dynamics) is that perturbations applied to a conservative oscillator will move it to another orbit or frequency, whereas a limit cycle oscillator will maintain its orbit or frequency when perturbed. An examination of Figure 7-5 helps clarify this point. In Figure 7-5A, we show the position versus time and velocity versus position functions for linear and nonlinear types of oscillators. In Figure 7-5B the spiral trajectory in the phase plane represents an oscillation that continuously decreases in amplitude until it comes to a standstill. This is the phase trajectory (velocity vs. position relation) of a stable, damped oscillation. A change in any parameter in the equation describing this motion—for example, the damping coefficient—would drastically change the form of the solution and thus the phase trajectory. In such linear systems there is then no *preferred* set of solutions in the face of parameter changes. In sharp contrast, nonlinear oscillators of the limit cycle type possess a family of trajectories that all tend asymptotically toward a *single* limit cycle despite quantitative changes in parameter values (see Figure 7-5C). Thus, a highly important property of limit cycle oscillators is their *structural stability* in the face of variations in parameter values.

We have shown, in a set of experiments on two-handed cyclical movements (Kelso et al., 1981), that the limbs (in this case the fingers) maintain their preferred frequency and amplitude relations no matter how they are perturbed. Perturbations took the form of brief (100 msec) or constant (applied at a variable point during the cycle and maintained throughout) torque loads unexpectedly applied to one hand or the other via direct-current (dc) torque motors situated above the axis of rotation of the metacarpophalangeal joints. In all four experiments there were no differences in amplitude or duration ($1/f$ msec) before and after perturbation (for many more details, see Kelso et al., 1981). Moreover, the fact that nonlinear oscillators must degrade a large amount of free energy in order to offset the energy lost during each cycle suggests that they will be quickly resettable following a perturbation. This was precisely the case in our experiments. The fingers were in phase in the cycle

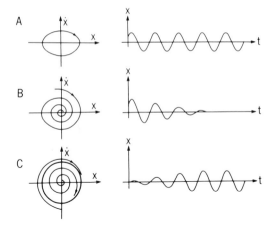

Figure 7-5. Phase plane trajectories (left) and corresponding position–time functions (right) for three different types of oscillation: A, idealized harmonic motion; B, damped harmonic motion; C, limit cycle oscillatory motion. (From Kelso et al., 1981.)

immediately following the perturbation, as revealed by cross-correlations between the limbs as a function of phase lag and by individual inspection of displacement–time waveforms. This capability to return to a stable, bounded phase trajectory despite perturbations, predicted by limit cycle properties, is an extension of our previous work (and that of others) on single trajectory movements (see Section III.B). The latter, it will be remembered, display the "equifinality" property in the face of perturbations, changes in initial conditions, and deafferentation (see Bizzi, this volume). The organization over the muscles is qualitatively like a nonlinear oscillatory system, regardless of whether one is speaking of discrete or cyclical movements (see Fel'dman, 1966; Fowler et al., 1980; Kelso & Holt, 1980; Kelso, Holt, Kugler, & Turvey, 1980).

B. Entrainment Properties

We have characterized coordination in biological systems as arising from cooperative relationships among nonlinear oscillator ensembles. As already intimated, the chief mode of cooperation among self-sustaining oscillators is entrainment or synchronization. Strictly speaking, the latter terms are not synonymous: Synchronization is that state which occurs when both frequency and phase of coupled oscillators are matched exactly; entrainment refers to the matching of frequencies, although one oscillator may lead or lag behind the other.

When coupled oscillators interact, *mutual entrainment* occurs (the "magnet" or "M" effect of von Holst, 1937/1973) with only a small frequency detuning

(Minorsky, 1962). Another form of mutual interaction occurs if the frequency of one oscillator is an integer multiple of another to which it is coupled, a property termed subharmonic entrainment or frequency demultiplication. These preferred relationships are ones that coupled oscillators assume under conditions of maximal coupling or phase locking. Years ago, von Holst discovered coordinative states in fish fin movements that correspond to the different types of entrainment discussed here (see von Holst, 1937/1973). The most common mode of coordination he termed *absolute coordination*, a one-to-one correspondence between cyclicities of different structures. The second and much less common interactive mode he called *relative coordination*. Here the fins exhibit different frequencies, although at least one corresponds to that seen in the absolute coordination state. In more recent times, Stein (1976, 1977) has elaborated on von Holst's work, using the mathematics of coupled oscillators to predict successfully patterns of neuronal activity for interlimb coordination. The oscillator theoretic approach to neural control, as Stein (1977) remarks, is still in an embryonic state. In our experiments we have taken a step in what we hope is a positive direction by examining the qualitative predictions of the theory without immediate concern for its neural basis. The results are intuitively apparent to any of us who have tried to perform different cyclical movements of the limbs at the same time. Thus the cyclical movements of each limb operating singly at its own preferred frequency mutually entrain when the two are coupled together (von Holst' "M" effect). When an individual is asked to move his or her limbs at different frequencies, low-integer subharmonic entrainment occurs. The waveforms of both limbs shown in Figure 7-6 also suggest amplitude modulation (von Holst's *superimposition* effect). Thus on some coinciding cycles a "beat" phenomenon can be observed (particularly in the 2:1 ratio) in which the amplitude of the higher frequency hand increases in relation to noncoincident cycles. These preferred relationships are *emergent* characteristics of a system of nonlinear oscillators; the collection of mutually entrained oscillators functions in a single unitary manner.

Entrainment properties are not restricted to movements of the limbs, but are also evident (as predicted by the principles of homeokinetic physics) in systems that share little or no common structural similarity. Returning to our analysis of the interrelationships between speaking and manual activity, we have shown that subjects, when asked to speak (again the familiar syllable /stak/) at a different rate from their preferred finger rate, do so by employing low-integer sub- or superharmonics (see Figure 7-7). The situation is reversed (although not necessarily symmetrically) when the individual is asked to move the finger at a different rate from speaking. The ratios chosen are always simple ones (e.g., 2:1 or 3:1; see Figure 7-8). The strict maintenance of cyclicity as predicted by homeokinetic theory is abundantly apparent. Entrainment ensures a stable temporal resolution of simultaneous processes throughout the whole system. Moreover, entrainment of oscillators is limited to a relatively restricted frequency range captured in Iberall and McCulloch's poetics as an "orbital constellation."

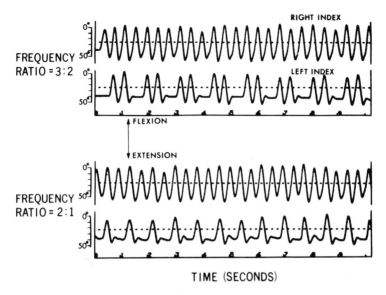

Figure 7-6.   An example of one subject's response to instructions to move the fingers at different frequencies. On some coinciding cycles, a "beat" phenomenon can be observed in which the amplitude of the higher frequency hand increases in relation to non-coincident cycles (see especially 2:1 ratio).

Homeokinetic theory requires a dynamic system analysis that, to be used optimally, requires a research decision as to the likely limiting conditions for the spectrum of effects of interest. In the continuum of cyclical processes, coherency is determined by the longest period over which "thermodynamic bookkeeping" is closed. For those interested in the production of speech, a possible candidate oscillation over which articulatory cycles of shorter periods may cohere is the "breath group" (Lieberman, 1967) or, more globally, the respiratory cycle (Fowler, 1977; Turvey, 1980). The latter, tied as it is to metabolic processes, may well be the organizing period for *all* the activity patterns of an animal. It is well known, for example, that during exercise, respiration is often synchronized with movements of body parts (Astrand & Rodahl, 1970). But even when metabolic demands are not altered from a resting state, preliminary data indicate entrainment between breathing and limb movements (see also Wilke, Lansing, & Rogers, 1975).

In Figure 7-9 we see data from the now familiar task of speaking and performing cyclical finger movements. In the first case the subject is instructed to move the left index finger at a different rate from speech. The finger waveform is highly regular (3 Hz) except at one point where a pause is evident. From the acoustic signal it is obvious that the pause in finger movement coincides perfectly with respiratory inhalation. In a parallel condition in which the subject is instructed to speak at a different rate from finger movement, we see exactly

CHANGE RATE OF SPEAKING

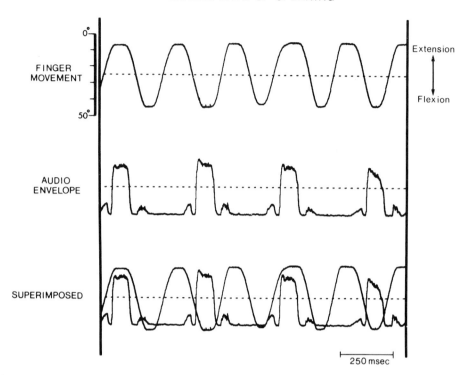

Figure 7-7. Simultaneous finger movement (top) and integrated speech waveform (center) produced by a subject asked to speak at a different rate from finger movement. The subject shown considered each flexion and extension as a separate finger movement. Thus, the finger-to-speech ratio is 3:1.

the same co-occurrence of breathing and a pause in the finger movements (see Figure 7-10). Aside from the fact that these data provide further and perhaps the most compelling evidence of entrainment in coupled systems, there is also the suggestion that *both* systems cohere to the longer time-scale activity, namely, breathing. Since the flow of oxygen constitutes a sustained temporal process in the system (the "escapement" for the thermodynamic power cycle), it seems reasonable to suppose that the respiratory cycle may play a cohering role around which other oscillations seek to entrain. But at this point the question is hypothetical in the face of nonexistent data.

We do not wish to give the impression, however, that the cohering role of the respiratory cycle gives it dominant status. On the contrary, it is well known that the respiratory cycle itself changes character to accommodate the demands of speech (e.g., Draper, Ladefoged, & Whitteridge, 1960). In fact, the entrainment of these systems cannot be explained solely on the basis of metabolic demands.

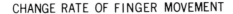

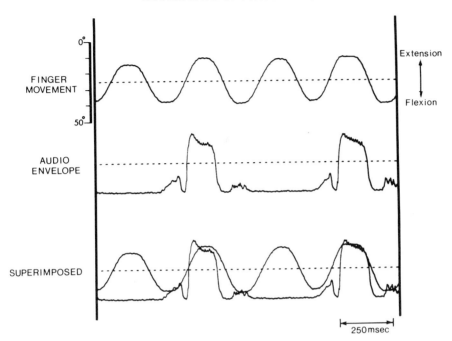

Figure 7-8. Simultaneous finger movement (top) and integrated speech waveform (center) produced by a subject when asked to move her finger at a different rate from her speaking. This subject shows a 2:1 ratio of finger movement to speech, each syllable synchronized with every second finger extension.

When subjects read silently (Conrad & Schönle, 1979), or when finger movements required are of minimal extent (Wilke, 1977), respiratory rhythms change in order to be compatible with the other activity. The point is that in an oscillator ensemble there is no fixed dominance relation. There are different modes of interaction (e.g., frequency and amplitude modulation) and there may be preferred phase relationships, as in the extreme case of maximal coupling or phase locking between two oscillators. A wide variety of behavioral patterns emerges from these interactions; there is structure and a complex network of interconnections but, strictly speaking, no dominance relation.

V. Concluding Remarks

The major problem confronting a theory of coordination and control (whether it be of speech or limbs) is the determination of how stable spatiotemporal organizations are realized from a neuromuscular basis of very many degrees of

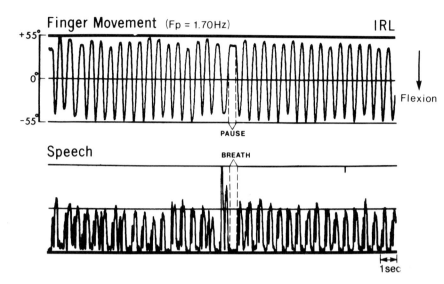

Figure 7-9. Simultaneous finger movement (top) and integrated speech waveform (bottom) produced by a subject when told to move her finger at a different rate from speaking. Pause in the finger movement and the simultaneous inhalation are indicated.

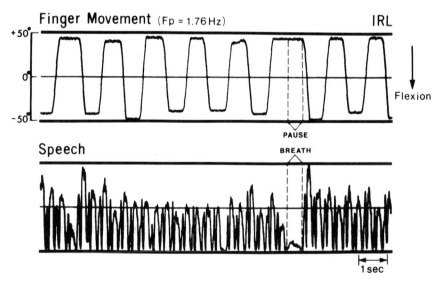

Figure 7-10. Simultaneous finger movement (top) and integrated speech waveform (bottom) produced by a subject when told to speak at a different rate from finger movement. A pause in the finger movement and the simultaneous inhalation are indicated.

freedom. Here we have offered the beginnings of an approach in which solutions to the degrees of freedom problem may lie not in machine-type theories but in the contemporary physical theories of dissipative structures and homeokinetics. A central characteristic of such theories is that complex systems consist of collectives of energy-flow systems that interact in a unitary way and, as a consequence, exhibit limit cycle oscillation. Many of the motor behaviors discussed in this chapter can be rationalized according to limit cycle properties. Common to all of them—including speech—is that certain qualitative properties are preserved over quantitative changes in the values of individual components (muscles, key-presses, kinematic attributes). This feature of coordinated activity exists across all scales of observation; it is as applicable to the microscale (e.g., physiological tremor) as it is to the gross movement patterns of locomotion. We suspect that the functional similarities observed across levels of analysis index the design of the motor system. Thus, even though the material composition varies dramatically from level to level, certain qualitative properties, like cycling, remain invariant (see Kugler et al., 1981; and for a similar view, Mandell & Russo, 1980).

Central to the view expressed here (see also Kelso, 1981; Kugler et al., 1980, 1982; Yates & Iberall, 1973) is that new forms of spatiotemporal organization are possible when scale changes and nonlinearities are present, and an energy supply is available. When a stable system is driven beyond a certain critical value on one of its parameters, bifurcation occurs and qualitatively new structures emerge (Guttinger, 1974). There are many examples of such phase transition phenomena in nature (see Haken, 1977; Prigogine, 1980; Winfree, 1980; for examples) and probably in movement as well. We know, for example, that at low velocities quadrupeds locomote such that limbs of the same girdle are always half a period out of phase. But as velocity is scaled up, there is an abrupt transition from an asymmetric to a symmetric gait (Shik & Orlovskii, 1976). The phase relations of the limbs change, but we doubt that a new "program" is required (Shapiro, Zernicke, Gregor, & Diestel, 1981) or that one needs to invoke a "gait selection" process (Gallistel, 1980). Emergent spatiotemporal order, in the view expressed here, is not owing to an a priori prescription, *independent of and causally antecedent to systemic behavior.* Rather it is an a posteriori fact of the system's dynamic behavior. As Gibson (1979) remarked, behavior is regular without being regulated.

The present perspective—with appropriate extensions (e.g., to a reconceptualization of "information" in naturally developing systems; Kugler et al., 1982)—is less antireductionistic than it is an appeal for epistemological change. Contemporary physics as characterized here does not assign priority to any privileged scale of analysis: There is no "fundamental unit" out of which one can construct a theory of systemic phenomena (see Buckley & Peat, 1979; Yates, 1978). Instead, homeokinetics and dissipative structure/dynamic pattern theory offer a single set of physical principles than can be applied at all levels of analysis. If there is reductionism, it is not in the analytical sense but rather to a minimum set of principles.

Acknowledgments. This work was supported by NIH Grants NS-13617, AM-25814 and NS-13870, and BRS Grant RR-05596.

Reference Notes

1. Greene, P. H. *Strategies for heterarchical control—an essay: I. A style of controlling complex systems.* Department of Computer Science, Illinois Institute of Technology, 1975.
2. Fentress, J. C. *Order and ontogeny: Relational dynamics.* Paper presented at the Interdisciplinary Study of Behavioral Development, Bielefeld, Germany, March 1978.
3. Patten, B. C. *Environs: Relativistic elementary particles for ecology.* Paper presented at the dedication of the Environmental Sciences Laboratory Building, Oak Ridge National Laboratory, Oak Ridge, Tennessee, February 26–27, 1979.

References

Adams, J. A. Feedback theory of how joint receptors regulate the timing and positioning of a limb. *Psychological Review,* 1977, *84,* 504–523.

Andranov, A., & Chaiken, C. E. *Theory of oscillations.* Princeton, N. J.: Princeton University Press, 1949.

Aschoff, J. Circadian rhythms: General features and endocrinological aspects. In D. Krieger (Ed.), *Endocrine rhythms.* New York: Raven Press, 1979.

Astrand, P. O., & Rodahl, K. *Textbook of work physiology.* New York: McGraw-Hill, 1970.

Bateson, P. P. G. & Hinde, R. A. (Eds.). *Growing points in ethology.* New York and London: Cambridge University Press, 1976.

Bellman, R. *Adaptive control processes: A guided tour.* Princeton, N. J.: Princeton University Press, 1961.

Bernstein, N. A. *The coordination and regulation of movements.* London: Pergamon Press, 1967.

Bizzi, E., Chapter 1, this volume.

Bizzi, E., Dev, P., Morasso, P., & Polit, A. Effect of load disturbances during centrally initiated movements. *Journal of Neurophysiology,* 1978, *41,* 542–555.

Bowers, D., Heilman, K. M., Satz, P., & Altman, A. Simultaneous performance on verbal, non-verbal and motor tasks by right-handed adults. *Cortex,* 1978, *14,* 540–556.

Boylls, C. C. A theory of cerebellar function with applications to locomotion, II: The relation of anterior lobe climbing fiber function to locomotor behavior in the cat. *COINS Technical Report* (Department of Computer and Information Science, University of Massachusetts), 1975, *76-1.*

Brindley, G. S., Goodwin, G. M., Kulikowski, J. T., & Leighton, D. Stability of vision with a paralyzed eye. *Journal of Physiology,* 1976, *258,* 65–66.

Buckley, P., & Peat, F. D. *A question of physics: Conversations in physics and biology.* Toronto: University of Toronto, 1979.

Cicone, M., Wapner, W., Foldi, N., Zurif, E., & Gardner, H. The relation between gesture and language in aphasic communication. *Brain and Language*, 1979, *8*, 324–329.

Conrad, B., & Schönle, P. Speech and respiration. *Archiv für Psychiatrie und Nervenkrankheiten*, 1979, *226*, 251–268.

Cooke, J. D. The organization of simple, skilled movements. In G. E. Stelmach & J. Requin (Eds.), *Tutorials in motor behavior*. Amsterdam: Elsevier/North-Holland, 1980.

Davis, G. Organizational concepts in the central motor networks of invertebrates. In R. M. Herman, S. Grillner, P. S. G. Stein & D. G. Stuart (Eds.), *Neural control of locomotion*. New York: Plenum, 1976.

Dellow, P. G., & Lund, J. P. Evidence for central timing of rhythmical mastication. *Journal of Physiology*, 1971, *215*, 1–13.

Denier van der Gon, J. J., & Thuring, J. Ph. The guiding of human writing movements. *Kybernetik*, 1965, *4*, 145–147.

Dennett, D. C. *Brainstorms: Philosophical essays on mind and psychology*, Montgomery, Vt.: Bradford Books, 1978.

Desmedt, J. E. (Ed.). *Progress in clinical neurophysiology* (Vol. 5): *Physiological tremor, pathological tremor and clonus*. Basel: Karger, 1978.

Draper, M. H., Ladefoged, P., & Whitteridge, D. Expiratory pressure and air flow during speech. *British Medical Journal*, 1960, *1*, 1837–1843.

Easton, T. A. On the normal use of reflexes. *American Scientist*, 1972, *60*, 591–599.

Emmett, K. Intentional systems: Dennett's philosophy of psychology. *Cognition and Brain Theory*, 1980, *3*, 109–111.

Engberg, I., & Lundberg, A. An electromyographic analysis of muscular activity in the hindlimb of the cat during unrestrained locomotion. *Acta Physiologica Scandinavica*, 1969, *75*, 614–630.

Fant, G., Stålhammar, U., & Karlsson, I. Swedish vowels in speech material of various complexity. In *Speech communication seminar, Stockholm, 1974*, Uppsala: Almqvist & Wiksell, 1974.

Fel'dman, A. G. Functional tuning of the nervous system with control of movement or maintenance of a steady posture, III: Mechanographic analysis of execution by a man of the simplest motor tasks. *Biophysics*, 1966, *11*, 766–775.

Fentress, J. C. Dynamic boundaries of patterned behavior: Interaction and self-organization. In P. P. G. Bateson & R. A. Hinde (Eds.), *Growing points in ethology*. New York and London: Cambridge University Press, 1976.

Folkins, J. W., & Abbs, J. H. Lip and jaw motor control during speech: Responses to resistive loading of the jaw. *Journal of Speech and Hearing Research*, 1975, *18*, 207–220.

Fowler, C. *Timing control in speech production*. Bloomington, Ind.: Indiana University Linguistics Club, 1977.

Fowler, C. Coarticulation and theories of extrinsic timing. *Journal of Phonetics*, 1980, *8*, 113–133.

Fowler, C. A., Rubin, P., Remez, R. E., & Turvey, M. T. Implications for speech production of a general theory of action. In B. Butterworth (Ed.), *Language production*. New York: Academic Press, 1980.

Fowler, C. A., & Turvey, M. T. Skill acquisition: An event approach with special reference to searching for the optimum of a function of several variables. In G. E. Stelmach (Ed.), *Information processing in motor control and learning*. New York: Academic Press, 1978.

Gallistel, C. R. *The organization of action: A new synthesis.* Hillsdale, N. J.: Lawrence Erlbaum Associates, 1980.

Gay, T. Effect of speaking rate on vowel formant movements. *Journal of the Acoustical Society of America,* 1978, *63,* 223–230.

Gay, T., Ushijima, T., Hirose, H., & Cooper, F. S. Effect of speaking rate on labial consonant-vowel articulation. *Journal of Phonetics,* 1974, *2,* 47–63.

Gelfand, I. M., Gurfinkel, V. S., Tsetlin, M. L., & Shik, M. L. Some problems in the analysis of movements. In I. M. Gelfand, V. S. Gurfinkel, S. V. Fomin, & M. L. Tsetlin (Eds.), *Models of the structural-functional organization of certain biological systems.* Cambridge, Mass.: MIT Press, 1971.

Gelfand, I. M. & Tsetlin, M. L. Mathematical modeling of mechanisms of the central nervous system. In I. M. Gelfand, V. S. Gurfinkel, S. V. Fomin, & M. L. Tsetlin (Eds.), *Models of the structural-functional organization of certain biological systems.* Cambridge, Mass.: MIT Press, 1971.

Gibson, J. J. *The ecological approach to visual perception.* Boston: Houghton-Mifflin, 1979.

Goodwin, B. Biological stability. In C. H. Waddington (Ed.), *Towards a theoretical biology.* Chicago: Aldine, 1970.

Greene, P. H. Problems of organization of motor systems. In R. Rosen & F. Snell (Eds.), *Progress in theoretical biology.* New York: Academic Press, 1972.

Grillner, S. Locomotion in vertebrates. *Physiological Reviews,* 1975, 55, 247–304.

Grimm, R. J., & Nashner, L. M. Long loop dyscontrol. In J. E. Desmedt (Ed.), *Progress in Clinical Neurophysiology* (Vol. 4): *Cerebral motor control in man: Long loop mechanisms.* Basel: Karger, 1978.

Gurfinkel, V. S., Kots, Y. A., Paltsev, E. I., & Fel'dman, A. G. The compensation of respiratory disturbances of the erect posture of man as an example of the organization of interarticular interaction. In I. M. Gelfand, V. S. Gurfinkel, S. V. Fomin, & M. L. Tsetlin (Eds.), *Models of the structural-functional organization of certain biological systems.* Cambridge, Mass.: MIT Press, 1971.

Guttinger, W. Catastrophe theory in physics and biology. In M. Conrad, W. Guttinger, & M. Dalcin (Eds.), *Lecture notes in biomathematics* (Vol. 4): *Physics and mathematics of the nervous system.* Berlin/Heidelberg/New York: Springer-Verlag, 1974.

Haken, H. *Synergetics: An introduction.* Heidelberg: Springer-Verlag, 1977.

Harris, K. S. Vowel duration change and its underlying physiological mechanisms. *Language and Speech,* 1978, *21,* 354–361.

Herman, R., Wirta, R., Bampton, S., & Finley, R. Human solutions for locomotion: Single limb analysis. In R. M. Herman, S. Grillner, P. S. G. Stein, & D. G. Stuart (Eds.), *Neural control of locomotion.* New York: Plenum, 1976.

Hicks, R. E. Intrahemispheric response competition between vocal and unimanual performance in normal adult human males. *Journal of Comparative and Physiological Psychology,* 1975, *89,* 50–60.

Hicks, R. E., Provenzano, F. J., & Rybstein, E. D. Generalized and lateralized effects on concurrent verbal rehearsal upon performance of sequential movements of the fingers by the left and right hands. *Acta Psychologica,* 1975, *39,* 119–130.

Hofstadter, D. R. *Gödel, Escher, Bach: An eternal golden braid,* New York: Basic Books, 1979.

Hollerbach, J. M. *An oscillation theory of handwriting.* Cambridge, Mass.: MIT Artificial Intelligence Laboratory, 1980.

Iberall, A. S. On nature, man and society: A basis for scientific modeling. *Annals of Biomedical Engineering,* 1975, *3,* 344–385.

Iberall, A. S. A field and circuit thermodynamics for integrative physiology, I: Introduction to general notion. *American Journal of Physiology,* 1977, *2,* R171–R180.

Iberall, A. S., & McCulloch, W. S. The organizing principle of complex living systems. *Transactions of the American Society of Mechanical Engineers,* 1969, pp. 290–294.

Katchalsky, A. K., Rowland, V., & Blumenthal, R. Dynamic patterns of brain cell assemblies. *Neurosciences Research Program Bulletin,* 1974, *12*(1).

Keele, S. W. Behavioral analysis of motor control. In V. Brooks (Ed.), *Handbook of physiology: Motor control.* Washington, D.C.: American Physiological Society, 1981.

Kelso, J. A. S. Motor control mechanisms underlying human movement reproduction. *Journal of Experimental Psychology,* 1977, *3,* 529–543.

Kelso, J. A. S. Contrasting perspectives on order and regulation in movement. In A. Baddeley & J. Long (Eds.), *Attention and performance* (Vol. 9). Hillsdale, N. J.: Lawrence Erlbaum Associates, 1981.

Kelso, J. A. S., & Holt, K. G. Exploring a vibratory systems account of human movement production. *Journal of Neurophysiology,* 1980, *43,* 1183–1196.

Kelso, J. A. S., Holt, K. G., & Flatt, A. E. The role of proprioception in the perception and control of human movement: Toward a theoretical reassessment. *Perception & Psychophysics,* 1980, *28,* 45–52.

Kelso, J. A. S., Holt, K. G., Kugler, P. N., & Turvey, M. T. On the concept of coordinative structures as dissipative structures: II. Empirical lines of convergence. In G. E. Stelmach & J. Requin (Eds.), *Tutorials in motor behavior.* Amsterdam: Elsevier/North-Holland, 1980.

Kelso, J. A. S., Holt, K. G., Rubin, P., & Kugler, P. N. Patterns of human interlimb coordination emerge from the properties of non-linear limit cycle oscillatory processes: Theory and Data. *Journal of Motor Behavior,* 1981, *13,* 226–261.

Kelso, J. A. S., Southard, D. L., & Goodman, D. On the nature of human interlimb coordination. *Science,* 1979, *203,* 1029–1031. (a)

Kelso, J. A. S., Southard, D. L., & Goodman, D. On the coordination of two-handed movements. *Journal of Experimental Psychology: Human Perception and Performance,* 1979, 5, 229–238. (b)

Kelso, J. A. S., & Tuller, B. Toward a theory of apractic syndromes. *Brain and Language,* 1981, *12,* 224–245.

Kimura, D. The neural basis of language *qua* gesture. In H. Whitaker & H. A. Whitaker (Eds.), *Studies in neurolinguistics* (Vol. 3). New York: Academic Press, 1976.

Kinsbourne, M., & Cook, J. Generalized and lateralized effects of concurrent verbalization on a unimanual skill. *Quarterly Journal of Experimental Psychology,* 1971, *23,* 341–345.

Kinsbourne, M., & Hicks, R. E. Functional cerebral space: A model for overflow, transfer and interference effects in human performance: A tutorial review. In J. Requin (Ed.), *Attention and performance* (Vol. 7). (Hillsdale, N. J.: Lawrence Erlbaum Associates, 1978. (a)

Kinsbourne, M., & Hicks, R. E. Mapping cerebral functional space: Competition and collaboration in human performance. In M. Kinsbourne (Ed.), *Asymmetrical function of the brain.* New York and London: Cambridge University Press, 1978. (b)

Kots, Ya. M. *The organization of voluntary movement.* New York: Plenum, 1977.

Kozhevnikov, V., & Chistovich, L. *Speech: Articulation and perception.* Moscow-Leningrad, 1965. (English translation: J.P.R.S., Washington, D.C. No. JPRS 30543.)

Kugler, P. N., Kelso, J. A. S., & Turvey, M. T. On the concept of coordinative structures as dissipative structures: I. Theoretical lines of convergence. In G. E. Stelmach (Ed.), *Tutorials in motor behavior.* Amsterdam: Elsevier/North-Holland, 1980.

Kugler, P. N., Kelso, J. A. S., & Turvey, M. T. On the control and coordination of naturally developing systems. In J. A. S. Kelso & J. E. Clark (Eds.), *The development of movement control and coordination.* New York: Wiley, 1982.

Lashley, K. The problem of serial order in behavior. In L. A. Jeffress (Ed.), *Cerebral mechanisms in behavior.* New York: Wiley, 1951.

Liberman, A. M. The specialization of the language hemisphere. In F. O. Schmitt & F. G. Worden (Eds.), *The neurosciences: Third study program.* Cambridge, Mass.: MIT Press, 1974.

Liberman, M., & Prince, A. On stress and linguistic rhythm. *Linguistic Inquiry,* 1977, *8,* 249–336.

Lieberman, P. *Intonation, perception, and language.* Cambridge, Mass.: MIT Press, 1967.

Lindblom, B. Spectrographic study of vowel reduction. *Journal of the Acoustical Society of America,* 1963, *35,* 1773–1781.

Lindblom, B. Motor control mechanisms. *Papers from the Institute of Linguistics, University of Stockholm,* 1974, *26,* 1–19.

Lomas, J., & Kimura, D. Intrahemispheric interaction between speaking and sequential manual activity. *Neuropsychologia,* 1976, *14,* 23–33.

Luschei, E. S., & Goodwin, G. M. Patterns of mandibular movement and jaw muscle activity during mastication in the monkey. *Journal of Neurophysiology,* 1974, *37,* 954–966.

Mandell, A. J., & Russo, P. V. Stochastic periodicity: Latent order in variance. *Totus Homo,* 1980, *12,* 23–36.

Mattingly, I. G. Epimenides at the computer. *The Yale Review,* Winter, 1980.

Miles, F. N., & Evarts, E. V. Concepts of motor organization. *Annual Review of Psychology,* 1979, *30,* 327–362.

Minorsky, N. *Nonlinear oscillations.* Princeton, N. J.: Van Nostrand, 1962.

Møller, E. Action of the muscles of mastication. In Y. Kawamura (Ed.), *Physiology of mastication.* Basel: Karger, 1974.

Morowitz, H. J. *Energy flow in biology.* Woodbridge, Conn.: Oxbow Press, 1979.

Nashner, L. M. Fixed patterns of rapid postural responses among leg muscles during stance. *Experimental Brain Research,* 1977, *30,* 13–24.

Oatley, K., & Goodwin, B. W. The explanation and investigation of biological rhythms. In W. P. Colquhoun (Ed.), *Biological rhythms and human performance.* New York: Academic Press, 1971.

Orlovskii, G. N. The effect of different descending systems on flexion and extensor activity during locomotion. *Brain Research,* 1972, *40,* 359–371.

Orlovskii, G. N., & Shik, M. L. Standard elements of cyclic movement. *Biophysics,* 1965, *10,* 935–944.

Patten, B. C., & Auble, G. T. Systems approach to the concept of niche. *Synthese,* in press.

Pearson, K. G. The control of walking. *Scientific American*, 1976, *235*, 72–79.

Perenin, M. K., Jeannerod, M., & Prablanc, C. Spatial localization with paralyzed eye muscles. *Ophthalmologica*, 1977, *175*, 206–214.

Polit, A., & Bizzi, E. Processes controlling arm movements in monkeys. *Science*, 1978, *201*, 1235–1237.

Prigogine, I. *From being to becoming*. San Francisco: W. H. Freeman, 1980.

Prigogine, I., & Nicolis, G. Biological order, structure and instabilities. *Quarterly Review of Biophysics*, 1971, *4*, 107–148.

Rashevsky, N. *Mathematical biophysics: Physico-mathematical foundations of biology* (Vol. 2). New York: Doyer, 1960.

Saltzman, E. Levels of sensorimotor representation. *Journal of Mathematical Psychology*, 1979, *20*, 92–163.

Schmidt, R. A. A schema theory of discrete motor skill learning. *Psychological Review*, 1975, *82*, 225–260.

Schmidt, R. A. On the theoretical status of time in motor program representations. In G. E. Stelmach & J. Requin (Eds.), *Tutorials in motor behavior*. Amsterdam: Elsevier/North-Holland, 1980.

Schrödinger, E. *What is life?* New York and London: Cambridge University Press, 1945.

Shaffer, L. H. Intention and performance. *Psychological Review*, 1976, *83*, 375–393.

Shapiro, D. C., Zernicke, R. F., Gregor, R. J., & Diestel, J.D. Evidence for generalized motor programs using gait pattern analysis. *Journal of Motor Behavior*, 1981, *13*, 33–47.

Shaw, R., & Turvey, M. T. Coalitions as models for ecosystems: A realist perspective on perceptual organization. In M. Kubovy & J. Pomerantz (Eds.), *Perceptual organization*. Hillsdale, N. J.: Lawrence Erlbaum Associates, 1981.

Shaw, R. E., Turvey, M. T., & Mace, W. Ecological psychology: The consequence of a commitment to realism. In W. Weimer & D. Palermo (Eds.), *Cognition and the symbolic processes* (Vol. 2), Hillsdale, N. J.: Lawrence Erlbaum Associates, 1982.

Shik, M. L., & Orlovskii, G. N. Neurophysiology of locomotor automatism. *Physiological Reviews*, 1976, *56*, 465–501.

Skavenski, A. A., Haddad, G., & Steinman, R. M. The extraretinal signal for the visual perception of direction. *Perception & Psychophysics*, 1972, *11*, 287–290.

Soodak, H., & Iberall, A. S. Homeokinetics: A physical science for complex systems. *Science*, 1978, *201*, 579–582.

Stein, P. S. G. Mechanisms of interlimb phase control. In R. M. Herman, S. Grillner, P. S. G. Stein, & D. G. Stuart (Eds.), *Neural control of locomotion*. New York: Plenum, 1976.

Stein, P. S. G. Application of the mathematics of coupled oscillator systems to the analysis of the neural control of locomotion. *Federation Proceedings*, 1977, *36*, 2056–2059.

Stein, P. S. G. Motor systems, with special reference to the control of locomotion. *Annual Review of Neuroscience*, 1978, *1*, 61–81.

Stevens, J. R. The corollary discharge: Is it a sense of position or a sense of space? *Behavioral and Brain Sciences*, 1978, *1*, 163–165.

Stevens, K. N., & House, A. S. Perturbation of vowel articulations by consonantal context: An acoustical study. *Journal of Speech and Hearing Research*, 1963, *6*, 111–128.

Stevens, P. S. *Patterns in nature.* Boston: Little Brown, 1974.

Studdert-Kennedy, M., & Lane, H. Clues from the differences between signed and spoken language. In U. Bellugi & M. Studdert-Kennedy (Eds.), *Signed and spoken language: Biological constraints on linguistic form.* Weinheim: Verlag Chemie, 1980.

Sussman, H. M. Methodological problems in evaluating lip/jaw reciprocity as an index of motor equivalence. *Journal of Speech and Hearing Research,* 1980, *23,* 699–702.

Taub, E. Movements in nonhuman primates deprived of somatosensory feedback. *Exercise Sports Sciences Review,* 1976, *4,* 335–374.

Terzuolo, C. A., & Viviani, P. The central representation of learned motor patterns. In R. E. Talbott & D. R. Humphrey (Eds.), *Posture and movement.* New York: Raven Press, 1979.

Teuber, H. L. Alteration of perception after brain injury. In J. C. Eccles (Ed.), *Brain and conscious experience,* New York: Springer-Verlag, 1966.

Thexton, A. T. To what extent is mastication pre-programmed and independent of peripheral feedback? In D. J. Anderson & B. Matthews (Eds.), *Mastication.* Bristol: Wright, 1976.

Thompson, D. A. W. *On growth and form* (2nd edn.). London: Cambridge Univ. Press, 1942.

Tsetlin, M. L. *Automata theory and modeling in biological systems.* New York: Academic Press, 1973.

Tuller, B., Harris, K. S., & Kelso, J. A. S. Stress and rate: Differential transformations of articulation. *Journal of the Acoustical Society of America,* 1982, *71,* 1534–1543.

Tuller, B., Kelso, J. A. S., & Harris, K. S. Interarticulator phasing as an index of temporal regularity in speech. *Journal of Experimental Psychology: Human Perception and Performance,* 1982, *8,* 460–472.

Turvey, M. T. Preliminaries to a theory of action with reference to vision. In R. Shaw & J. Bransford (Eds.), *Perceiving, acting and knowing: Toward an ecological psychology.* Hillsdale, N. J.: Lawrence Erlbaum Associates, 1977.

Turvey, M. T. Clues from the organization of motor systems. In U. Bellugi & M. Studdert-Kennedy (Eds.), *Signed and spoken language: Biological constraints on linguistic form.* Weinheim: Verlag Chemie, 1980.

Turvey, M. T., & Shaw, R. The primacy of perceiving: An ecological reformulation for understanding memory. In N. -G. Nillson (Ed.), *Perspectives in memory research: Essays in honor of Uppsala University's 500th anniversary.* Hillsdale, N. J.: Lawrence Erlbaum Associates, 1979.

Turvey, M. T., Shaw, R. E., & Mace, W. Issues in the theory of action: Degrees of freedom, coordinative structures and coalitions. In J. Requin (Ed.), *Attention and performance* (Vol. 7). Hillsdale, N. J.: Lawrence Erlbaum Associates, 1978.

Viviani, P., & Terzuolo, V. Space-time invariance in learned motor skills. In G. E. Stelmach & J. Requin (Eds.), *Tutorials in motor behavior.* Amsterdam: Elsevier/North-Holland, 1980.

von Holst, E. *The behavioral physiology of animal and man: The collected papers of Erich von Holst* (Vol. 1; R. Martin, trans.). London: Methuen, 1973. (Originally published, 1937.)

Webb, D. W. The swimming energetics of trout: I. Thrust and power output at cruising speeds. *Journal of Experimental Biology,* 1971, *55,* 489–520.

Weiss, P. Self-differentiation of the basic patterns of coordination. *Comparative Psychology Monographs,* 1941, *17*(4).

Wilke, J. T. Ultradian biological periodicities in the integration of behavior. *International Journal of Neuroscience*, 1977, *7*, 125–143.

Wilke, J. T., Lansing, R. W., & Rogers, C. A. Entrainment of respiration to repetitive finger tapping. *Physiological Psychology*, 1975, *3*, 345–349.

Winfree, A. *The geometry of biological time.* New York/Heidelberg/Berlin: Springer-Verlag, 1980.

Wing, A. M. Response timing in handwriting. In G. E. Stelmach (Ed.), *Information processing in motor control and learning.* New York: Academic Press, 1978.

Yates, F. E. Complexity and the limits of knowledge. *American Journal of Physiology: Regulatory, Integrative, and Comparative,* 1978, *234,* R201–R204.

Yates, F. E. Physical causality and brain theories. *American Journal of Physiology,* 1980, *238,* R277–R290.

Yates, F. E., & Iberall, A. S. Temporal and hierarchical organization in biosystems. In J. Urquart & F. E. Yates (Eds.), *Temporal aspects of therapeutics.* New York: Plenum, 1973.

Part II

Production Constraints and
Sound Patterns of Languages

Chapter 8

Cross-Linguistic Studies of Speech Production

PETER LADEFOGED

We are all tempted to think that the normal is what we do. Cross-linguistic studies of speech are a healthy corrective to this attitude in that they demonstrate that what is commonplace for us is exotic for others. We may think that there is nothing very unusual about American English, but in fact the vowels in words such as *beard, bard*, and *bird* are most peculiar, and occur in few, if any, of the other languages in the world. Conversely, words with clicks in them sound curious to us, but they are nothing special to speakers of Bushman languages, in which the majority of words begin with clicks. Studying the speech production mechanisms that occur in other languages enables us to realize the full, extraordinary capabilities of the human vocal apparatus.

We are, in fact, at a time in history that is probably the most advantageous for cross-linguistic studies. The range of languages spoken is almost as great as it has ever been. About 10,000 years ago, when the world's population was very much smaller, there may have been no more than a dozen languages spoken in Europe; now there are over 100. Similar multiplication has no doubt occurred all over the world, as groups of people have become more widespread and diversified. But now, with wider communications making it possible for one group to extend its influence and dominate larger regions, speakers of the smaller, less politically powerful languages are disappearing. The process of language loss has been accelerating in recent times. We are now soon after a peak in the number of languages in the world, and thus have an unrivaled opportunity to observe the greatest possible range of human linguistic capabilities. In a few hundred years, when the accidents of history may have resulted in Russian, Chinese, and English being the only living languages, linguistics will not be so fortunate.

When linguists describe the languages of the world, they often limit themselves to specifying just the linguistic contrasts—the sounds that can be used to change the meanings of words. The phonemic contrasts that occur in most languages can be specified by reference to a fairly limited set of categories. The contrasts among the consonants of English (or Swedish, or German, or Japanese, for that matter) can be adequately specified by saying whether they are voiced or voiceless, and where and how they are articulated. Thus, each consonantal segment in these languages can be characterized by taking one term from each of the three columns at the left in Table 8-1.

The vowels of most languages can also be described by means of two or three terms, in these cases specifying what are traditionally called the degrees of height and backness of the tongue, and the position of the lips, as shown at the right in Table 8-1. Linguists differ slightly in the labels that they use, but the notion of a three-term specification is generally valid for all descriptions of contrasts except those using binary features; and even these can usually be reduced to three-term descriptions by taking into account the constraints on possible combinations of values of features that can occur. This chapter examines the extent to which the contrasts in some less well-known languages can be categorized by means of sets of terms such as those in Table 8-1. It will also discuss whether these ways of classifying contrasts provide a valid picture of the capabilities of the speech production mechanism.

Speech sounds that do not occur in English are of two types: those that use different combinations of the terms in Table 8-1, and those that necessitate the use of additional descriptive terms. The latter may be further split into those that require simply an additional possibility in one of the three columns, and those that require an additional column with terms that can be combined with one from each of the existing three columns.

There are numerous examples of sounds in other languages that can be described as combinations of the consonant terms in Table 8-1 that do not

Table 8-1. Three-term Descriptions for the Specification for English Speech Sounds

Consonants			Vowels		
voiceless	bilabial	stop	high	front	rounded
voiced	labiodental	nasal	mid-high	central	unrounded
	dental	fricative	mid-low	back	
	alveolar	approximant	low		
	palatoalveolar	trill			
	retroflex	flap			
	palatal	lateral			
	velar				

occur in English. Thus Burmese has not only voiced nasals and laterals as in English, but also the corresponding voiceless sounds (symbolized by a subscript [̥], as illustrated in [1]).

[1]   ma (healthy)   na (pain)   la (moon)   ŋa (fish)

    m̥a (order)   n̥a (nostril)   l̥a (beautiful)   ŋ̥a (rent)

Melpa, a language spoken in Papua New Guinea, has, in addition to the alveolar lateral familiar to us, both dental laterals (symbolized by adding [̪] to form [l̪]) and velar laterals (symbolized by ʟ], as in [2]. These sounds may be allophonically voiced or voiceless. Illustrative spectrograms are given in Ladefoged, Cochran, and Disner (1977).

[2]   kialtim (fingernail)   lola (speak improperly)   paʟa (fence)

    wal̥ (knitted bag)   bal̥ (apron)   raʟ̥ (two)

Kele, another Papua New Guinea language, has voiced bilabial trills (symbolized by [B]), as well as the more familiar alveolar trills, as in [3]. Ladefoged, Cochran, and Disner report that the rate of vibration of the lips is typically about 30 Hz, and is not significantly different from that for lingual or uvular trills.

[3]   ᵐBin (vagina)   ᵐBulim (face)   ᵐBuwen (testicle)
    ⁿril (song)   ⁿruwin (bone)   ⁿrikei (leg)

Margi, a Chadic language spoken in northern Nigeria, has a voiced labiodental flap (symbolized by [ⱱ]) as in [4]. Photographs of the lip action in this sound have been given in Ladefoged (1968).

    [4]   bəⱱú (ideophone descriptive of sudden appearance and flight)

Considering all these (to our ears) unusual sounds, it becomes a challenging exercise to find physiologically possible combinations that do *not* occur. It is not, however, always easy to say which combinations of categories can be ruled out as physiologically impossible. Is it, for example, possible to make labiodental stops and nasals? I would say that these sounds can be made only by people with exceptional dentition, such that there are no gaps between the teeth. Others, however, call the allophone of /m/ that occurs in *symphony* a voiced labiodental nasal. (I prefer to think of it as a voiced nasalized labiodental fricative; but in any case discussion of this sound need not detain us further, since it has not been found to be contrastive in any language.)

Some of the other combinations are more obviously impossible. Thus, although it is possible to make a trill by using both lips, as in Kele, or a flap by using only one lip, as in Margi, a labiodental trill using only the lower lip is beyond my capabilities, and a bilabial flap is not at all easy. Physiological constraints on trills and flaps also apply in the retroflex and palatoalveolar regions. I can curl the tip of my tongue up and back and then let it strike the back of the alveolar ridge as it goes forward, thus forming a retroflex flap; and I think I can make a trill in the retroflex position, but I do not know of one in any language. If we take palatoalveolar to imply raising of the tongue blade in the postalveolar region, then the fricative *r* sound that occurs in Czech may be categorized as a voiced palatoalveolar trill. But from a physiological point of view, it is difficult to get the blade of the tongue to form a flap in this area. Tongue tip trills and flaps in the palatal and velar regions also seem to be impossible. But are bilabial laterals (the two lips meeting at the center, but not at the side) viable linguistic possibilities? Similarly, how about labiodental laterals? They can be made (with a bit of a grimace), but they have not been observed in any known language.

Apart from the sounds discussed in the preceding paragraph, all the other combinations of consonantal terms in Table 8-1 are symbolized in Table 8-2. It is instructive to try to find pairs of items that do not contrast. Since it is usually fairly easy to find examples of contrasts between sounds with different manners of articulation, or with very different places of articulation, we will limit this discussion to an assessment of the contrasts between sounds that are very similar to one another. In Table 8-2, parentheses enclose all those items that do not contrast with one of the adjacent sounds in the same row. In some cases an arbitrary choice has to be made as to which of two symbols should be parenthesized. Thus, considering the lateral symbols in the bottom row, either the palatal lateral [ʎ] or the velar lateral [ʟ] could have been put in parentheses. There are languages such as Melpa, illustrated earlier in [2], which have velar laterals [ʟ] contrasting with alveolar laterals [l] and dental laterals [l̪]. There are also Arandic languages spoken in Australia, such as Kaititj, that have palatal laterals contrasting with dental, alveolar, and retroflex laterals. Examples of contrasts in final position are given in [5].

[5]   il̪ bal (smoke)   irmal (fire)   aldimal̠ (saw)   kuraʎ (star)

But as far as I know, no language contrasts velar laterals and palatal laterals, and accordingly either [ʎ] or [ʟ] has to be parenthesized. There are also problems in determining which items can be said to contrast in that there are no well-defined boundaries between each of the eight places of articulation that have been listed. Thus Yanuwa, another Australian language, contrasts seven out of the eight places of articulation, missing only a contrast between bilabial and labiodental sounds. Examples of oppositions between nasals in intervocalic position are given in [6].

[6]   umuwaḍala   wununu   wunala   waṇura   nanalu   luwaɲu

(in the   (cooked)   (kangaroo)   (white   (tea)   (strips
canoe)   crane)   of fat)

waŋulu

(big boy)

Table 8-2. Symbols for Combinations of Terms in Table 8-1[a]

	1	2	3	4	5	6	7	8
1(a)	p	*	t̲	t	t̪	ṭ	c	k
(b)	b	b	d̲	d	(d̪)	ḍ	ɟ	g
2(a)	m̥	*	(n̥̲)	n̥	(n̥̪)	(n̥̣)	(ɲ̥)	ŋ̥
(b)	m	m	n̲	n	n̪	ṇ	ɲ	ŋ
3(a)	Φ	f	θ	s	ʃ	ṣ	ç	x
(b)	β	v	ð	z	ʒ	ẓ	jʌ	γ
4(a)	ʍ	ʊ̥	(θ ᵥ)	ɹ̥	(ʃᵥ)	(ɻ̥)	j̊	(xᵥ)
(b)	w	ʊ	(ðᵥ)	ɹ	(ʒᵥ)	ɻ	j	γᵥ
5(a)	B	(r̥)	(r̥̲)	(ɾ̥)	(ɽ̥)	*	*	*
(b)	B	(r̲)	r̲	ɾ	(ɽ)	*	*	*
6(a)	*	(ѵ̥)	(r̥̲)	(ɾ̥̲)	*	(ɽ̥)	*	*
(b)	*	ѵ	(r̲)	ɾ̣		ṛ	*	*
7(a)	*	*	(l̥̲)	l̥	(l̥̪)	(l̥̣)	(ʎ̥)	(ɫ̥)
(b)	*	*	l̲	l	l̪	ḷ	ʎ	(ɫ)

[a] Alternate rows: (a) voiceless (b) voiced; pairs of columns: eight places of articulation as in Table 8-1; pairs of rows: seven manners of articulation as in Table 8-1. Asterisks denote combinatorial possibilities that do not and/or cannot occur, as discussed in the text. Parenthesized symbols denote possibilities that have not been observed as contrasting with at least one of the unparenthesized adjacent sounds in the same row.

It must also be remembered that the categories that we have been using do not distinguish between the different parts of the tongue that may be involved in an articulation. A more detailed analysis, as in Kirton and Charlie (1978), would show that the differences include tip of the tongue (apical) and blade of the tongue (laminal) distinctions, as well as what might more properly be called a prevelar rather than a palatal articulation.

In the light of this more detailed analysis it might be thought somewhat procrustean to use the data in [6] to demonstrate that the items in Table 8-2, Row 2a can be said to contrast. But it is inevitable, if we are simply specifying contrasts, that we either have to postulate a very large number of features, or we have to admit that the terms for different features have to be interpreted in different ways in different languages. Linguists invariably try to describe contrasts in terms of a small number of simple properties. Despite the earlier claims of Chomsky and Halle (1968), it now seems completely clear that such a small set of features cannot be regarded as designating phonetic properties definable in terms of physical scales. Instead, each value of a feature (and it does not really matter whether we are talking about traditional features such as place of articulation, or Chomsky–Halle innovations such as coronal) designates a cluster of related properties. In some languages some of these properties are necessary (e.g., the fact that certain sounds are laminal as opposed to being apical in Yanuwa); in other languages other properties are more important (e.g., in making Malayalam contrasts what matters is the precise part of the upper surface of the vocal tract contacted by the tip or the blade of the tongue). Sounds with the same values of the features have a family resemblance to one another in the Wittengensteinian sense, rather than being alike in their values on some simple physical scale.[1]

I will not try to illustrate all the possible contrasts between adjacent items in the rows in Table 8-2. Examples of contrasts involving some of the more unfamiliar sounds have been given earlier. Examples of contrasts between adjacent items for nearly all the other unparenthesized sounds have been given elsewhere (Ladefoged, 1968, 1971).

There are several points that are worthy of note concerning the distribution of the parenthesized items in Table 8-2. First, the fricative symbols form the only sets for which a full range of contrasts has been observed. In some ways this is surprising in that fricatives are fairly complex sounds to make. They necessitate more precise positioning of the tongue than, say, stops, in which the lower articulator can be raised against the upper articulator with varying degrees of force as long as a closure is formed. In the case of fricatives the degree of narrowing of the vocal tract has to be very precisely controlled. Second, and conversely, there are considerably fewer contrasts among approximants. Indeed, many of these sounds have no special symbol, and I have had to use the corresponding fricative symbol followed by a lowering mark $[_v]$, indicating that the articulation involves a lesser degree of stricture. Third, 21 of the 28 parenthesized items that do not contrast with adjacent sounds are voiceless. All these (and several similar) facts are hard to explain simply from the point of view of avoiding difficulties in speech production. Fricatives are certainly no easier to produce than approximants; and there is certainly not much more physiological difficulty in making any of these sounds voiceless rather than voiced (although it may be significant that more air is used up when making voiceless sounds, so that they require more respiratory effort).

Full explanations of the distribution of the parenthesized and nonparenthesized items lie outside the realm of speech production. Voiceless sounds are less often contrastive, perhaps in part because they are in some way less distinct. Conversely, there may be more oppositions among fricatives than there are among stops or nasals because fricatives may be more distinct. Differences among stops or nasals are often marked by only very small differences in the formant transitions. At this point in time, when languages are so numerous and diverse, the observed linguistic phenomena probably reflect a natural balance

---

[1]This view of features as designating Wittgensteinian family resemblance types is considered further by Lindau (1980) and is also mentioned by Anderson (1980).

between the demands of speech production, perception, learnability, memory, and other cognitive factors, all these conflicting demands being tempered by the stresses put on the system by foreign borrowings and other influences resulting from contacts between languages.

We must now consider sounds that cannot be described in terms of the categories in Table 8-1. Even if we limit ourselves to simply adding terms to each column, the number of possibilities becomes too great to try to represent the observed contrasts as in Table 8-2. Instead of alternate rows indicating just voiced and voiceless sounds, we would have to take into account at least two other states of the glottis: murmur (breathy voice) as observed in Marathi and other Indo-Aryan languages; and laryngealization (creaky voice) as in Hausa and other Chadic languages. I used to think that no language contrasted all four of the possibilities: voiced, voiceless, murmured, and laryngealized. But now I have observed all these states of the glottis and an additional fifth state involving a tightening of the upper part of the larynx to produce what may be called ventricular voice in !Xóõ, a Bushman language fully described by Traill (1981). Ventricular phonation is probably more associated with vowels than with consonants, and therefore need not be considered as an extra category in the terms for consonants in Table 8-1. But since we will not be considering vowels further in this chapter, examples of different phonation types in !Xóõ are listed in [7] in order to demonstrate another aspect of the range of the speech production mechanism. The examples also illustrate a phonation type involving a combination murmur followed by laryngealization in the form of a brief glottal catch.

[7] voiced   ‖áa   camelthorn tree
     laryngealized   g‖à'je   bend
     murmured   !ao̤   slope
     ventricular   !ào   base
     murmured laryngealized ‖a̤'je   wait for him

There is some evidence from Traill's work that speakers of particular languages may overdevelop certain muscles so that they take on an appearance that is not normal in speakers of other languages. The !Xóõ sounds with ventricular phonation are produced by constricting the upper part of the larynx so that the posterior portion of the aryepiglottic muscle nearly contacts the root of the epiglottis. Traill has been able to examine two speakers of this language using both cineradiology and fiberoptic techniques. Both these speakers have abnormally (from an ethnocentric point of view) enlarged muscular pads just above the larynx. Traill, who is himself a fairly fluent speaker of this language, had also been examined in the same way, prior to the recording of the !Xóõ speakers. The X-ray photographs revealed such curious enlargements of the posterior part of his larynx that it was feared that he might have a tumor, a worry that was finally laid to rest only when the X-rays of the !Xóõ speakers showed similar results.

Additional phonation types are far from the only extra terms needed in Table 8-1. There must be further terms in the list of places of articulation. The contrastive use of glottal stops (as in Javanese) requires recognition of the glottis as a place of articulation. We must also add terms to account for uvular stops and nasals (as in Eskimo), uvular fricatives (as in French), and pharyngeal sounds (as in Arabic). It has recently been shown (Laufer & Condax, 1981) that pharyngeal fricatives involve the active use of the epiglottis as an articulator, thus demonstrating one more degree of complexity in the use of the speech production mechanism in the formation of linguistic contrasts. Other sounds made at unusual places of articulation include apicolabials in languages such as Big Nambas. According to Fox (1979), this language has stops, nasals, and fricatives in which "the apex of the tongue comes into contact with the upper lip." Additional manners of articulation must also be provided (or a fourth column added) to account for central versus lateral distinctions among fricatives (as in Zulu) and taps (as in Chaga). All these contrasts are illustrated in Ladefoged (1971).

Extra columns are needed to describe sounds in which the primary source of energy is not just lung air moving outward. I will not attempt to discuss all the ways in which acoustic energy can be generated without the use of the respiratory system forcing air out the lungs. Even linguists who are concerned only with classifying contrasts have to complicate the set of categories quite considerably at this point. In this chapter I will simply exemplify the range of the speech production mechanism by giving a more detailed account of what goes on in the formation of a sound that may be classified as a voiced uvular ejective dental click. This sound has been chosen for illustrative purposes as it is perhaps the most complicated of the 80 contrasting clicks that occur in !Xóõ (Traill, 1979).

Figure 8-1 is a composite of data related to the !Xóõ word [g|q'àã] (chase). The upper part of the figure shows the estimated positions of the vocal organs at two different moments in time. These diagrams are based on cineradiology data reported in Traill (1981). The original tracings are actually of a different word, and do not show the position of the larynx. Cineradiology data illustrating the articulatory movements that occur in a voiced uvular ejective dental click are not available to me. There may, therefore, be some inaccuracies in the positions I have reconstructed; but the general picture is fully validated by Traill's cineradiology data on a large number of similar sounds. The lower part of the figure shows actual data on the pressure of the air in the pharynx, and on the acoustic components of this sound, recorded by means of techniques described in Ladefoged and Traill (1980).

This sound begins with the raising of the back of the tongue to the soft palate, forming a velar closure, and the closing of the nasopharyngeal port so that the pressure of the air in the pharynx begins to rise. As the spectrogram shows, the vocal cords continue to vibrate during this period. At about the same time as the velar closure is formed, the tip, blade, and sides of the tongue contact the hard

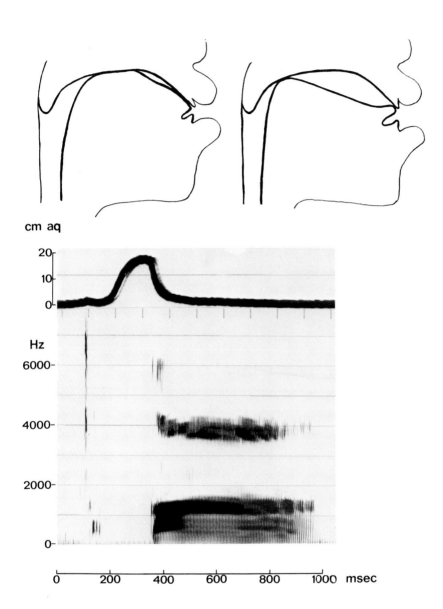

Figure 8-1. The pronunciation of a voiced uvular ejective dental click in the !Xóõ word g|q'àã (chase). The upper part of the figure shows the estimated positions of the vocal organs at approximately times 0 and 100 msec. The curve in the middle is the pressure of the air in the pharynx. The lower part of the figure is a wide-band spectrogram.

palate, so that a very small volume of air is enclosed in the mouth, as shown in the left-hand diagram of the vocal organs. The tongue then moves down and back to the position in the right-hand diagram, with the air in the mouth being rarefied within a considerably larger cavity. The spectrogram shows the small burst of noise that occurs when the tip of the tongue is lowered and air rushes into the mouth cavity. Shortly after this the glottis is constricted so that there are three slow irregular vibrations of the kind that occur in creaky voice. Since the pressure in the pharynx goes down slightly at this moment, we may infer that the pharyngeal cavity is being enlarged, perhaps by a slight downward movement of the constricted glottis. Shortly after the irregular vibrations cease we can deduce that the glottis must be completely closed and moving upward so that the air in the pharynx behind the uvular closure is compressed. The pharyngeal pressure record shows that the pressure rises to nearly 20 cm aq, which is about double the pressure of the air in the lungs in this speaker's other utterances in the same set of recordings. This pressure increase can only be due to the pistonlike action of the closed glottis. There is a small burst of noise that occurs when the uvular closure is released, which is followed fairly rapidly by the release of the glottal stop and the start of regular vocal cord vibrations for the vowel.

The complex timing of the events just described cannot be inferred from the classificatory label "voiced uvular ejective dental click" (or the equivalent set of distinctive feature values), which the linguist ascribes to the sound. Nor, for that matter, are the actions of the speech production mechanism adequately specified by the much simpler set of terms discussed earlier in this chapter. Even the different combinations of the terms in Table 8-1 can be considered only as labels, specifying linguistic contrasts and grouping them into classes that are appropriate for phonological rules. They are not descriptions that enable speech scientists to know, without further information, the required movements of the vocal organs. Thus describing Burmese as having voiceless alveolar nasals as exemplified in [1] does not make it clear that in a typical production of a word such as [n̥à] (nostril) the tip of the tongue is raised to contact the alveolar ridge, and air escapes through the nose for the first part of this sound; then, about 20 msec before the tip of the tongue comes down, the glottis narrows and voicing begins. Finally, about 40 msec after the vocal cords have begun to vibrate, and 20 msec after the lowering of the tip of the tongue, the soft palate is raised to form a velic closure, so that air can no longer go out through the nose.

As a further example of the inadequacy of linguistic specifications of the speech production mechanism consider the description "voiced velar lateral" as applied to the sounds in Melpa exemplified in [2]. Given only this specification, there is no way in which one could set up a computer model of the tongue along the lines suggested by Fujimura (1977) so as to form this sound. Both the term *velar* and the term *lateral* have to be given special definitions that apply only when they occur together if we want to use them to provide a precise specification of what part of the tongue is narrowed, and where (and for how long) there is contact with the roof of the mouth.

Furthermore, the inadequacies of linguistic specifications are not just a matter of filling in detail in a mechanical way. There cannot be an algorithm that, given the co-occurrence of three terms such as *voiceless dental fricative*, enables a full description of the speech production mechanism to be given. These three terms specify different sounds when, for example, they refer to different dialects of English. A typical speaker of Californian English makes the voiceless dental fricative in words such as *thin* with the tip of the tongue protruding below the upper front teeth (Ladefoged, 1979). But most speakers of British English make this sound with the tongue behind the upper teeth (Jones, 1956). Linguistic descriptions must be accompanied by a detailed, language-specific set of algorithms before they can be interpreted in terms of actual sounds.

As we noted at the beginning of this chapter, cross-linguistic studies are useful in drawing our attention to the wide range of phenomena that occur in the languages of the world. But we must always remember that linguists are usually more concerned with classifying contrasts than with describing different actions of the vocal organs. Unless cross-linguistic studies are supported by detailed phonetic investigations, they do not give a valid indication of the capabilities of the speech production mechanism.

References

Anderson, S. Why phonology isn't "natural." *UCLA Working Papers in Phonetics*, 1980, *51*, 36–93.

Chomsky, N., & Halle, M. *The sound pattern of English*. New York: Harper & Row, 1968.

Fox, G. J. Big Nambas grammar. *Pacific Linguistics*, 1979, *B-60*. (Australian National University, Canberra).

Fujimura, O. Model studies of tongue gestures and the derivation of vocal tract area functions. In M. Sawashima & F. S. Cooper (Eds.), *Dynamic Aspects of Speech Production*. Tokyo: University of Tokyo Press, 1976, pp. 225–232.

Jones, D. *An outline of English phonetics*. Cambridge, England: Heffer, 1956.

Kirton, J., & Charlie, B. Seven articulatory positions in Yanuwa consonants. *Pacific Linguistics*, 1978, *A-51*, 179–197.

Ladefoged, P. *A phonetic study of West African languages*. New York and London: Cambridge University Press, 1968.

Ladefoged, P. *Preliminaries to linguistic phonetics*. Chicago: University of Chicago Press, 1971.

Ladefoged, P. Review of *Fundamental Problems in Phonetics*, by J. C. Catford. Language, 1979, 55(4), 904–907.

Ladefoged, P., Cochran, A., & Disner, S. Laterals and trills. *Journal of the International Phonetic Association*, 1977, *7.2*, 46–54.

Ladefoged, P., & Traill, T. Instrumental phonetic fieldwork. *UCLA Working Papers in Phonetics*, 1980, *49*, 28–42.

Laufer, A., & Condax, I. The function of the epiglottis in speech. *Language and Speech*, 1981, *24*, 39–62.

Lindau, M. Phonetic differences in Nigerian languages. *UCLA Working Papers in Phonetics*, 1980, *51*, 105–113.

Traill, A. Another click accompaniment in !Xhóõ. *Khoisan Linguistic Studies*, 1979, 5, 22–29.

Traill, A. *Phonetic and phonological studies in !Xhóõ Bushman*. Ph.D. thesis, University of Witwatersrand, Johannesburg, S. Africa, 1981.

Chapter 9

The Origin of Sound Patterns in Vocal Tract Constraints

JOHN J. OHALA

I. Introduction

The ultimate task of phonology is to discover the causes of the behavior of speech sounds. To do this phonologists must refer to the way speech is created and used by humans, including how it is stored in the brain, retrieved, executed, perceived, and used to facilitate social interaction among humans. The domain of phonology is therefore mind, matter, and manners. This chapter is about matter: some aerodynamic and anatomical properties of the vocal tract and how they influence the shape and patterning of speech sounds. A secondary aim of this chapter is to show not only that the study of the physical aspects of speech assists phonology but also that phonology can return the favor: A careful, perhaps inspired, analysis of sound patterns in language can help us to discover and understand some of the complexities of speech production (Ohala, 1975a, 1975b, 1978a, 1978b, 1980, 1981; Ohala & Riordan, 1979; Shattuck-Hufnagel, Chapter 6, this volume; MacKay, 1972).

Language is a very complex human activity and, as mentioned, sound patterns can be determined by psychological and social factors as well as physical factors. But such nonphysical factors tend to vary widely from one community to another or even from one individual to another. Thus, their influence on speech sound behavior should be quite different when viewed over widely divergent languages. Physics and human physiology, however, represent a universal substrate on which all speech is built. Therefore, to be sure we are dealing with sound patterns that are due primarily to these universal factors, it is necessary to look for them repeated in several unrelated languages.

In fulfilling this task I will cite what might seem like quite dissimilar pieces of data from different languages: allophonic variation, sound change, dialect variation, morphophonemic alternation (i.e., contextually determined variation in the phonetic shape of a given morpheme within a single language), and patterns in segment inventories. In fact, I believe it is safe to regard all of these as manifestations of the same phenomenon caught at different stages or viewed from slightly different angles. I assume that the allophonic variations cited arise from constraints of the vocal tract, the topic of interest. Some of these allophonic variations become sound changes. If a sound change affects words in one linguistic community but not another, dialect variation results. If the sound change affects a given morpheme in one phonetic environment but not another, then morphophonemic variation results. If one consequence of the sound change is to eliminate a segment from or introduce a segment into the language, then it would influence the language's total segment inventory.

It might be thought that if the same physical factors have been at work shaping all human speech, then all languages should be tending toward the same phonological state. It is true that the more we look at diverse languages' phonologies, the more we find very similar patterns or metapatterns. Thus, although it is surprising to learn from Ladefoged (chapter 8, this volume) that one language has some 80 click phonemes in addition to nonclick sounds, in general, none of the phonemes or features utilized in the Khoisan languages requires us to stretch the conceptual and descriptive framework laid down for other languages' sound systems. Nevertheless, languages' phonologies differ very much in details, and there is no detectable trend toward convergence. One reason for this is that there are many degrees of freedom in the design of a vocal–auditory signaling system and that several designs (i.e., phonologies) can serve the primary function of communication and still stay within the bounds set by articulatory (and auditory) constraints. Another reason for diversity in languages is that the psychological and social factors shaping speech may run counter to the influence of purely physical factors.

II. Speech Aerodynamics

A. Preliminaries

The speech production mechanism can be viewed as a device that converts muscular energy into acoustic energy. It does this by creating within the vocal tract direct-current (dc) pressure differences that, when allowed to equalize with atmospheric pressure, create turbulence in the rapidly moving air which in turn produces the alternating-current pressure variations we call sound. It is therefore useful to consider how these dc pressure changes are made.

Figure 9-1 gives a schematic representation of the vocal tract as a collection

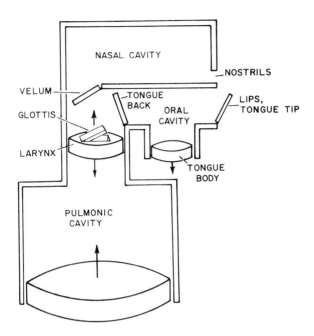

Figure 9-1. Schematic representation of the vocal tract as a device for the production of local dc pressure variations.

of pistons, valves, and piston chambers that can produce slowly varying localized pressure changes. There are three pistonlike structures in the vocal tract: the chest wall, the larynx, and the tongue. Sounds created with these three mechanisms as the initiator of the pressure change are called *pulmonic, glottalic,* and *velaric* sounds, respectively. If these pistons compress air in the chamber they are associated with, the sound is said to be *egressive*; if they rarefy the air, that is, create a negative pressure vis-à-vis atmospheric pressure, the sound is called *ingressive* (Ladefoged, 1971; Catford, 1977a).

B. Preferred Segment Types

Although it is physically possible for these three pistons to move in both directions to create both ingressive and egressive sounds, in fact, as indicated by the arrows near these structures in Figure 9-1, only four of the six possible sound types are found in human languages: pulmonic egressives, for example, [p, 1, a, ʔ, s];[1] glottalic egressives, or "ejectives," for example, [p', t'];

---

[1]The phonetic transcription used throughout, except as noted to the contrary, is that approved by the International Phonetic Association as of 1979. Forms in square brackets [. . .] represent detailed or narrow phonetic transcriptions, those bounded by slashes / . . . / represent broad or
(continued next page)

glottalic ingressives or "implosives," such as [ɓ, ɗ, ɠ]; and velaric ingressives or "clicks," such as [ʇ, ʖ]. Pulmonic ingressive vocalization is not found except as a stylistic variant of pulmonic egressive speech, for example, Swedish [ja] (on ingressive voice) "yes" (emphatic), French [wi] (ingressive voice) "yes" (used primarily by females). Velaric egressive sounds are even rarer, being found only (as far as I know) as imitations of animal sounds or flatulence, the latter used for mockery or insults.

Why should two of the possible six sound types not be used? The lack of pulmonic ingressive sounds, if I may speculate, is probably due to the shape of the vocal cords in normal voice (modal register), which, in coronal section (see Figure 9-2), are seen to be asymmetric about the plane that is normal to the airflow and that passes through them at the point of closest approximation. The vocal cords have more bulk below this plane than they do above it. If airflow is egressive, that is, has greater sub- than supraglottal pressure, the upward movement of the vocal cords will necessarily also involve their lateral movement, thus smoothly and effectively opening the valve that vents the subglottal air. If airflow is ingressive, however, it would seem that a downward movement of the vocal cords would involve a slight bulging of the lower tissues, which would not move laterally as easily in order to release an excess of supraglottal pressure. (This argument would not apply to falsetto voice, where the vocal cords are considerably thinned and thus have a more symmetric coronal profile. Accordingly, I find that I can phonate in falsetto voice about as well ingressively as egressively.)

Of course, it is also true that some fricatives, notably sibilants such as [s, ʃ], cannot be produced as well ingressively as egressively. No doubt this is because during ingressive airflow the primary location of the noise source (the point where the air exits and expands from the narrow channel it is forced through) is on the wrong side—the inside—of the oral constriction, which, because it has very high acoustic impedance, does not permit the sound generated to radiate to the atmosphere.

Velaric egressives may not make good speech sounds, I would speculate, because the characteristics of the tongue blade as a valve permit higher negative pressures (but not positive pressures) to develop and to be released in a suitably abrupt fashion before the seal fails.

Many other constraints on the form of speech stem from the properties of the speech system represented in Figure 9-1. It is evident, for example, that a chamber in which an appreciable pressure change is created ($\Delta p = \pm 5$ cm

---

phonemic transcriptions, and the remainder, including those in italics, are purposely ambiguous as to the level of phonetic detail that they represent (in some cases they represent the standard orthographic form of the word). Forms marked with an asterisk (*) are hypothetical, and in most cases are reconstructed. The symbols (>) and (<) stand for "became" and "derived from," respectively. A tilde (~) between cited forms means "freely alternates with." Tone and stress are not marked, and vowel length is marked with a macron (¯) in the Latin examples.

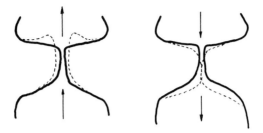

Figure 9-2. Hypothetical coronal sections of the vocal cords showing the pattern of vibratory movement during egressive voice (left) and ingressive voice (right) (arrows show direction of airflow). Solid lines show positions of vocal cords when transglottal pressure is relatively low; dotted lines represent their position as the transglottal pressure builds up to a maximum, that is, as the excess pressure is being vented. Egressive voice, but not ingressive voice, allows lateral movement of the vocal cords and thus easy venting of the excess pressure.

H_2O), and that has to be vented through one valve in order to create an audible sound, must have all other valves closed. Thus there can be no nasalized [p]. Also, there can be no glottalic sonorants, for example, ejective [m], implosive [l]. This is because any pressure change created by the larynx acting as a piston would equalize immediately by leakage across the rather large valvular openings characteristic of sonorants. For similar reasons, all oral obstruents that are released at the uvular region or farther forward (except clicks) must have the soft palate elevated (i.e., the velopharyngeal valve closed). Pharyngeal or glottal obstruents (the latter including, from a physical point of view, all vowels and voiced sonorants) would not require soft palate elevation—the open velopharyngeal valve does not connect to, and therefore does not vent air pressure in, the pharyngeal or subglottal cavities. (This assumes, of course, that these sounds are not distinctively nasal, e.g., [ĩ].) I will explore below some phonological consequences of this point.

Another sound pattern deducible in part from aerodynamic considerations is that evident in languages' segment inventories. Tables 9-1 and 9-2 give the consonant inventories of Abkhaz and Yala, respectively. On the basis of such data, Hockett (1955, pp. 104ff.) offered the generalization that the more consonants a language has, the greater is the ratio, r, of obstruents to nonobstruents. Yala has 28 consonants, of which 18 are obstruents, giving an r of 1.8. In Abkhaz, which has 58 consonants, $r = 7.3$. Salient acoustic signals are those that involve rapid spectral modulations (Stevens, 1980). Obstruents, especially those that involve a transient burst due to the rapid equalization of an appreciable difference in air pressure, create more rapid spectral changes and thus are able to carry more information and make many more distinctive sounds than can nonobstruents. This accounts for Hockett's observation.

Table 9-1. Consonant Inventory of Abkhaz

m	n													
b	d	dʷ				gʲ	g	gʷ						
p	t	tʷ				kʲ	k	kʷ						
p'	t'	tʷ'				kʲ'	k'	kʷ'	qʲ'	q'	qʷ'			
	dz	dzʷ	dʒ		dʐ									
	ts	tsʷ	tʃ		tɕ									
	ts'	tsʷ'	tʃ'		tɕ'									
v	z		ʒ		ʐ	ʐʷ								
f	s		ʃ		ɕ	ɕʷ				ʁʲ	ʁ	ʁʷ		
w			l	r	j	ɥ				χʲ	χ	χʷ	ħ	hʷ

Note. From Catford (1977b).

C. Constraints on the Voicing or Devoicing of Stops

Voicing—vibration of the vocal cords—has two physiological requirements: First, the vocal cords must be in a suitable configuration—typically, lightly adducted; and second, there must be sufficient air flowing past them. If either one or both of these conditions are missing, there will be no voicing. To the extent that both of these conditions are approached during a voiceless segment, the chance of that segment becoming voiced is greater.

There is a well-recognized difficulty in maintaining voicing during a stop (in which, by definition, all exit valves are closed) because the air flowing through the glottis accumulates in the oral cavity, causing oral pressure to approach subglottal pressure. When this happens the air flowing through the glottis gradually diminishes and voicing is extinguished.

In view of this, it is not surprising to find that of the 706 languages whose segment inventories were surveyed by Ruhlen (1975) 166 have only voiceless stops and 4 have only voiced stops (the remainder using both voiced and voiceless stops). Even if the reliability of such large-scale surveys may be questioned, the decisive "tilt" toward voicelessness in the stops could not be reversed by a few inaccuracies.

Table 9-2. Consonant Inventory of Yala (Ikom)

m	n	ɲ	ŋ		ŋ͡w
m͡b				ŋmgb	
b	d	ɟ	g	g͡b	g͡w
p	t	c	k	k͡p	k͡w
f	s		x		
	s͡j				
l	r				
		j	ɥ	w	

Note. From Armstrong (1968).

The longer the stop closure is held, the greater is the likelihood that voicing will be extinguished. Thus the tendency for long voiced stops (so-called geminates) to become voiceless is particularly strong. Phonological data from Mõrė, which illustrates this, are given in Table 9-3. (See also Jaeger, 1978, for further evidence on this point.) Conversely, the shorter a stop closure is, the more likely it is to remain voiced, or if originally voiceless, to become voiced. There is, therefore, a very widespread tendency among languages to have voiced stops (or voiced obstruents in general) shorter than their voiceless counterparts (Lehiste, 1970, pp. 27ff.).

There is also extensive evidence that voicing sits more comfortably on stops, pulmonic or implosive, made at some places of articulation rather than at others (Greenberg, 1970; Gamkrelidze, 1975; Sherman, 1975). Table 9-4 provides some representative data, the stop inventories from three languages. Sherman conducted one of the most extensive surveys on this pattern; out of over 570 languages whose stop inventories were examined (these did not include implosives), he found 87 that had gaps. The distribution of these "stop gaps" are shown in Table 9-5 (some languages had more than one gap). From such data it is clear that velar stops and voicing show the greatest incompatibility, labial stops and voicing the greatest compatibility. (These data also show that voicelessness does not sit well on bilabial stops. Although to some extent this may be a reflection of the greater hardiness of [b] over [p], or that [p] has a greater tendency to become voiced and thus merge with [b], it is also likely that acoustic–auditory factors are a more important determinant of this pattern: as Stevens (1980) has pointed out, [p] has the lowest amplitude and spectrally most diffuse burst of any of the voiceless stops and is thus less salient auditorily.)

It was once thought that the relative volumes of the oral cavities of the stops [b, d, g] were responsible for this pattern of stop gaps (Greenberg, 1970; Smith, 1977). It was reasoned that the larger volume of the oral cavity for [b] would accommodate more glottal airflow before pressure built up to the point where the transglottal pressure drop fell below the level necessary to maintain voicing, and conversely, that the smaller oral volume for [g] would accommodate less air, thus causing voicing to cease relatively soon. This reasoning is technically

Table 9-3. Morphophonemic Variation in Mõrė

Morphophonemic form	Phonemic form	French gloss
pabbo	> papo	*frapper*
daw-ba	> dapa	*hommes* (w < b, cf. dibla, *petit mâle*)
bad + do	> bato	*corbeilles*
lug + gu	> luku	*enclos*
boɣ + ɣo	> boko	*trou* (ɣ < g)

Note. From Alexandre (1953); transcription simplified.

Table 9-4. Stop Inventories of Thai (Abramson, 1962), Kalabari (Ladefoged, 1964), and Efik (Ward, 1933) Showing Absence of Voiced Velars

Thai			Kalabari					Efik			
p	t	k	p	t	k	k͡p			t	k	kʷ	k͡p
pʰ	tʰ	kʰ	b	d	ɟ	g	g͡b		b	d		
b	d		ɓ	ɗ							

correct but the magnitude of the effect of initial oral cavity volume on the length of voicing during stops is negligibly small. Calculations suggest that if the oral volume does not change during the stop closure, voicing can be maintained for approximately 10 msec during [g] and 15 msec during [b] (Catford, 1977a, p. 74; Ohala & Riordan, 1979).

Such periods of voicing are negligible in comparison with the typical duration of voiced stops (ca. 70 msec; Lehiste, 1970, pp. 27ff.). Clearly, initial oral volume by itself cannot explain why [b] is more common than [g] (Ohala, 1975a, 1976; Javkin, 1977). Voicing can be maintained beyond the limits cited if the oral volume increases *during* the stop closure, that is, expands to accommodate the accumulating glottal airflow (Ohala, 1975a, 1976). Such oral cavity enlargement can be accomplished *passively*, that is, as a result of the natural compliance of the walls of the oral cavity; or *actively*, by lowering the larynx, the mandible, and so on (see Chao, 1936; Javkin, 1977; Catford, 1977a).

Ohala and Riordan attempted to determine how long voicing would last if only passive expansion of the vocal tract took place. They had an adult male American English speaker say $V_1C:V_2$ utterances where $V_1 = V_2 = $ [i, u, e, a] and C: was an abnormally prolonged voiced stop [b, d, g]. The stop could be prolonged indefinitely because the oral pressure built up during the stop was vented through a nasal catheter. At unpredictable moments, however, a solenoid-activated valve closed the catheter so that oral air pressure would rapidly rise and voicing would be extinguished. The duration of voicing beyond the moment of complete closure was measured on signals from a throat microphone and an air pressure transducer that sensed oral air pressure. The results are presented graphically in Figure 9-3. Over all conditions the median

Table 9-5. Incidence of Stop Gaps According to Place or Articulation and Voicing in 87 Languages

	Labial	Apical	Velar
Voiceless	34	0	0
Voiced	2	21	40

Note. From Sherman (1975).

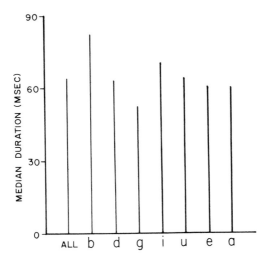

Figure 9-3. Median duration of voicing during stops when only passive expansion of the vocal tract occurs (data from Ohala & Riordan, 1979).

duration of voicing was 64 msec, but it was greatest for [b] (82 msec), least for [g] (52 msec). Moreover, with one exception, the stops coarticulated with the high vowels [i, u] permitted voicing to continue longer than those coarticulated with low vowels. The one exception was that [b] coarticulated with [a] had the longest stretch of voicing (91 msec), presumably because only this combination of consonant and vowel involved passive oral cavity expansion by the highly compliant cheeks.

These results can be accounted for by considering the net compliance of the surfaces on which oral air pressure impinges during the production of the stops. For velar stops only the pharyngeal walls and part of the soft palate can yield to the air pressure; in dentals, these surfaces plus the greater part of the tongue surface and all of the soft palate are involved; and in labials, these surfaces plus all of the tongue surface and some parts of the cheeks participate (see Houde, 1968; pp. 88–92; Rothenberg, 1968). Moreover, as Smith (1977) has indicated, the high vowels [i, u], by virtue of their greatly enlarged pharyngeal cavity, have greater oral volume (and thus greater surface area) than do the nonhigh vowels.

If active expansion were to be investigated in a similar way, presumably roughly similar patterns could be expected: Voicing could be extended several hundred milliseconds in this case, but still longer for labials than for velars, as with passive expansion. As Chao remarked:

> Between the velum and the glottis, there is not much room to do any of the tricks that can be done with the larger cavity for a **b** or a **d**.

(See also Javkin, 1977.)

In view of the preceding discussion it is interesting to note that one of the sources of voiced implosives (sounds involving active expansion of the oral cavity) may be former voiced geminates. This is the case, for example, with the implosives of Sindhi, an Indo-Aryan language; see Table 9-6.

Khubchandani (1969) reports that not all dialects of Sindhi have the same number of implosives. The pattern of gaps is entirely consistent, however, with our expectations regarding which places of articulation can most easily support voicing during stops: The B'ani dialect has the maximum number, four, / ɓ, ɗ, ʄ, ɠ/; Maṇḍvi has two, / ɓ, ɗ/; and Vagdi has only one, / ɓ /.

A morphophonemic alternation in Nubian (Bell, 1971; Ohala & Riordan, 1979) also exemplifies two of the tendencies discussed; see Table 9-7. In Nubian the noun inflection that means "and" involves the gemination of the stem-final consonant and the addition of the sequence /—ɔn/. When a final /b/ is geminated it remains voiced; /d, dʒ, g/, however, the stops (and affricate) with farther-back points of articulation, become devoiced to /t, tʃ, k/.

Given the evidence cited here from Ohala and Riordan, we would predict that stops coarticulated with high vowels would more readily retain voicing than those coarticulated with nonhigh vowels. I have not found much support for this in the phonological literature, however. The one bit of data that may be a reflection of this effect (as well as the effect of place of articulation of the stop) is given in Table 9-8. These data show that of the original Proto-Bantu initial voiced stops (column 1), it is the */b/ which seems to preserve both voicing and stoppedness in the modern reflexes in Duala and Ngɔm (albeit as implosives), whereas */g/ loses voicing and/or stoppedness. In the case of */d/, its fate depends on the height of the following vowel: Before the high vowels /i, u/ it behaves similarly to */b/ in preserving both voicing and the stop character (the forms above the dashed line), whereas before other vowels it loses one or both of these features, as was the case with */g/ (the forms below the dashed line).

It should be mentioned at this point that, as illustrated by the Bantu data in Table 9-8, the resolution of the "conflict" between voicing and stops is not always done by devoicing the stop—it may also be accomplished by unstopping the stop, that is, changing it to a voiced fricative or, better, a voiced approximant. (The phonetic symbols [v, β, ð, γ] are often used for either fricatives or frictionless continuants.)

Table 9-6. Origin of Sindhi Implosives from Prakrit Voiced Geminate Stops

Prakrit		Sindhi	English gloss
*pabba	>	paɓuṇi	lotus plant fruit
gaddaha	>	gaɗahu	donkey
-(g)gamᵗʰi*	>	ɗaɳɗʰi	knot
bʰagga	>	bʰaːɟu	fate

Note. From Varyani (1974).
*This "ṁ" is the conventional transliteration of the Devanagari *anusvara*, best regarded as symbolizing a nasal homorganic to the following obstruent.

Table 9-7. Morphophonemic Variation in Nubian

Noun stem	Stem + "and"	English gloss
/fab/	/fab:ɔn/	father
/sɛgɛd/	/sɛgɛt:ɔn/	scorpion
/kadʒ/	/katʃ:ɔn/	donkey
/mʊg/	/mʊk:ɔn/	dog

Note. From Bell (1971) and Ohala and Riordan (1979).

The evidence presented so far suggests that the farther forward in the vocal tract a stop is articulated, the better able it is to accommodate voicing. From my own reading of the phonological literature I think this is the dominant pattern. There are complications, however, which could override this generalization. The probability of a voiced stop remaining voiced (or a voiceless one becoming voiced) depends in a major way on the duration of the stop closure, a shorter duration allowing voicing to be maintained for all of, or a majority of, the stop duration. Stop closure duration may be affected by such factors as articulator mobility. A less massive and therefore faster articulator such as the tongue tip may be capable of making and then breaking a stop closure in a very brief interval.

In American English, for example, it is the apical stop /t/ (and not /p/ or /k/) that has become voiced in certain environments, for example [fæt] "fat" but [fæɾɚ] "fatter." But the duration of this [ɾ] is extremely short (ca. 30–40 msec), whereas /p/ and /k/ in the same environment are usually much longer (Fox & Terbeek, 1977).

Also, the particular trajectory the articulator makes may affect the probability of voicing being maintained during the stop closure. Velar stops in English have been shown to have a forward-moving component to them (Houde, 1968, pp.

Table 9-8. Bantu Sound Changes Showing Modification of Initial Voiced Stops as a Function of Place of Articulation of Stop and Quality of Following Vowel

Proto-Bantu		Reflex in Duala	Reflex in Ngom	English gloss
*-bi	>		-ɓ e	bad
*-bod	>	-ɓ ɔ-	-ɓ o	become rotten
*-dib-	>	-ɗ i	-ɓ iɗ	shut
*-dug	>	-ɗ u-	-ɗ uk-	paddle
*-dob-	>	-ɔ ɓ -	-ðɔ ɓ -	fish with line
*-daad-	>		-ðað-	lie down
*-godi	>	m-ɔɗ i	ŋ-kɔli	string
*-gag-	>		-kak-	go bad

Note. From Guthrie (1967–1970); transcription simplified.

93ff). (See Figure 9-4.) Such a movement constitutes a very marked form of active cavity enlargement and could more than compensate for the other factors which disfavor voicing on velars. This may, in fact, be the reason why velar stops are articulated in this way. Voiced apical stops could be voiced longer if the tongue body lowered during the stop closure. This gesture has been found in the production of /d/ in English and Japanese (Ohala & Kawasaki, 1979). This may be the reason why so many of the voiced apical implosives are retroflex (Greenberg, 1970; see also Table 9-6, where one of the Sindhi retroflex implosives comes from an earlier *dental* geminate): Retroflex stops are distinguished from nonretroflex primarily by having an enlarged oral cavity immediately behind the point of constriction—this cavity, an effective low-pass filter, is what gives retroflex sounds their characteristic "dark" auditory quality.

Some languages solve the problem of how to maintain voicing on stops by skirting the aerodynamic constraints and producing something that *sounds* like a voiced stop but that is not wholly a stop, namely, a prenasalized stop, for example, [^{m}b, ^{n}d]. The air that would accumulate in the oral cavity is vented through the velic opening during the initial part of the consonant closure. Both a fully voiced stop and a prenasalized stop will create an abrupt attenuation of the speech amplitude, will have voicing throughout the closure, and will be released with a burst. It is easy to imagine that through sound change a voiced stop could be replaced by a prenasalized stop.

An otherwise puzzling aspect of the phonology of Japanese verbs may be accounted for in part by this pattern. As shown in Table 9-9, the conjunctive form of Japanese strong verbs involves replacing the last consonant in the verb stem by a geminate dental consonant whose voicing agrees with the replaced consonant (except that /r/ is replaced by /tt/). However, where a voiced

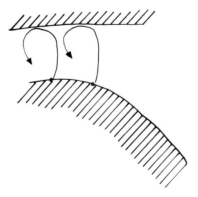

Figure 9-4. Trajectory of two points on the surface of the tongue (lower contour) during the approach to and break of contact with the palate (upper contour) in the production of the sequence [aga] (left is front, right is back) (redrawn from Houde, 1968, p. 114). The forward movement of the tongue during the closure constitutes active enlargement of the vocal tract.

Table 9-9. Morphophonemic Variation in Japanese Strong Verbs

Non-past indicative verb stem	Conjunctive		English gloss
	Standard dialect	Hachijojima dialect	
tatu	tatte		stand up
uru	utte		sell
but:			
asobu	asonde	asudde	play
jomu	jonde	jodde	read

Note. From Kawasaki (1981).

geminate consonant would be expected (and is, in fact, found in a remote conservative dialect spoken on the island Hachijojima), the standard dialect has a *nasal + stop* sequence. There is evidence that the NC sequence was once a prenasalized stop (Shevelov & Chew, 1971; Kawasaki, 1981). As we have seen, prenasalized stops avoid the problems associated with maintaining voicing in stops.

The stop inventory of Quileute is reported by Andrade (1933–1938) to be /b, d, p, t, k/. In addition to the lack of a /g/, the most difficult stop to voice, Andrade reports that the /d/, the second most difficult stop to voice, is phonetically [^{n}d].

D. Constraints on Voicing in Fricatives

If the problem with stops and voicing is that the accumulation of air in the oral cavity eventually quenches voicing, then this constraint should be less evident with fricatives since they have a continuous venting of oral air pressure. So much for a priori prediction, since this turns out not to be true. Table 9-10 provides tabulations of the interaction of voicing with stops (including affricates) and fricatives for the 706 languages surveyed by Ruhlen. Considering languages that utilize voicing with one of the obstruent types but not the other, the table shows that there is more than twice the probability of voicing being absent on fricatives ($p = 192/536 = .358$) as on stops ($p = 63/391 = .16$).

Two factors probably account for this pattern. First, voiced fricatives have more exacting aerodynamic requirements than do voiced stops: For the sake of continued voicing the oral pressure should be low, but for the sake of frication the oral pressure should be high, that is, the difference between oral pressure and atmospheric pressure should be high enough to cause high air velocity through the consonantal constriction. Meeting both of these requirements simultaneously may be difficult. To the extent that the segment retains voicing it may be less of a fricative, and if it is a good fricative it runs the risk of being

Table 9-10. Tallies from 706 Languages on Use of Voicing with Obstruents

No. of languages that have	No fricatives	Voiced/voiceless fricatives	Only voiceless fricatives	Only voiced fricatives	Total
Voiced/voiceless stops, affricates	15	327	192	2	536
Only voiceless stops	19	63	79	5	166
Only voiced stops	3	1	0	0	4
Total	37	391	271	7	706

Note. From data in Ruhlen (1975).

devoiced. In fact, the noise component of voiced fricatives is much less than that for voiceless fricatives (Pickett, 1980, p. 155) and on nonsibilant voiced fricatives ([β, v, ð, j, γ, ʁ]) is often so weak as to be barely detectable.

The second reason why the arguments presented above for stops do not apply to fricatives is that there is evidence that the state of the glottis may not be the same during voiced fricatives as it is during voiced stops. Hirose and Ushijima (1978) report electromyographic (EMG) data for laryngeal muscles which suggest that, at least for medial consonants, [z] has a less constricted glottis than [b, d, g]. If so, this may be necessitated by the fact that voiced fricatives, but not voiced stops, require greater glottal airflow for the sake of maintaining the trans-oral constriction pressure differential. Quantitative aerodynamic modeling of these sounds is necessary to clarify this point.

As a possible manifestation of this greater incompatibility of voicing with fricatives than stops, I have the impression, from listening to speech and examining acoustic records of speech, that in American English the "voiced" fricatives /v, z/ are more likely to be devoiced in word-final position than are the stops /b, d, g/.

E. Frication and Devoicing of Glides, Vowels

1. Mathematical Simulation of Close versus Open Vowels' Aerodynamics To illustrate some of the aerodynamic constraints that govern the phonological behavior of nonobstruents, a quantitative simulation of some of the relevant parameters was performed using a simple mathematical model of speech aerodynamics (Ohala, 1975a, 1976). Figure 9-5 shows superimposed the simulation of two V_1CV_2 utterances where C is a voiceless unaspirated stop (e.g., [p]), V_1 is an open vowel (e.g., [æ]), and V_2 is either the same open vowel (solid line) or a close vowel (e.g., [i]: broken line). The bottommost function shows the single independent parameter—area of the oral constriction—that varied between the two utterances. The top two functions, oral air pressure and

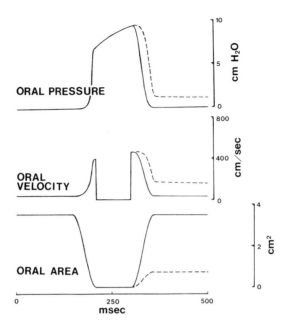

Figure 9-5. Mathematical simulation of two VCV utterances such as [æpæ] (solid line) and [æpi] (broken line). Oral area is an independent parameter, that is, input to the aerodynamic model; oral pressure and oral (particle) velocity are two dependent parameters, that is, output of the model (from Ohala, 1976).

oral (particle) velocity, are dependent parameters. There are four observations to make about the aerodynamic differences between close and open vowels. These will be taken up separately in the next four sections.

2. Devoicing of Vowels, Glides Figure 9-5 shows that a close vowel creates an appreciable back pressure (ca. 1 cm H_2O) in comparison with open vowels. Thorsen (cited by Fischer-Jørgensen, 1963) demonstrated this empirically. Although the magnitude of the oral back pressure is not very great, it does reduce the transglottal pressure drop and could, in conjunction with other factors (see below), contribute to vowel devoicing. Greenberg (1969) and Jaeger (1978) surveyed a total of 30 languages that allophonically devoiced a subset of their total vowel inventory and found a strong tendency for high vowels to exhibit devoicing as opposed to low vowels. Table 9-11 presents a sample of the data they surveyed.

The other factors that contribute to vowel devoicing are (1) partial assimilation to adjacent voiceless segments or pause (i.e., the vocal cords become slightly abducted), (2) lowered subglottal pressure, as would be encountered on unstressed vowels and/or vowels following consonants characterized by heavy airflow (e.g., English *potato* as [pʰətʰeɪroŭ]), and (3) the shortness of the vowel, since the shorter it is, the more it can be influenced by the first two factors.

Table 9-11. Distribution of Voiceless and Voiced Vowels

Language	Voiceless and voiced	Voiced only
Awadhi	i, u, e	a, o
Campa	i	o, e, a
Chatino	i, u	o, e, a
Dagur	i, u, ə	o, a
Huichol	i, ɨ, e	u, a
Serbo-Croatian	i, u	e, o, a
Tadjik	i, u, a	e, o, ú
Tunica	u	i, e, ɛ, a, ɔ, o
Uzbek	i, u	e, ɔ, o, a

Note. Sample from Greenberg (1969).

3. Frication of Vowels, Glides A second point to note about the difference between close and open vowels as revealed in Figure 9-5 is that close vowels give rise to a higher velocity of the oral airflow. The greater the velocity of the airflow, the greater is the turbulence and thus the frication of the segment (Stevens, 1971). Close glides, because they often have a constriction smaller than vowels, should be particularly subject to the development of frication. Phonological data support this.

According to Millardet (1911), the long high vowels of Swedish, which are diphthongized, may end in fricated glides, these glides being voiceless before a final voiceless obstruent, otherwise voiced. No frication, however, was found for the nonhigh vowels. See Table 9-12 (where modern IPA transcription has been substituted for that used by Millardet, except for [jˆ], a voiced palatal fricative; these data may not be representative of Modern Swedish). Similar data have been reported for the Jutish dialect of Danish (Andersen, 1972).

A well-known variation among Spanish dialects attests the sound change [j]→[ʒ]: Andalusian [kabajo] "horse," Argentine [kabaʒo]. Similarly, Latin *iugam* and Sanskrit *yugam* "yoke" corresponds to Classical Greek *dzugon*, from which we get the stem of the English word *zygomatic*. In American English, one can find the following dialectal or even ideolectal variation among [tj—], [tʃ—], and [tʃ(ɹ)—]: [tʰjuzdi]~[tʃuzdi] "Tuesday" (Kurath & McDavid, 1961), [tʰɹʌk] ~ [tʃʰɹʌk] "truck." Benjamin Franklin's (1806) phonetic transcription of his speech reveals that he pronounced *natural* as [nætjuɹəl]; today the pronunciation is [nætʃɚəl].

4. Affrication of Stops Before High Vowels There is also a strong tendency for stops to develop an affricated release when they precede simple close vowels, since (as Figure 9-5 shows) the high velocity of the airflow created upon release of a stop lasts longer when the stop precedes a close vowel as opposed to an open vowel. Table 9-13 presents evidence of a sound change from Proto-Bantu

Table 9-12. Fricated Glides in Swedish

Swedish orthography	Phonetic	English gloss
vit	viçt	white
krig	kri:jˆg	war
plog	pluβg	plow
bro	bruβ	bridge
gud	gɯβd	God
fru	frɥβ	madame
knyta	knyjˆçta	to tie, knot
by	byjˆ	village
but:		
tack	tak:	thanks
dö	dø:	to die
tåg	to:g	train
lag	lɑ:g	team

Note. From Millardet (1911).

to Mvumbo, which is based on this tendency. (In these data, the changes in place of articulation of the initial stop, although interesting for what they reveal about acoustic–auditory constraints, are irrelevant to the point being made.) In Japanese the dental stop phonemes are realized as affricates before the high vowels /i, ɯ/ (e.g., /tɯti/ = [tsɯtʃi] "ground"). Similar patterns can be found in other languages.

5. *Aspiration of Stops* Figure 9-5 reveals that after the release of a stop the time required to reduce oral pressure to a given level, say 4 cm H_2O, is greater when a close vowel follows (ca. 38 msec) than an open vowel (ca. 17 msec). Insofar as voicing requires some minimum transglottal pressure drop, it follows that voice onset should be appreciably delayed when a close as opposed to an open vowel follows a stop. In other words, stops preceding close vowels should be more aspirated than those preceding nonclose vowels. Several phonetic studies show this to be the case (Ohala, 1981, and references cited there). There are many reports in the phonological literature of languages having stops with more aspiration (allophonically) before high vowels than nonhigh vowels (Cook, 1969; Vogler, 1968).

F. Nasalization Blocks Devoicing and Affrication

Earlier I mentioned that if air under pressure is to be released through one of the vocal tract's valves, then all other valves that would vent that air must be closed. If another valve is open, then a noisy audible flow of air through the intended

Table 9-13. Sound Change in Bantu Showing Development of Affricated Release to Stops at a Function of Following Vowel

Proto-Bantu		Mvumbo	English gloss
*-buma	>	bvumo	fruit
*-dib-	>	dʒiwo	shut
*-dut	>	-bvure	pull
*-tiitU	>	tʃir	animal
*-tud-	>	-pfule	forge
*-gida	>	ma-tʃie	blood
*-gubU	>	m-bvuu	hippopotamus
*-kiŋgo	>	tʃiuŋ	neck, nape
*-kuba	>	pfuwo	chicken
but:			
*-bod	>	-buo	become rotten
*-dɪ	>	-di	eat
*-toog	>	-tuog	boil up
*-gada	>	-kala	mat
*-konde	>	kwande	banana

Note. From Guthrie (1967–1970).

valve will be lessened or eliminated. From this we would predice that the devoicing and frication of vowels and glides discussed in the preceding section should be blocked by nasalization—the open velopharyngeal port acting to reduce the oral pressure that contributed to these effects. This prediction (which I made, by the way, before knowing whether there was phonological evidence for it) is borne out (Ohala, 1978b). In English /h/ becomes the voiceless palatal fricative [ç] before the palatal glide /j/, for example, "human" /hjumən/ is [çjūmə̃n]. But in a heavily nasalized environment the palatal frication is apparently blocked and the /h/ is manifested simply as a glottal fricative: "unhuman" is [ʌ̃nhjūmə̃n], not *[ʌnçjūmə̃n].

Similarly, in Fante (Schachter & Fromkin, 1968) the word with "underlying" form /hɪ/ "border" is realized phonetically as [çɪ] but the word /hĩ/ "where" is [hĩ], not *[çĩ].

Beasely and Pike (1957) report that in Jivaro voiceless vowels appear in word-final position when unstressed but voiceless nasal vowels were not found to occur.

In Yuchi, according to Wagner (1933–1938), voiceless spirants appear predictably between all vowels and following lingual stops but not if the vowel is nasalized.

In Chinese, dialectal data reveal the existence of a sound change by which the palatal vowel /i/ develops into some kind of voiced apical fricative, for example, */siəp/, /siəj/, and so on → */si/ → [sz]. However, if the original syllable ended in a nasal and the vowel became nasalized, the frication of the vowel does not occur: */siən/ ↛ [sz̧] (unless, of course, the nasalized vowel first became denasalized; Steve Baron, personal communication).

G. Stop Epenthesis

The valves we have been discussing—the lips, tongue, and glottis—do not open and close instantaneously; they take an appreciable amount of time to switch from one state to another. This is because (1) they have some inertia, (2) some muscular slack needs to be taken up before the articulators can move, and (3) the neuromuscular control system may have some limited temporal resolution. Assimilation is probably the neuromuscular control system's way of compensating for these constraints. Occasionally assimilation of one valvular state to another has rather dramatic effects on the shape of words. The production of a sequence of nasal consonant followed immediately by an oral segment having an articulation different from the nasal may result in partial denasalization of the nasal due to anticipatory assimilation of the velic closure required by the oral segment. A segment may be "oral" because it is required for aerodynamic reasons (e.g., [s, θ, k]), or for acoustic-auditory reasons, that is, nasalization would distort the acoustic characteristics of the sound (e.g., any distinctively oral sonorant or in some cases any segment, distinctively oral or not, that has a low first formant—the formant that would be most distorted by nasalization, such as [l, w, i, u]; Ohala, 1975b). Thus in English, one finds so-called intrusive or epenthetic stops in words such as those in Table 9-14. Similar data exist for other languages; see Table 9-15.

Although it is more common to find anticipatory assimilation (Javkin, 1979), perseveratory assimilation may occur, and this accounts for the variants /kr̥ṣṇa/ ~ /kr̥ṣṭṇa/ "Krishna" in the Indo-Aryan languages (Varma, 1961, p. 123).

Much the same phenomenon underlies a phonological process misnamed "nasal strengthening." Table 9-16, columns 1 and 2, provides representative data from Kongo (Bentley, 1887). A common analysis of this alternation is that the nasal prefix "strengthens" the stem-initial consonant by increasing its degree of obstruency. This, however, is not the correct analysis (as was explicitly pointed out by Jacottet, 1927, in his analysis of this phenomenon in Sesuto). As the fourth column in Table 9-16 shows (from Guthrie, 1967–1970), these words originally started out with obstruents, which have been retained following the nasal but which have undergone sound changes turning them into nonobstruents in word-initial position. We may imagine that whatever forces acted on these initial stops to change them in this way did so in both environments. However, a preceding nasal consonant, as we saw above, will have the effect of carving out a stop from the nasal preceding the oral segment. In this way the stop will be preserved when there is a preceding nasal. "Nasal preservation" may be a better name for this process. The phonological literature

Table 9-14. Epenthetic Stops in English

Orthographic representation	Phonetic	Source
warmth	[wɔɹmpθ]	< warm + [θ]
something	[sʌmpθɪŋ]	< some + thing
Thompson	[tʰampsən]	< Thom + son
glimpse	[glɪmps]	< gleam + s
teamster	[tʰimpstɚ]	< team + ster
youngster	[jʌŋkstɚ]	< young + ster
length	[lɛŋkθ]	< long + [θ]

contains abundant examples of this process. For example, in most dialects of
Spanish an original set of medial and final voiced stops have become cognate
voiced spirants except after nasals. See Table 9-17. This, of course, is precisely
the same phenomenon exemplified diachronically in Kongo (Table 9-16).
Similar patterns may be found in Gadsup (Frantz & Frantz, 1966) and Camsa
(Howard, 1967).

In Latin the reflex of original Indo-European *gʷ and *ghʷ is usually /w/ (or
written v). However, the stop element is most often preserved after a nasal;
see Table 9-18.

H. Nasal Prosody

The incompatibility between obstruents and velic opening has consequences for
the phonology of languages like Sundanese (Robins, 1957) and Trique
(Hollenbach, 1977), which have a remarkable type of perseveratory nasalization. In general, these "nasal prosodies" work as follows: After a nasal
segment all following segments are nasalized, with nasalization spreading all the
way to the end of the word unless blocked by an oral obstruent. See Table 9-19,
which gives data from Sundanese. As would be predicted, the glottal obstruents
[h,ʔ] do not block spreading nasalization, since in their case the air under
pressure could not be vented by the velic valve. Schourup (1973) has documented several cases of this sort.

Tereno, one of the Arawakan languages of South America, also has perseveratory spreading of nasalization as part of the first-person inflection (where
the nasalization is started at the beginning of the word). In this case voiceless
stops block spreading nasalization but become prenasalized voiced stops in the
process. Again, nonobstruent consonants and [ʔ] do not block nasalization but,
contrary to our expectations, [h] does, and in the process becomes [ⁿz]. See
Table 9-20. We could dismiss this exception as just a language-specific
peculiarity but there is no need to: There is comparative evidence (Bendor-
Samuel, 1966; Noble, 1965, pp. 49–50) that at least some of Tereno's [h]'s
derive from earlier dental obstruents (e.g., Tereno /ɨhɨ/, Piapoco /izipi/, Ipeca

Table 9-15. Examples of Assimilatory Denasalization of Nasal Consonants.

Language	Source	Example	English gloss
Spanish	Spaulding (1965)	vendre (<Latin *ven(i)re*)	sell
		temblar (<Latin *trem(u)lar*)	tremble
		Alhambra (<Arabic *al hamra*)	the red (house)
Ulu Muar Malay	Hendon (1966)	ban ~banᵈ_U	doorsill
Korean	Chen and Clumeck (1975)	mul ~ mᵇul	water
Telefol	Healey (1964)	/suːm/ = [suːᵇm]	banana
Parintintin	Pease and Betts (1971)	/õmoapɨ/ = [õᵐboapɨ]	he cooks
		/ɲãnu/ = [ɲãⁿdu]	spider
Tenango Otomi	Blight and Pike (1976)	/mohi/ = [mᵇohi]	plate
		/nĩne/ = [nĩnᵈe]	your mouth

Table 9-16. So-Called Nasal Strengthening in Kongo

Verb stem	Gerund	English gloss	Proto-Bantu	English gloss
mona	mbona	a sight	< *-bon-	see
vunda	mpunda	a resting	<? *-puum-	breathe, rest
landa	ndanda	a following	< *-dand-	follow

Note. From Bentley (1887) and Guthrie (1967–1970).

/itsipi/, Rio Icanna Baniva /itipi/ "tail"). Rather than being an exception to the phonetically based principles of which sounds should and should not block spreading nasalization, it is very probably a regular example of another phonetically based process: nasal preservation. (See also Court, 1970, who cites cases in Indonesian languages where spreading nasalization does *not* pass through nasals *m*, *n*, etc.—a surprising pattern on the surface but not when it is made clear that these nasals derived from earlier *mb*, *nd* and that the spreading nasalization is a historical relic.)

III. Conclusion

Liljencrants and Lindblom (1972) have challenged those who ask, "Why do speech and language have the form and behavior that they do?" to attempt to derive the answers deductively by considering the real-world constraints— physical, physiological, psychological, and social—within which language is used. This chapter is offered as a modest addition to the growing number of contributions, including those of Lindblom and his colleagues, that have taken up this challenge. I have attempted to show how certain cross-language regularities in the behavior of speech sounds stem from universal physical phonetic properties of the speech mechanism, in particular its aerodynamic properties.

Such work should be viewed as but one aspect of a much larger effort recently undertaken in biology and related disciplines to explain the behavior, especially the social behavior, of animals and man by reference to the ecological situation in which the species exist (Maynard Smith, 1974; Wilson, 1975; Krebs & Davies, 1978; Morton, 1975). Within phonology, as in biology, prior qualitative work has shown us the great promise of this approach (Passy, 1890; Martinet, 1955). Nevertheless, if we can learn anything from the recent work in biology, the real breakthroughs will come only when we can employ reliable, formal, but empirically motivated, quantitative models of the complex "ecological" forces that shape speech and language.

Acknowledgments. This work was supported in part by the National Science Foundation and by the Committee on Research of the University of California at Berkeley. I am also grateful to my friends and colleagues for help and advice, especially Mariscela Amador, Jeri Jaeger, Carol Justus, Haruko Kawasaki, Björn Lindblom, Yakov Malkiel, Manjari Ohala, Steve Pearson, and Carol Riordan. I assume responsibility for the accuracy of the data and for the ideas presented here.

Table 9-17. Preservation of Voiced Stops After Nasals in Spanish

Phonemic	Phonetic	English gloss		Phonemic	Phonetic	English gloss
/sobra/	[soβra]	surplus	*but:*	/sombra/	[sombra]	shadow
/rodaɾ/	[roðar]	to roll	*but:*	/rondaɾ/	[rondaɾ]	to go around
/mago/	[maɣo]	magician	*but:*	/mango/	[maŋgo]	handle

Table 9-18. Preservation of Stop Element of Indo-European *g(h)ʷ Following a Nasal Consonant in Latin

Proto-Indo-European		Latin	English gloss
*gʷiōu–		vivus	living
*tergʷ̄–		torvus	wild
*wegʷ–		ūvidus	moist
but:			
*dn̥ghʷā		lingua	tongue
*engʷ–		inguen	abdomen
*ongʷ–		unguō	to anoint
cf. also:			
*sneighʷ–		nivis	snow (noun, genitive)
	But:	ninguit	snows (verb with nasal infix)

Note. From Pokorny, (1959) and Poultney (1963).

Table 9-19. Perseveratory Assimilation of Nasalization in Sundanese

Example	English gloss
[ɲãĩãn]	to wet
[bɣŋ̄hãr]	to be rich
[ɲãhõkɣn]	to inform
[mĩʔãsih]	to love

Note. From Robins (1957).

Table 9-20. Perseveratory Spreading of Nasalization in Tereno

Third person (no nasalization)	English gloss	First person (spreading nasalization)	English gloss
[piho]	he went	[ᵐbiho]	I went
[ahjaˀaʃo]	he desires	[ãⁿʒaˀaʃo]	I desire
[iso]	he hoed	[ĩⁿzo]	I hoed
[owoku]	his house	[õw̃õⁿgu]	my house
[ajo]	his brother	[aĵõ]	my brother
[emoˀu]	his word	[ẽmõˀũ]	my word
[iha]	his name	[ĩⁿza]	my name

Note. Data from Bendor-Samuel (1960, 1966).

References

Abramson, A. S. The vowels and tones of Standard Thai: Acoustical measurements and experiments. *International Journal of American Linguistics*, 1962, Publication *No. 20.*

Alexandre, R. P. *La langue mō̌rě.* Dakar: Mémoires de l'Institut français d'Afrique noire, 1953, *No. 34.*

Andersen, H. Diphthongization. *Language*, 1972, *48*, 11–50.

Andrade, M. J. Quileute. In F. Boas (Ed.), *Handbook of American Indian languages* (Part 3). New York: Columbia University Press, 1933–1938, pp. 154–292.

Armstrong, R. G. Yala (Ikom), a terraced-level language with three tones. *Journal of West African Languages*, 1968, *5*, 49–58.

Beasley, D., & Pike, K. Notes on Huambisa phonemics. *Lingua Posnaniensis*, 1957, *6*, 1–8.

Bell, H. The phonology of Nobiin Nubian. *African Language Review*, 1971, *9*, 115–159.

Bendor-Samuel, J. T. Some problems of segmentation in the phonological analysis of Tereno. *Word*, 1960, *16*, 348–355.

Bendor-Samuel, J. T. Some prosodic features in Terena. In C. E. Bazell, J. C. Catford, M. A. K. Halliday, & R. H. Robins (Eds.), *In memory of J. R. Firth.* London: Longmans, 1966, pp. 30–39.

Bentley, W. H. *Dictionary and grammar of the Kongo language.* London: Trübner & Co., 1887.

Blight, R. C., & Pike, E. V. The phonology of Tenango Otomi. *International Journal of American Linguistics*, 1976, *42*, 51–57.

Catford, J. C. *Fundamental problems in phonetics.* Bloomington: Indiana University Press, 1977. (a)

Catford, J. C. Mountain of tongues: The languages of the Caucasus. *Annual Review of Anthropology*, 1977, *6*, 283–314. (b)

Chao, Y. R. Types of plosives in Chinese. *Proceedings of the 2nd International Congress of Phonetic Sciences.* Cambridge: Cambridge University Press, 1936, pp. 106–110.

Chen, M., & Clumeck, H. Denasalization in Korean: A search for universals. In C. A. Ferguson, L. M. Hyman, & J. J. Ohala (Eds.), *Nasálfest: Papers from a symposium on nasals and nasalization.* Stanford: Language Universals Project, 1975, pp. 125–131.

Cook, T. L. *The pronunciation of Efik for speakers of English.* Bloomington: African Studies Program and Intensive Language Training Center, Indiana University, 1969.

Court, C. Nasal harmony and Indonesian sound laws. In S. A. Wurm & D. C. Laycock (Eds.) *Pacific linguistic studies in honour of Arthur Capell.* Canberra: Australian National University, 1970. pp. 203–217.

Fischer-Jørgensen, E. Beobachtungen über den Zusammenhang zwischen Stimmhaftigkeit und intraoralem Luftdruck. *Zeitschrift für Phonetik, Sprachwissenschaft und Kommunikationsforschung*, 1963, *16*, 19–36.

Fox, R. A., & Terbeek, D. Dental flaps, vowel duration and rule ordering in American English. *Journal of Phonetics*, 1977, *5*, 27–34.

Franklin, B. A scheme for a new alphabet and reformed mode of spelling. In *The complete works of Dr. Benjamin Franklin* (Vol. 2). London, 1806, pp. 357–366.

Frantz, C. I., & Frantz, M. E. Gadsup phoneme and toneme units. *Linguistic Circle of Canberra Publications* (Series A), 1966, *7*, 1–11.

Gamkrelidze, T. V. On the correlation of stops and fricatives in a phonological system. *Lingua*, 1975, *35*, 231–261.

Greenberg, J. H. Some methods of dynamic comparison in linguistics. In J. Puhvel (Ed.), *Substance and structure of language.* Los Angeles: Center for Research in Languages and Linguistics, 1969, pp. 147–204.

Greenberg, J. H. Some generalizations concerning glottalic consonants, especially implosives. *International Journal of American Linguistics*, 1970, *36*, 123–145.

Guthrie, M. *Comparative Bantu* (4 vols.). Farnborough: Gregg, 1967–1970.

Healey, A. Telefol phonology. *Linguistic Circle of Canberra Publications* (Series B), 1964, Monograph No. 3

Hendon, R. S. The phonology and morphology of Ulu Muar Malay. *Yale University Publications in Anthropology*, 1966, *No. 70.*

Hirose, H., & Ushijima, T. Laryngeal control for voicing distinction in Japanese consonant production. *Phonetica*, 1978, *35*, 1–10.

Hockett, C. F. A manual of phonology. *International Journal of American Linguistics*, 1955, *Memoir 11.*

Hollenbach, B. E. Phonetic vs. phonemic correspondence in two Trique dialects. In W. R. Merrifield (Ed.), *Studies in Otomanguean phonology.* Arlington: Summer Institute of Linguistics, 1977, pp. 21–33.

Houde, R. A. *A study of tongue body motion during selected speech sounds.* Speech Communication Research Laboratory (Santa Barbara), 1968, Monograph *No. 2.*

Howard, L. Camsa phonology. In V. Waterhouse (Ed.), *Phonemic systems of Colombian languages.* Norman, Okla.: Summer Institute of Linguistics, 1967, pp. 73–87.

Jacottet, E. *A grammar of the Sesuto language.* [*Bantu studies*, Vol. 3, Special Number.] Johannesburg: University of Witwatersrand Press, 1927.

Jaeger, J. J. Speech aerodynamics and phonological universals. *Proceedings of the Annual Meeting of the Berkeley Linguistics Society*, 1978, *4*, 311–329.

Javkin, H. Towards a phonetic explanation for universal preferences in implosives and ejectives. *Proceedings of the Annual Meeting of the Berkeley Linguistics Society*, 1977, *3*, 559–565.

Javkin, H. R. Phonetic universals and phonological change. *Report of the Phonology Laboratory (Berkeley)*, 1979, *No. 4.*

Kawasaki, H. *Voicing in Japanese.* Unpublished manuscript, University of California at Berkeley, 1981.

Khubchandani, L. M. Sindhi. *Current trends in linguistics*, 1969, 5, 201–234.

Krebs, J. R., & Davies, N. B. (Eds.). *Behavioural ecology: An evolutionary approach.* Oxford: Blackwell, 1978.

Kurath, H., & McDavid, R. I. *The pronunciation of English in the Atlantic States.* Ann Arbor: University of Michigan Press, 1961.

Ladefoged, P. *A phonetic study of West African languages.* Cambridge: Cambridge University Press, 1964.

Ladefoged, P. *Preliminaries to linguistic phonetics.* Chicago: Chicago University Press, 1971.

Ladefoged, P. Chapter 8, this volume.

Lehiste, I. *Suprasegmentals.* Cambridge, Mass.: MIT Press, 1970.

Liljencrants, J., & Lindblom, B. Numerical simulation of vowel quality systems: The role of perceptual contrast. *Language*, 1972, *48*, 839–862.

MacKay, D. G. The structure of words and syllables: Evidence from errors in speech. *Cognitive Psychology*, 1972, *3*, 210–227.

Martinet, A. *Économie des changements phonétiques.* Berne: Francke, 1955.

Maynard Smith, J. *Models in ecology.* New York and London: Cambridge University Press, 1974.

Millardet, G. Insertions de consonnes en suédois moderne. *Revue de Phonétique*, 1911, *1*, 309–346.

Morton, E. S. Ecological sources of selection on avian sounds. *American Naturalist*, 1975, *108*, 17–34.

Noble, G. K. Proto-Arawakan and its descendants. *International Journal of American Linguistics*, 1965, Publication No. 38.

Ohala, J. J. A mathematical model of speech aerodynamics. In G. Fant (Ed.), *Speech communication* (Vol. 2: *Speech production and synthesis by rule*). Stockholm: Almqvist & Wiksell, 1975, pp. 65–72. (a)

Ohala, J. J. Phonetic explanations for nasal sound patterns. In C. A. Ferguson, L. M. Hyman, & J. J. Ohala (Eds.), *Nasálfest: Papers from a symposium on nasals and nasalization.* Stanford: Language Universals Project, 1975, pp. 289–316. (b)

Ohala, J. J. A model of speech aerodynamics. *Report of the Phonology Laboratory (Berkeley)*, 1976, *1*, 93–107.

Ohala, J. J. The production of tone. In V. A. Fromkin (Ed.), *Tone: A linguistic survey.* New York: Academic Press, 1978, pp. 5–39. (a)

Ohala, J. J. Phonological notations as models. In W. U. Dressler & W. Meid (Eds.), *Proceedings of the 12th International Congress of Linguists.* Innsbruck: Innsbrucker Beiträge zur Sprachwissenschaft, 1978, pp. 811–816. (b)

Ohala, J. J. The application of phonological universals in speech pathology. In N. J. Lass (Ed.), *Speech and language: Advances in basic research and practice* (Vol. 3). New York: Academic Press, 1980, pp. 75–97.

Ohala, J. J. Articulatory constraints on the cognitive representation of speech. In T. Myers, J. Laver, & J. Anderson (Eds.), *The cognitive representation of speech.* Amsterdam: North-Holland, 1981, pp. 111–122.

Ohala, J. J., & Kawasaki, H. *The articulation of [i]'s.* Paper presented at the 98th meeting of the Acoustical Society of America, Salt Lake City, November 1979.

Ohala, J. J., & Riordan, C. J. Passive vocal tract enlargement during voiced stops. In J. J. Wolf & D. H. Klatt (Eds.), *Speech communication papers.* New York: Acoustical Society of America, 1979, pp. 89–92.

Passy, P. *Étude sur les changements phonétiques.* Paris: Librairie Firmin-Didot, 1890.

Pease, H., & Betts, L. Parintintin phonology. In D. Bendor-Samuel (Ed.), *Tupi studies I.* Norman, Okla.: Summer Institute of Linguistics, 1971, pp. 1–14.

Pickett, J. M. *The sounds of speech communication.* Baltimore: University Park Press, 1980.

Pokorny, J. *Indogermanisches etymologisches Wörterbuch.* Berne: Francke, 1959.

Poultney, J. W. Evidence for Indo-European alternation of initial /gʷ/ and /w/. *Language.* 1963, *39*, 398–408.

Purnell, H. C., Jr. *Phonology of a Yao dialect spoken in the province of Chiengrai, Thailand.* Hartford Studies in Linguistics, 1965, *No. 15.*

Robbins, F. E. Quiotepec Chinantec syllable patterning. *International Journal of American Linguistics*, 1961, *27*, 237–250.

Robins, R. H. Vowel nasality in Sundanese. In *Studies in Linguistic Analysis.* Oxford: Blackwell's, 1957, pp. 87–103.

Rothenberg, M. *The breath-stream dynamics of simple-released-plosive production. Bibliotheca Phonetica*, 1968, *No. 6.*

Ruhlen, M. *A guide to the languages of the world.* Stanford, 1975.

Schachter, P., & Fromkin, V. A phonology of Akan: Akuapem, Asante, and Fante. UCLA Working Papers in Phonetics, 1968, *No. 9.*

Schourup, L. C. A cross-language study of vowel nasalization. *Ohio State University Working Papers in Linguistics*, 1973, *15*, 190–221.

Shattuck-Hufnagel, S., Chapter 6, this volume.

Sherman, D. Stop and fricative systems: A discussion of paradigmatic gaps and the question of language sampling. *Stanford Working Papers in Language Universals*, 1975, *17*, 1–31.

Shevelov, G. Y., & Chew, J. J., Jr. Open syllable languages and their evolution: Common Slavic and Japanese. In G. Y. Shevelov, *Teasers and appeasers. Essays and studies on themes of Slavic philology.* München: Wilhelm Fink Verlag, 1971, pp. 15–34.

Smith, B. L. *Effects of vocalic context, place of articulation and speaker's sex on "voiced" stop consonant production.* Paper presented at West Coast Phonetics Symposium, March 1977, Santa Barbara, California.

Spaulding, R. K. *How Spanish grew.* Berkeley: University of California Press, 1965.

Stevens, K. N. Airflow and turbulence noise for fricative and stop consonants: Static considerations. *Journal of the Acoustical Society of America*, 1971, *50*, 1180–1192.

Stevens, K. N. Discussion during symposium on phonetic universals in phonological systems and their explanation. *Proceedings of the 9th International Congress of Phonetic Sciences*, 1980, *3*, 185ff.

Varma, S. *Critical studies in the phonetic observations of Indian grammarians.* Delhi: Munshi Ram Manoharlal, 1961.

Varyani, P. L. Sources of implosives in Sindhi. *Indian Linguistics*, 1974, *35*, 51–54.

Vogler, P. Esquisse d'une phonologie du baoulé. *Annales de l'université d'abidjan* (Series H): Linguistique, 1968,*1*, 60–65.

Wagner, G. Yuchi. In F. Boas (Ed.), *Handbook of American Indian languages* (Part 3). New York: Columbia University Press, 1933–1938, pp. 300–384.

Ward, I. C. *The phonetic and tonal structure of Efik*. Cambridge, Mass.: Heffer, 1933.

Wilson, E. O. *Sociobiology: The new synthesis*. Cambridge, Mass.: Belknap Press, 1975.

Chapter 10
Economy of Speech Gestures

BJÖRN LINDBLOM

I. Introduction

A. Theoretical Issues

Normal language acquisition and adult verbal behavior presuppose speech production. This fact makes it reasonable to assume that languages tend to evolve sound patterns that can be seen as adaptations to biological constraints of speech production. This reasoning seems valid also for speech perception and speech development, which presumably introduce their own boundary conditions on linguistic form. The constraints of speaking, listening, and learning thus interact in complex ways to delimit humanly possible sound patterns.

If we accept this hypothesis we may do so because we view optimistically the prospects of accounting for significant portions of language form and language behavior in terms of language-independent information on, for example, the brain (mind), the ear, the speech organs, and variables of social interaction. Or we may accept the idea because we believe that such an account, successful or not, would in principle represent the scientifically most satisfactory type of explanation in linguistics.

A lack of interest in the hypothesis, on the other hand, may arise out of the conviction that such attempts will be fruitless, since the secrets of much linguistic regularity are hidden deep in human biology and prehistory, and in most cases should be regarded as genetic idiosyncracies and frozen accidents

(Chomsky, 1972[1]). Or they are by and large culturally determined and are therefore best described as arbitrary social conventions.

The former "functionalist" position implies theories of language whose explanations are substantively (biologically and socially) motivated. The latter "nonfunctionalist" attitude leads to theories in which the primitives of explanation are abstract and formal[2]. Whereas the former derives the fundamental units and process of linguistic structure *deductively* from independent premises anchored in psychological and physical realities, the latter postulates them *axiomatically* for formal reasons. Structuralism and transformational grammar belong to the latter category. They represent the traditional paradigm of linguistics, which is stronger and more extensively formalized than functionalistic approaches.[3]

Important empirical information on these issues can be expected to come from various sources (e.g., the recently initiated comparative studies on sign language and spoken language; Bellugi & Studdert-Kennedy, 1980). The aim of the present study is to contribute to their discussion by drawing attention to some of the constraints of speech production and by considering their role in shaping phonological structure.

---

[1]Chomsky (1971) on the topic of "structure-dependent operations" in syntax:

"I have stressed throughout that in the cases discussed there appeared to be no general explanation for the observed phenomena in terms of communicative efficiency or simplicity. In other words, there seems to be no 'functional explanation' for the observations in question." He continues: "Where properties of language can be explained on such 'functional' grounds they provide no revealing insight into the nature of mind. Precisely because the explanations proposed here are 'formal explanations,' precisely because the proposed principles are not essential or even natural properties of any imaginable language, they provide a revealing mirror of mind (if correct)." (p. 41)

[2]Halle (1975):

"One of the competing themata which I personally have found particularly intriguing is the non-functionalist conception of language as playful activity, as a kind of a game. In the words of the late 18-century German poet and mystic, Novalis: 'das rechte Gespraech ist ein blosses Wortspiel. . . . Wenn man den Leuten nur begreiflich machen konnte, dass es mit der Sprache wie mit den mathematischen Formeln sei— Sie machen eine Welt fuer sich aus—Sie spielen nur mit sich selbst, druecken nicht als ihre wunderbare Natur aus, und eben darum sind sie so ausdrucksvoll—eben darum spiegelt sich in ihnen das seltsame Verhaeltnisspiel der Dinge. . . . So ist es auch mit der Sprache' (Sprachwissenschaftlicher Monolog)." (p. 527)

[3]Some recent phonetic examples of the latter approach include the quantal theory of speech (Stevens, 1972); the paradigm of phonetic explanation in phonology (Ohala, forthcoming); and attempts to deduce phonological systems from phonetic universals (Liljencrants & Lindblom, 1972; Lindblom, 1982).

B. Pronounceability: Physical Limits and Physiological Economy Constraints

The most general and obvious requirement that any potential speech sound, or speech sound sequence, must meet is physical: It must fall within the limits of pronounceability inherent in the human speech apparatus. How can these limits be determined?

Empirically, by gathering data from the world's languages, it might be suggested. Such an approach would clearly shed valuable light on the question. However, it provides no basis for determining when sufficient amounts of data have been collected and when the limits have been established. This would be true even in the event of a highly extensive search.

Alternatively they could be studied theoretically in attempts to simulate speech production as a physical system. This would in principle be the more satisfactory alternative provided that the composite (neuromotor and bio-mechanical) degrees of freedom and their acoustic consequences could be exhaustively modeled. It would provide phonetic theory with a way of defining *pronounceability* and making predictions about notions such as "possible speech sound" and "possible sound sequence" in terms of a universal phonetic signal space. How is this space used?

A major point of this chapter is that languages tend to behave rather "fastidiously" with respect to the total set of physical capabilities of the speech apparatus. In normal speech the production system is rarely driven to its limits. Typically we speak at a "comfortable" volume or rate and we use a degree of articulatory precision that seems "natural." On the other hand, we are of course occasionally perfectly capable of hyperarticulating (and hypoarticulating), that is, of adjusting the loudness, tempo, clarity, etc. of our speech to the needs of the situation, thereby exploiting more of the full range of phonetic possibilities. As we hope to show, this style of behavior can be observed not only phonetically in the pronunciation of individual utterances but also phonologically in the properties of segment inventories, sequences, and rules. We shall conclude that when we examine gestures in relation to the potential capacity of the system we note a tendency toward underexploitation. What does this observation tell us about the physiology of speech production?

It is our guess that the underexploitation of the phonetic space reflects not only speech production constraints but the *concurrent* demands of speech perception as well. These conditions interact to yield a subset of signals which are sufficiently adapted to their communicative purpose but at the same time put reasonable demands on the expenditure of physiological energy. In other words underexploitation is, among other things, related to a criterion of physiological economy which participates in, as it were, a biological "cost–benefit" con-spiracy. Wilson (1975) presents

> a picture of extreme opportunism in the evolution of communication systems, in which signals are molded from almost any biological process convenient to the

species. It is therefore legitimate to analyze the advantages and disadvantages of the
several sensory modalities as though they were competing in an open marketplace for
the privilege of carrying messages. Put another, more familiar way, we can
reasonably hypothesize that species evolve towards the mix of sensory cues that
maximizes either energetic or informational efficiency, or both. (p. 231)

This speculative account has important implications for the development of
linguistically useful theories of speech production. It says that languages build
their sound patterns within the physical limits of pronounceability and under
conditions of motor optimization. Thus if a better understanding of these
physical and physiological constraints were available, a more powerful
definition of pronounceability and the phonetic signal space might be achieved,
couched in terms of notions such as "possible and favored speech sound"
and "possible and favored phonetic sequence." It appears clear that negative
and positive results obtained within such a research program would be valuable
in the evaluation of the theoretical issues raised earlier in this introduction and
in determining whether deductive rather than axiomatic definitions can be given
for concepts such as the distinctive feature, the segment, the syllable, and other
linguistic constructs.

This chapter gives two fairly detailed instances of phonetic "motor e-
conomy": consonant–vowel coarticulation and vowel reduction. These analyses
will suggest two physiologically based conditions: a *synergy constraint*
governing static spatial relations among articulators, and a *rate constraint*
operating dynamically on articulatory movements. A final section will
demonstrate some phonological consequences of motor economy. Several sets
of data will be used to exemplify language adaptations to the synergy and rate
constraints: *assimilation rules* and the *patterning of consonant and vowel
segments* within the syllable. Moreover, an attempt will be made to elucidate the
topic of economy in a more general context by using observations of both speech
and nonspeech motor behavior.

II. Coarticulation

The motor events of a sequence of phonemes overlap in space and time. In
pronouncing, for example, [ku], the speaker begins to round and protrude his
lips in anticipation of [u] before the release of the tongue closure for [k]. This
spatial and temporal overlap of adjacent gestures is a very general phenomenon
and can be observed in all languages. The term for it is *coarticulation*.

Figure 10-1 summarizes some observations reported by Öhman (1966). In
the left column we see stylized spectrograms of [d] in three symmetric vowel
contexts. Note the systematic variation of formant positions at the boundaries of
the [d] segment. Consider in particular the second formant frequency. Its value
at these points appears to be correlated with its location at the vowel steady

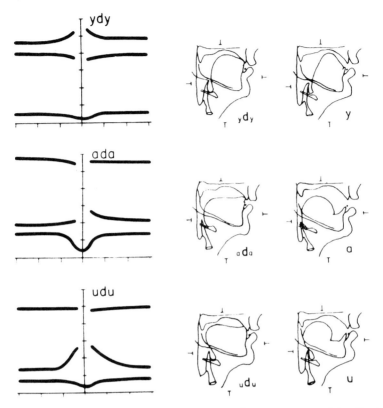

Figure 10-1. Coarticulation. Vowel–consonant–vowel utterances containing the dental stop [d]. Left column: Averages of pencil tracings of the formant center lines obtained from spectrograms. Time along abscissa; frequency along ordinate. Time marks are 100 msec apart; frequency marks are 500 Hz apart. Middle and right columns: Contour tracings from X-ray motion pictures. Samples taken at the middle of [d] occlusions and at vowel steady states. (Adapted from Öhman, 1966.)

states. Such dependencies can be described in terms of linear "locus" equations (see below). Beside these formant patterns in Figure 10-1 are the articulatory configurations that underlie the acoustic facts. We note that while the point of contact of the tongue tip remains invariant for [d] the tongue-body contour varies and bears a strong resemblance to its shape in the adjacent vowel. It is thus clear how the spectrographic patterns of Figure 10-1 arise. They come about because the geometry of the cavities behind the occlusion for [d] influences formant frequency locations, particularly F_2 in this case, and because the tongue tip gesture for [d] is *coarticulated* with the tongue-body position for the vowel environment.

Having thus presented an introduction to our first topic, we can now proceed to more quantitative considerations of it. We shall examine observed *degrees of coarticulation* in relation to the general motor capabilities of speech production. In order to do so we shall use a numerical model developed by Lindblom and Sundberg (1971) and Lindblom, Pauli, and Sundberg (1974) as an empirically based first approximation of the natural degrees of freedom of the articulatory system.

The model input parameters are as follows:

1. Lips:
   (a) distance between mouth corners ("width");
   (b) vertical midsagittal separation between lips ("height").
2. Mandible:
   (a) position (relative to clench) along single path.
3. Tongue body (mandibular reference):
   (a) degree of deviation from neutral shape;
   (b) location of tongue.
4. Tongue blade (defined relative to tongue body):
   (a) elevation of tip;
   (b) location of tip (protrusion/retraction).
5. Larynx:
   (a) vertical position.

For the remainder of this discussion the lips and the larynx will be disregarded. A fixed position of the jaw will be assumed ($j = 7$mm). The tongue parameters are illustrated in Figure 10-2. For the tongue tip the location parameter (protrusion) is held constant while elevation is varied stepwise (left). Tongue-body contours are shown for a given degree of displacement from neutral shape at various locations (top right). The class of all possible model tongue-body contours can be conveniently described in terms of a semicircle (bottom right). Any given point within the semicircle indicates a pair of values pertaining to the two tongue-body dimensions and is consequently associated with a unique contour. For a justification of these choices see Lindblom (1975).

The model uses input specifications of these parameters and a set of geometric rules to generate an articulatory profile providing the necessary information for acoustic calculations. Our present interest in it will be limited to the tongue parameters. We shall explore the various ways in which it can produce tongue tip stops in order to shed some further light on coarticulation.

Let us first investigate all possible ways of making a retroflex (postdental) stop, more specifically, all possible combinations of parameter values that are compatible with a point of contact between the tip and the palate located 12 mm behind the upper incisors. The result is summarized in Figure 10-3 (left) in terms of iso-retroflexion contours. A given contour indicates that subclass of tongue body contours which are all compatible with the required place of articulation as well as a single value of the retraction parameter. It makes intuitive sense that the high numbers (= marked degree of retroflexion) should occur near the palatal or [i]-like region and that smaller and even negative (protrusive) values should be obtained for more posterior or [o]-like tongue

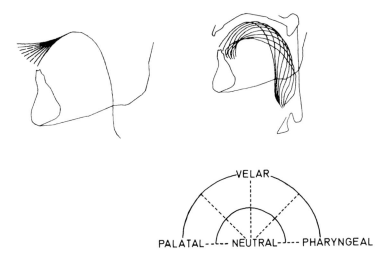

Figure 10-2. Parameters of articulatory model. Tongue tip and tongue body are two-dimensional. The two numbers specifying tongue-body contours are *position* (= angle of semicircle radius) and *displacement from neutral* (= location along radius). The numbers specifying tongue tip articulation are analogous: *protrusion/retraction* and *elevation*.

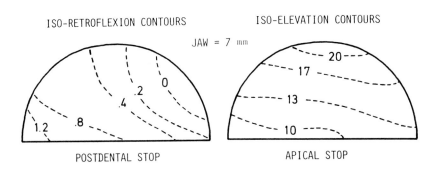

Figure 10-3. Left: Iso-retroflexion contours. The diagram can be used to find the answer to: Given an arbitrary tongue-body contour (= an arbitrary point within semicircle), what value of the retraction parameter will produce an apical stop 12 mm behind the upper incisors? Right: Iso-elevation contours. A given contour represents that subclass of tongue bodies which are compatible with occlusion and the indicated degree of elevation (in millimeters).

bodies. In summary, the question that the left semicircle provides the answer to is: Given an arbitrary tongue-body contour, what value of the retraction parameter will produce an apical stop 12 mm behind the incisors?

As a second exercise let us examine the elevation parameter, keeping the degree of retraction constant at the neutral value. How far does the tongue tip have to be raised to produce a stop at any point along the palate? The right semicircle of Figure 10-3 contains the answer. A given contour indicates that subclass of tongue bodies which are all compatible both with the required manner of articulation (stop) and with a single value of the elevation parameter. Again the results make good sense. For example, it appears reasonable to find that for a palatal configuration such as [i] the tip is close to the alveolar ridge and the tip–palate contact is accordingly within shorter reach than it is for a velar or [u]-like contour, for which the tongue is back and the tip near the floor of the mouth.

Our experience from comparing the model configurations with X-ray data on VCV utterances shows that although the model is a simplification, it is nevertheless capable of providing quite realistic descriptions of real articulatory profiles. However, the main impression from such comparisons is that the model overgenerates. It is by far too rich in that the majority of its output configurations are not at all seen in speech data. In human speech, extreme values of the parameters are avoided. To appreciate more fully that claim, consider for a moment the following easily testable and rather compelling case. It is perfectly possible for most normal speakers to produce a stop (e.g., [d]) in spite of a large bite block and an abnormally low jaw. They can do so evidently by invoking compensatory tongue tip elevation, in analogy with their ability to produce bite block vowels by tongue-body compensation (Lindblom, Lubker, & Gay, 1979). This fact leads us to state once more the main point of the chapter: Normal speech seems to exploit no more than a fraction of the degrees of freedom that are in principle available for articulation. It also makes us conclude that models of the speech structures that are based on purely physical speech-independent principles (Perkell, 1974; Kiritani, Miyawaki, & Fujimura, 1976) *should* in fact—if correctly and consistently constructed—possess considerable overcapacity in relation to phonetic facts.

At this point we shall summarize the preceding discussion by trying to describe the production of a VCV sequence in terms of the present model. Let us consider the production of a moderately retroflex stop (point of contact $= 12$ mm postdentally) in a front and a back vowel environment, [i-i] and [o-o]. In view of our conclusions above it is natural to introduce a rule implying that extreme parameter values are avoided. This could be done, for instance, by selecting threshold values in approximate agreement with their ranges in speech. The maximal limit of retraction could then be set at 0.4 and that of elevation at 12 mm. What are the tongue-body contours that are compatible with those constraints? In our presentation so far we have imposed: jaw opening $= 7$ mm; place of articulation $= 12$ mm postdentally; manner $=$ stop; maximum elevation $= 12$ mm; maximum retraction $= 0.4$. Our procedure for finding the answer to this question is as follows. We start out from the 0.4 contour of the diagram at left in Figure 10-3, derive the values of elevation along it and take note of the threshold value. Then this procedure is repeated for smaller degrees of retraction, keeping the point of contact unchanged. Eventually an area will be identified containing only those tongue bodies that will generate the intended postdental stop at no more than 12 mm elevation and at no more than the required degree of retraction. That area is shown in black in Figure 10-4. We see that the maximum retraction criterion (0.4) precludes any tongue body that is too front (cf. also Figure 10-3, left). The elevation limit disfavors configurations that are extreme along the back and low dimensions. The class of compatible tongue bodies is seen to be neutral and somewhat displaced toward low and back vowels [o, a]. This result will perhaps make phonologists think of the lowering effect on vowels of [r] and other retroflex consonants in many languages. This is the result we need in order to be able to return to an interpretation of the data of Figure 10-1 and to examine sample generations by the model of VCV sequences. The initial tongue-body configurations for the vowels are marked by the solid dots in Figure 10-4. As the medial consonant is produced the tongue body moves toward the area labeled "class of compatible tongue bodies." There is a simultaneous retraction and elevation of the tongue tip. At the moment of closure the tongue body has reached the compatibility area. The configurations underlying [iɖi] and [oɖo] are now both compatible with the closure condition but differ since each retains features of its vowel environment. There is an overriding constraint on the place of tongue tip closure that remains constant but there is no invariance of underlying tongue-body shape. It reaches a state of "sufficient compatibility" and then begins to anticipate the final vowel.

We have thus developed a bit further our account of how and why consonant–vowel coarticulation arises. It arises because of a *synergy constraint* on tip–body coordination. The degree of coarticulation is manifested in the extent to which the vowel environment is allowed to color the formant frequency pattern of the consonant and to influence the tongue-body shape underlying tip closure.

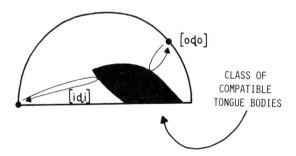

Figure 10-4. Restricting elevation and retroflexion to certain maximum values. The class of tongue-body contours that are compatible with these constraints are indicated by the black area. Their effect on consonant–vowel coarticulation is shown by the arrows.

Evidently the degree of coarticulation is related to the severity of the rule saying that extreme displacements are avoided. As a consequence of the "sufficient compatibility" condition on tongue-body movement our model predicts that a slackening or elimination of the tongue tip constraints would lead to an increase in the degree of coarticulation: Any tongue body would then tend to become compatible. If, on the other hand, these constraints are made more severe, the black area of Figure 10-4 would shrink: The degree of coarticulation would decrease, there being fewer compatible tongue bodies.

The present view stresses that although vowel–consonant coarticulation appears to be a ubiquitous phonetic phenomenon, there is nothing inevitable about its presence or degree of manifestation. We interpret it as a result of motor control optimization processes contributing, whenever other contingencies permit, toward making speech gestures more economical. This treatment is consistent with the observation that the degree of coarticulation can vary in a given individual's speech. Quantifying this parameter in terms of locus e-quations, Lindblom (1963a) found coarticulation (vowel dependence) at VC boundaries more extensive than CV coarticulation:

$$\left. \begin{array}{ll} \text{at CV boundary:} & F_{2i} = 1225 + .278 \cdot F_{20} \\ \text{at VC boundary:} & F_{2f} = 640 + .549 \cdot F_{20} \end{array} \right\} \quad \text{for C} = [d]$$

where F_{20} refers to the second formant of the vowel and F_{2i} and F_{2f} represent CV and VC samples, respectively. Our account is also consistent with the fact that degree of coarticulation can be phonologically controlled. A case in point is the "clear" and "dark" British English varieties of [l], which are produced with palatal (Figure 10-5, top left) and velar (top right) tongue bodies, respectively. According to the present model, the dark velarized variant involves a greater departure from neutral tongue tip position than the clear one. In historical phonology (and present-day American English) we find many examples of vocalization into non-syllabic [u] of dark [l] (English, French, Polish). A related case is the velarization of consonants in Arabic (emphasis). The plain or nonemphatic consonants (bottom left) are opposed to consonants with a velar tongue constriction superimposed (bottom right). Our model assigns lower naturalness to velarized dentals than to plain ones. Supportive of that result is the fact that velarization as a secondary articulation seems to be a rare (marked) attribute in the languages of the world.

III. Vowel Reduction

Our second topic is introduced in Figure 10-6. The spectrograms to the right show two Swedish nonsense words: [ˈdʊdːː] and [ˈdʊdːalal]. The first syllables both have main stress but differ in vowel duration. This shortening, a characteristic of words in many languages, increases with the number of

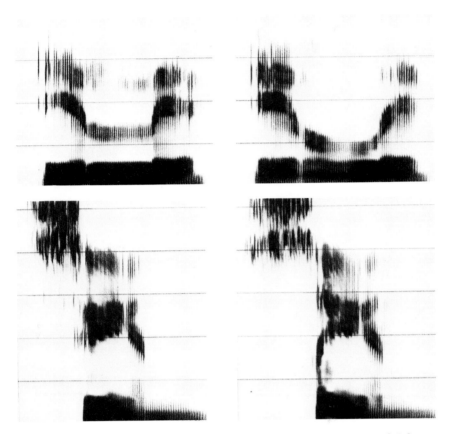

Figure 10-5. Phonologically controlled degree of coarticulation. Top row: [ɪ l ɪ], more velarization (lower F_2) in the right utterance (American English phonetician). Bottom row: plain (left) versus velarized (right) [s] in Arabic words meaning "the letter s" and "China."

following syllables (Lyberg, 1981). There is also a formant pattern difference most evident in F_2 which is several hundred hertz higher in the polysyllable. Some time ago (Lindblom, 1963a, 1963b) we demonstrated that in CVC syllables formant frequencies tend to vary systematically as a function of vowel duration and consonant context. The reduced extent of formant movement here exemplified by [ˈd ʊ d:alal] is often referred to as formant undershoot (Stevens & House, 1963) and is an acoustic manifestation of vowel reduction.

   Our original interpretation of this phenomenon was inspired by comparing the articulators to a mechanical system made up of mass, damping, and spring components (Figure 10-7A). The solid curve of Figure 10-7B shows how such a system behaves if sufficiently damped. It moves sluggishly in response to a force that is applied and removed abruptly (dashed line, arbitrary ordinate scales). If

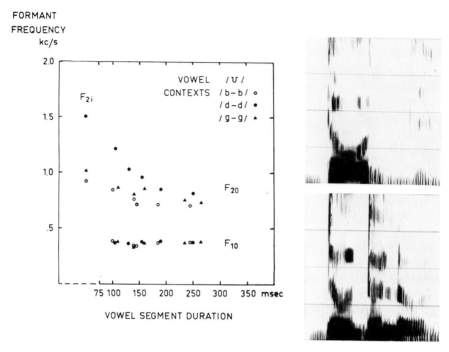

FORMANT
FREQUENCY
kc/s

Figure 10-6. Vowel reduction. Dependence of formant frequencies, especially F_2, on vowel duration is illustrated spectrographically for [ʊ] in test words [dʊd:] and [dʊd:alal]. Diagram from Lindblom (1963a).

the application and removal of the force occur within an interval that is short compared with the response characteristics of the system there will not be sufficient time for it to reach its target (i.e., the state corresponding to the initial step) before the second step occurs. As a consequence it will fall short of, or "undershoot," the steady-state target (Figure 10-7C). If the mass, spring, and damping are constant, then the response to the forcing function and the extent of the undershoot depend exclusively on the duration of the event.

The movement of articulators in a CVC syllable resembles the displacement of the mass in our example. Attributing biomechanical inertia to the articulators and idealizing the forces underlying the consonant–vowel–consonant sequence as a rectangular step function (cf. Figure 10-7B), we would make the following prediction on the basis of the mechanical analogy: As the duration of the vowel decreases, there will be less and less time to complete the approach to the vowel target. The vowel gesture will be more and more reduced. It will exhibit undershoot. In the formant domain the value observed for the vowel will show the influence of the adjacent consonants more and more strongly. This prediction is consistent with a great deal of data on vowel formant frequencies (Figure 10-6, right diagram) and on articulatory movement (Lindblom 1963a,

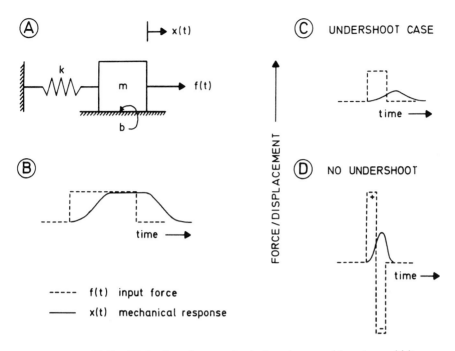

Figure 10-7. Undershoot in a mechanical system—and how to avoid it.

1963b, 1964). One major conclusion of previous work was that it appeared to offer a way of reconciling the conflict arising out of the following two basic facts:

1. Phonemes are by definition invariant units.
2. Their phonetic correlates are characterized by considerable and often ambiguous variability.

The proposed resolution of this dilemma consisted in saying that the intended articulatory configuration, or the underlying vowel target, remains invariant, whereas the lack of constancy at the articulatory and acoustic levels is due to constraints on speech production dynamics.

Another conclusion later rejected (Lindblom, 1968) was that vowel duration is the main determinant of reduced movement and formant undershoot. It has since been challenged by a number of investigators who have produced both articulatory and acoustic evidence (Kuehn, 1973; Gay, Ushijima, Hirose, & Cooper, 1974; Gay, 1978) demonstrating that undershoot is *not* an inevitable consequence of short duration. Thus Kuehn and Moll (1976) interpreted their results to mean that, at a rapid speaking rate, "speakers have the option of either increasing velocity of movement or decreasing articulatory displacement." In other words, undershoot can be, and sometimes is, avoided by making more rapid approaches to targets.

Let us return to Figure 10-7D to see how movement might be speeded up to counteract the effect of short duration. This diagram shows that the displacement of the mass can be as extensive as in Figure 10-7B if the driving force (and thus the acceleration) is compensatorily increased and an opposite negative force is introduced to bring the system back on time. In the light of Figure 10-7D the phonetic behavior observed by Kuehn and Moll accordingly implies that the muscular forces underlying speech produced more rapidly may have to be reorganized not only temporally but with respect to amplitude as well. That talkers are indeed capable of such behavior will be suggested also by the following results.

Figure 10-8 shows average jaw movement data plotted against gesture duration for three speakers, A, B, and C. Measurements were made of maximum jaw excursion in the vowel of the stressed syllable ['dad:] whose duration was systematically manipulated by varying the number of syllables of the word in which it occurred (Lyberg, 1981). The talkers were instructed to produce the test words under three conditions: with soft, normal, and loud voice effort. The results indicate that the extent of mandibular displacement depends on two factors: duration and vocal effort. Since it seems reasonable to assume that vocal effort is correlated with the muscular force driving the jaw, these observations provide some additional justification for applying the simplified mechanical model of Figure 10-7 (10-7D in particular) to the complexities of speech. The data of Figure 10-8 cluster around falling exponential curves and accordingly demonstrate a tendency toward duration-dependent undershoot behavior at all levels of vocal effort. On the other hand, the undershoot relative to the normal target (= asymptote of normal curves) can evidently be avoided (and turned into overshoot) by invoking a more forceful gesture.

Phonetic observations indicate that for many languages vowel reduction is a common phenomenon. It appears in spontaneous speech. It surfaces in formalized form in phonologies. It is similar to coarticulation in that its degree can be to some extent independently controlled. It is an example of a general process of reduction that can apply not only to vowels but also to other units such as consonants and syllables. The degree to which this process is manifested is language dependent but its occurrence is general and widespread presumably because of our universal tendency as speakers to hypo- rather than hyperarticulate.

If the analogy of Figure 10-7 is pursued somewhat further we can formulate an explanation of this behavior in terms of mechanics. Physics teaches us that work equals force times distance and that power is work per unit time. With these definitions in mind we now look at Figures 10-7C and 10-7D. We find that in comparison with Figure 10-7B the undershoot case is characterized by an unchanged value of the driving force but a reduced distance, whereas the case of no undershoot requires increased force to produce the desired displacement. Consequently, in the undershoot situation less work is being done over time as compared with the reorganized movement.

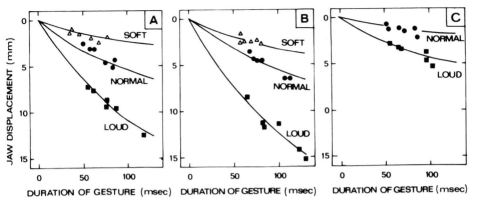

Figure 10-8. Jaw excursion for stressed vowel in [′dad:] is seen to depend on two factors: duration of jaw opening gesture and degree of vocal effort (three speakers: A, B, C).

Summarizing, we can say that the frequent occurrence of reduction processes in speech, here typified by vowel observations, provides additional evidence that extremes are avoided. Extreme displacements and extreme velocities are avoided. The system is indeed capable of raising the level of its performance, but as any phonetician will testify, it "prefers" not to. Generalizing from the physics of the spring–mass system to speech, we find that speech production appears to operate as if physiological processes were governed by a *power constraint* limiting energy expenditure per unit time.

IV. Speech and General Motor Behavior

The preceding analysis of coarticulation was presented to draw attention to what we have called the synergy constraint which governs static *spatial* relations among articulatory components. Vowel reduction was introduced to suggest a power constraint which also operates dynamically in the *temporal* domain. The claim that spatial and temporal extremes are avoided finds extensive additional support in research on motor behavior in general, and in many areas of phonetic observation too vast to receive a detailed treatment here.[4] Some reference to this evidence is nevertheless necessary.

---

[4]Pike (1943):

> ... extreme displacements do not occur in speech (e.g., the tongue tip against the uvula) ... spasmodic forms (e.g. belches, sneezes, hiccoughs, and some kinds of laughter) ... do not produce speech norms. (pp. 149–151)

It is easy to observe the synergy constraint at work in our everyday life outside the laboratory. Consider for instance the cleaning of a window, a task that can be accomplished in natural as well as unnatural ways (Figure 10-9). The window cleaner's two approaches may be compared with two analogous ways of producing the vowel [i]: by lowering the jaw and compensatorily raising the tongue (above) or by raising both in synergistic interaction (normal case, below).

The window cleaner tells us that the explanation of coarticulation proposed earlier cannot be specific to speech since the coordination of articulators parallels the organization of nonspeech gestures. Our examples show the following analogous relationships:

$$\frac{\text{tongue tip}}{\text{tongue body}} \simeq \frac{\text{tongue body}}{\text{jaw}} \simeq \frac{\text{arm} + \text{body}}{\text{feet}}$$

$$\text{(coarticulation)} \qquad \text{[i]} \qquad \text{(window cleaner)}$$

In the phonetic literature "ease of articulation" has often been criticized as an explanation for historical sound changes and the modifications that phonetic segments undergo in speech development (Kiparsky, 1970; Jakobson, 1941, 1962). Equally frequently one comes across positive treatments (Kiparsky, 1975; Donegan, 1978). There are several reasons why this principle has failed to attract the serious attention of theoretically oriented linguists. One difficulty is no doubt the circumstance that articulatory "economy" interacts in complex ways with other demands and functions shaping speech.

It is important to bear in mind that, if there is such a thing as an economy of effort criterion in speech, it must be assumed to be *teleologically* controlled. In other words, speech is similar to other motor behaviors in that muscular force levels are tailored to the needs of the situation (Granit, 1977). Economizing occurs only insofar as it is purposeful. Thus in speech it occurs only insofar as communicative, listener-oriented goals permit. EMG records of the muscles of respiration, mastication, and swallowing are rather "quiet" during normal speech but become by comparison very "loud" in chewing[5] and eating and breathing during hard physical work. Speech prefers the *physiological pianissimo*—so long as the purpose of the utterance is served and the linguistic job gets done.

---

[5]Carlsöö (1952):

Some anatomists, e.g. Benninghoff (1949, maintain that, when the mandible performs its closing movement, the masseter muscle comes into action probably only when the mandible has to overcome resistance, as, for instance, in mastication. On the other hand, when the movement takes place without any resistance, as, in speech, the movement is, in all likelihood, performed by the temporal muscle alone. (p. 13)

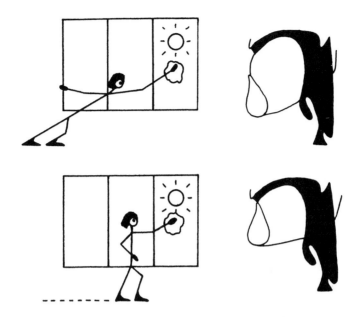

Figure 10-9. Analogy between speech and nonspeech gestures.

Speech movements are strikingly effortless and highly automatized but so are other movements (e.g., handwriting, the gestures of sign language, and piano playing). "Thus, in man learning to manipulate tools all muscles of a limb are fired during the training period, while in the end only agonists and antagonists act in harmonious alternation . . . " (Granit, 1970, p. 216). What motor control parameters are optimized in skilled and voluntary movements? What are the mechanisms? Grillner (1975) has said, "During ambulation the four limbs of a tetrapod have to be moved in such a manner that they can jointly provide the suitable forward force at a minimal energy expenditure. This must be carried out with a maintained equilibrium." Cavagna, Heglund, and Taylor (1977) observe that "What at first seemed a bewildering array of models of locomotion— bipedal walking in humans and in birds, quadrupedal walking in mammals, trotting, galloping and hopping—can all be reduced to two general mechanisms, a pendulum and a spring which have been utilized either singly or in combination, to minimize the expenditure of chemical energy by the muscles for lifting and reaccelerating the center of mass within each stride." There is, moreover, evidence indicating that energy expenditure is greater than normal when human subjects are forced to walk in a way that interferes with normal arm movements (e.g., with their backs immobilized and the rotation movements of the shoulders and the pelvis eliminated; Chapman & Ralston, 1964).

Comparing speech and nonspeech movements, we find many similarities. They both obey the rule that, if possible, extremes are avoided. This in turn reflects the fact that energy expenditure tends to be minimized. Consequently there is strong evidence for the existence of physiological mechanisms that automatically generate such behavior, but so far there appears to be only limited understanding of their precise nature in speech.

V. Phonological Adaptations

A. Assimilation

When we study descriptions of how languages have changed historically we often find developments that seem to be phonetically motivated. A large class of such changes are called *assimilations*. This term is used to describe phonetic sequences where the production of a segment (vowel or consonant) becomes more similar to the production of an adjacent (preceding or following) segment. When the modification occurs as a result of the following segment we speak of *regressive* assimilation. When it happens under the influence of a preceding segment it is a *progressive* assimilation. The term may be used in several domains of linguistic description, for example, phonologically with reference to a historical change or a grammatically determined rule (synchronic phonological rule), and phonetically about fortuitous pronunciation effects in individual utterances.

   In the following we shall present a systematic list of phonological assimilations. The logical possibilities of regressive and progressive assimilatory interaction between vowels and consonants are indicated in Table 10-1. The point of this presentation, which will follow the order indicated in Table 10-1, is to show that there appears to be no logical possibility that languages leave unexploited (although certain statistical biases may no doubt exist—regressive cases occur more often than progressive ones, for instance).

Table 10-1. Logical Possibilities of Assimilation[a]

	Influenced by			
	Vowel		Consonant	
Segment	PRO	REG	PRO	REG
Vowel	1	2	3	4
			7a	8a
Consonant	5	6		
			7b	8b

[a]Key: PRO stands for progressive, REG for regressive, a for articulatory assimilation, and b for voicing assimilations.

1. A vowel is influenced by a preceding vowel.

a. Progressive i-umlaut (Old Swedish):

$$hialpa > hiælpa \qquad \text{(to help)}$$
$$biorn > biørn \qquad \text{(to bear)}$$

b. Progressive vowel harmony:

gül	(rose)	*at*	(horse)
güller	(roses)	*atlar*	(horses)

The plural ending is *-ler* or *-lar*, depending on preceding front or back stem vowel (cf. also Hungarian, Finnish).

2. A vowel is influenced by a following vowel.

	Old Norse		Old Swedish	
Umlaut:	γastiR	>	gæster	(guests)
	*xelpan	>	hialpa	(help)
Breaking:	*βernuR	>	biorn	(bear)

3. A vowel is influenced by a preceding consonant.

Old English		Middle English		Modern English	
a:	>	o:	>	u:	/CCV (two, who)
		a	>	ɔ	/CV (was, swan, quarrel)

Modern Chinese (standard Mandarin) has a phoneme /ï/ whose apicalized allophones [iᶻ] and [ɚ] obey the rule:

$$/\ddot{\text{i}}/ \rightarrow \left\{ \begin{array}{c} [\text{i}^z] \\ [\text{ɚ}] \end{array} \right\} \Big/ \left\{ \begin{array}{c} \text{dental} \\ \text{retroflex} \end{array} \; \text{sibilant} \right\} \underline{\qquad}$$

4. A vowel is influenced by a following consonant.

/ɪ/ → [ʊ]/_____ [ɫ]   in English *children*

/ε,ø/ → [æ, œ]/_____ [r]   in Swedish *ära, öra*

5. A consonant is influenced by a preceding vowel.

$$/x/ \rightarrow \left\{ \begin{array}{l} [\text{x}]/ \left\{ \begin{array}{l} +\text{back} \\ \text{vowel} \end{array} \right\} \underline{\qquad} \\ [\text{ç}]/\text{elsewhere} \end{array} \right\} \quad \text{German } \textit{Licht, acht}$$

Note *rauchen* [x] and *Frauchen* [ç], which indicate the necessity of including morpheme boundary information in a more accurate version of this rule.

6. A consonant is influenced by a following vowel.

$$/h/ \rightarrow \left\{ \begin{array}{l} \emptyset / \underline{\quad} u \\ \text{ç}/ \underline{\quad} i \\ h/ \underline{\quad} e, o, a \end{array} \right\} \text{Japanese}$$

A combination of 5 and 6 and voicing assimilation are found in:

[bʌt̮ɚ]   *butter*

                 in American English

[sɪt̮ɪŋ]   *sitting*

Latin		Spanish	cf. French	
rīpam	>	riba [β]	*rive*	(bank)
sētam	>	seda [ð]	*soie*	(silk)
focum	>	fuego [γ]	*feu*	(fire)

These cases, in particular the Spanish, could be regarded as instances of "phonological undershoot" relative to Latin.

7a. The articulation of a consonant is influenced by the articulation of a preceding consonant.

[haːbm, ziːbm̩]	German *haben, sieben*
[hæpm̩, beɪkŋ]	English *happen, bacon*
[Fœʂːt̮ ŋaːvadahanː]	Swedish *först snavade han*
cf. /føʂːtsnaː-/	(All dental consonants following /ʂː-/ get modified.)

7b. The voicing feature of a consonant is influenced by the voicing feature of a preceding consonant.

[-pl̥yj], [kr̥yj]	in Swedish	*paraply, kry*
[gɔtʃə]	in English	*got you!*
cf. [tj] > [tʃ]	in English	*feature, nature*

8a. The articulation of a consonant is influenced by the articulation of a following consonant.

English		Swedish	
improper	[-mʹp]	*Lin(d)blom*	[-mb-]
intolerable	[-nʹt-]	*Lin(d)dahl*	[-nd-]
incomplete	[-ŋʹk-]	*Lin(d)gren*	[-ŋg-]

Latin		Italian
scriptum	>	*scritto*
octō	>	*otto*
ruptum	>	*rotto*
somnus	>	*sonno*

8b. The voicing feature of a consonant is influenced by the voicing feature of a following consonant.

French:

[nɛʒ fɔ̃dy]	*neige fondue*
[sak̬ dɔR]	*sac d'or*
[yntRup̬dəsɔlda]	*une troupe de soldats*

German "Auslautverhärtung":

[taːk], [taːgə]	*Tag, Tage*
[gaːp], [gaːbən]	*gab, gaben*

The examples show devoicing of final consonant in anticipation of the abducted state of the glottis associated with normal breathing and silence.

Swedish adjectives (adverbs):

[trygːt]	*tryggt*	(secure(ly))	[trygː]	*trygg*
[snabːt]	*snabbt*	(quick(ly))	[snabː]	*snabb*

The majority of the illustrations are phonological assimilations at the supraglottal level. They demonstrate that the modification results in a sequence of segments between which the distance in articulatory space is reduced. In the case of the voicing assimilations (7b, 8b) aerodynamic factors must be considered in addition to the abduction–adduction movements of the vocal cords. The voicing changes nevertheless reinforce the overall conclusion to be drawn from the assimilation data: An assimilation—whether phonological (a historical fact or a grammatically significant pronunciation rule), or phonetic (a grammatically nonsignificant attribute of an individual utterance)—invariably implies shortened movement (glottal or supraglottal). If once more we compare speech production to a second-order mechanical system (Figure 10-7) and examine the efficiency of such a system in terms of its energy expenditure, we see that assimilation, defined as reduced distance between two sequentially timed articulatory targets, implies less work per unit time. In a mechanical system such a restructuring of a frequently used sequence of targets will obviously, in the long run, lower energy costs. Since languages do in fact restructure vowel and consonant targets in patterns of assimilation, it does not seem unreasonable to hypothesize by way of analogy that they do so to optimize motor control by minimizing physiological energy expenditure. When it appears in the phonology of a language, assimilation, we accordingly conclude, represents an adaptation to constraints that speech production shares with many other biological processes.

B. The Syllable: Segmental Organization

With the aid of the synergy and rate constraints we can make some qualitative predictions about favored phonotactic patterns of segment sequences in syllables: consonant–vowel sequences and consonant clusters. To do so we need an argument that we shall present in three steps: first a few comments on average syllable duration; second, some remarks on how the inherent characteristics of segments influence their ability to be coarticulated with other segments; and third, brief reference to concurrent demands for perceptual salience or distinctiveness.

Why is the *average* duration of syllables around 160–200 msec? Is it physiologically determined? If more culturally than physiologically determined, why then is it not more strongly influenced by the language spoken? These questions were raised by Lenneberg (1967, pp. 109–120), who reviewed evidence on various psychological and neurological "clocks" and proposed that speech timing was based on an underlying "physiological rhythm consisting of periodic changes of states at a rate of 6 ± 1 cps."

An alternative idea (Brodda, 1979) is that 160–200 msec represents an adaptation to speech biomechanics and that this is related to the "resonant frequency" of the structures performing the opening–closing movement typical of the syllable (i.e., principally the mandible). Preliminary attempts to obtain approximate information on the frequency response of the mandible (Sorokin, Gay, & Ewan, 1980) have been made and are not incompatible with Brodda's suggestion. Driving a system at a rate close to its natural frequency of vibration is an energy-saving arrangement (cf. pushing a swing). Perhaps other gross timing universals of speech could be understood along similar lines. The respiratory system and phonatory structures would on this view condition utterance length and the duration of tonal (fundamental frequency) events. The response characteristics of the lips, tongue tip, and tongue body would influence inherent segment durations and contribute toward determining intrasyllabic temporal organization (cf. the rapid flaps and trills of the tongue tip and uvula vs. the slower vowel- and consonant-related movements of the tongue body). It thus appears justified to conclude that in all probability the average duration of a syllable, or a segment, is not an arbitrary but to a significant extent a biomechanically and physiologically conditioned figure. The syllable thus provides a fairly fixed time frame within which consonant and vowel events are constrained to take place. (It is true on the one hand that the presence of large clusters in a syllable does indeed increase its duration. On the other hand, there is clear evidence of compensatory shortening of a given segment as a function of cluster size, reflecting an adjustment toward constant syllable duration; Lindblom, Lyberg, & Holmgren, 1976.)

The second point is the observation that pairs of arbitrary speech sounds differ in terms of articulatory compatibility. The previous treatments of co-articulation, vowel reduction, and assimilation were developed from that observation. For example, assimilations were analyzed as reductions of distance in the articulatory space, that is, as developments toward greater articulatory compatibility of sequential gestures.

Third, it was pointed out earlier that motor optimization must not be assumed to operate in isolation but only along with other factors. There is the obvious requirement on any communicative code that semantically distinct information (syllables and words meaning different things) remain perceptually distinct for the listener. This constraint—let us term it the *distinctiveness condition*—is in conflict with the forces bringing about assimilations, reductions, and omissions. In evolving their inventories of syllabic structures languages have thus had to make compromises.

Against the background of the preceding three points it appears natural to ask whether syllables can be seen as such perceptual–motor compromises. One might for instance expect that syllabic structures are sequences that have evolved to facilitate coarticulation (i.e., meet the synergy constraints) given (a) the conflicting distinctiveness condition and (b) the physiological limitations on articulatory rate (the rate constraint), as well as (c) the factors restricting the variation of syllable duration.[6] With this expectation in mind let us see what we find in consonant–vowel sequences and in consonant clusters. More precisely, how does "facilitation of coarticulation" manifest itself?

Normal vowels appear to be primarily tongue-body or dorsal articulations. Occasionally vowels become apicalized (cf. Section V.A. 3). Vowel systems containing a subset of retroflex vowels have been reported (Crothers, 1978; Sedlak, 1969) but are apparently rare. In a universal phonetic study of consonant inventories Nartey (1979, p. 37) states that the "preferred set of consonants in a given language is:

```
        p           t    tʃ    |    k
            f    s              |
        m        n              |
```

As we compare this inventory with the IPA symbols for nasals, voiceless stops, and fricatives:

---

[6]Consider this hypothesis in the light of tongue twisters and the phonetic problems of a student beginning to learn a second language.

Nasals	m	ɱ	n	ɳ			ɲ	ŋ	N
Stops	p		t	ʈ			c	k	q
Fricatives	ɸ	f	θs	ʂ	ʃ	ɕ	ç	x	χ	ħ
Extremes of vowel space							i	u	a

Nondorsal   Dorsal

we note a striking preference in Nartey's data for anterior, nondorsal places of articulation. It appears possible to conclude that there are universal place-of-articulation preferences that are different for consonants and for vowels. These results imply then that the preferred consonant–vowel (CV) sequence is one that uses independent, spatially compatible articulators and that makes temporal overlap of adjacent gestures possible. Note incidentally that the alternation between anterior (nondorsal) and posterior (dorsal) articulations reinforces the partly source-dependent tendency for consonants to exhibit high-pass and vowels to have low-pass spectral characteristics. Perceptual benefits no doubt accrue from such sequential acoustic contrast (Kawasaki & Ohala, 1980). We see then that the typical CV syllable does indeed seem to be built to facilitate coarticulation within the limits of the synergy and rate constraints and the perceptual salience condition.

The consonant sequences of Swedish have been thoroughly investigated (Sigurd, 1965; Elert, 1970; Brodda, 1979). It is of interest to note here that initial clusters, and to some extent final clusters, show differentiation with respect to both manner and place of the consonants. There is, for instance, a marked tendency for /j/, /v/, and /l/ to be preceded by inhomorganic consonants. In agreement with this rule the permissible Swedish three-consonant clusters that contain these segments are /spj/, /spl/, and /skv/. This tendency toward place and manner differentiation provides support to a generalized version of our previous interpretation of the CV results: The preferred syllabic organization is one with segments that use independent, spatially compatible articulators and that make temporal overlap of adjacent gestures possible.

We should also mention here the absence of rapid intrasyllabic alternations of inspiration and expiration. The universally preferred airstream mechanism appears to be expiratory (with marginal exceptions). A similarly no doubt energy-saving arrangement is observed in the distribution of phonation types (e.g., voicing–devoicing). Clusters do not allow *[+voiced C] [−voiced C]V initially, nor its mirror image finally. However, they do allow the other possible combinations of voicing states. These observations, which are valid not only for Swedish, provide additional evidence of phonotactic consequences of the rate and synergy constraints.

As a further example of the systematic nature of consonant cluster data consider what has been called the *vowel adherence* (Sigurd, 1965) or *sonority principles* (Jespersen, 1926; Hooper, 1976). These terms refer to the fact that consonants in clusters vary with respect to their preferred distance to the sonority peak (vowel). Elert (1970) proposed the following hierarchy for Swedish initial and final consonant groups:

Sonority class:	I	II	III	IV	V
		p t k	m		
	s				
	ɦ	b d g	n	j	r
				v	l
	f		ŋ		

This grouping implies that in a typical two- or three-consonant cluster the expected order of consonants is such that in positions successively closer to the vowel a monotonic increase (decrease) in sonority is observed in an initial (final) cluster. Thus the data show [skr-, skv-, str-, spj-, spr-, spl-] but not *[rks-, vks-, etc.]. In the usage of Swedish linguists [r] and [l] show greater vowel adherence than, for instance, stops and fricatives. Such phonotactic patterns do not seem to be a peculiarity of Swedish but seem to have some generality across languages. We find that Jespersen (1926) built his definition of the syllable around the concept of sonority and saw it as a determinant of syllable structure. Hooper (1976) has tried to describe similar regularities in many languages in terms of universal "strength" hierarchies. Do these findings support the hypothesis that syllable structures tend to evolve to facilitate coarticulation while maintaining sufficiently functional perceptual properties?

In the context of applying the constraints developed so far to cluster data the following hypothesis suggests itself:

> *Segments that are more difficult to coarticulate show up in positions remote from each other, whereas more compatible sounds tend to be relatively more adjacent in the syllable.*

We can throw light on this assumption with the aid of the following experiment to investigate the extent to which the Swedish consonants mentioned in Elert's sonority hierarchy are coarticulated with adjacent vowels. Examples of the observed parameter (jaw movement) and some test words are shown at the top of Figure 10-10. Measurements were made of the position of the jaw relative to clench during the consonant. Observations were made in stressed syllables and for both final and initial positions of the consonants [a'Cɑ:, 'ɑ:C, 'aC:], at least six repetitions of each test item. The graph at the bottom in Figure 10-10 shows a plot of sonority as defined phonotactically by Elert versus jaw position for the consonant averaged over all repetitions and test frames. There is a clear correlation between sonority and jaw position. In other words, rank in the sonority hierarchy and the extent of mandibular coarticulation parallel each other. This result is not incompatible with our idea that segments that are articulatorily relatively incompatible tend to show up in positions more distant from each other, whereas segments that permit more extensive coarticulation tend to assume more adjacent positions. It is also

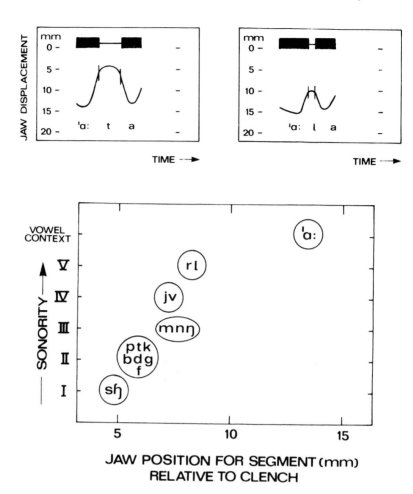

Figure 10-10. Top: Jaw movement records. Curves sampled at peaks during consonants—a measure taken to indicate the propensity of the consonant to be influenced by adjacent vowels. Bottom: Phonotactically based sonority categories plotted against jaw position (coarticulation "propensity").

compatible with the fact that initial and final patterns are close to mirror images of each other. Extending these results beyond jaw movement to all other articulatory parameters, we see that the sonority or vowel adherence hierarchy is a matter of coarticulation propensity,[7] which in turn results from the interplay of the rate and synergy constraints and the inherent characteristics of speech segments.

---

[7]Lack of space prevents our expanding on this point. It would be possible to use this hypothesis to explain the special status of [s] as the minimally vowel-adherent consonant in Germanic clusters with reference to its inherent coarticulatory properties. For evidence on the special resistance to coarticulation that a British [s] offers see Bladon and Nolan (1977).

VI. Summary

The goal of this chapter has been to show that languages tend to evolve sound patterns that can be seen as adaptations to the motor mechanisms of speech production. Evidence for such adaptations was obtained from studies of assimilations and the segmental organization of the syllable, for example, the phonotactic patterns of consonant–vowel sequences and consonant clusters. It was hypothesized that the phonological regularities discussed arise out of biological processes that are not unique to speech but are characteristic of motor behavior in general. They interact with concurrent perceptual demands on the speech code and serve the purpose of minimizing the expenditure of physiological energy. This interpretation was preceded by demonstrating that an analysis of the phonetic facts on vowel reduction and coarticulation is possible and can be made insightfully if a criterion of motor "economy" is introduced. It is hoped that these results may be of some use in the context of a biological theory of language that aims at deriving linguistic elements and processes deductively rather than postulating them axiomatically.

Acknowledgments. The author gratefully acknowledges the collaborative efforts of Judith Hutchison, Richard Schulman, and Johan Sundberg in the experimental and modeling projects, and has profited from numerous discussions of the present topic with Tom Gay, Sten Grillner, Tore Janson, Jim Lubker, Peter MacNeilage, and Michael Studdert-Kennedy.

References

Bellugi, U., & Studdert-Kennedy, M. (Eds.) *Sign language and spoken language: Biological constraints on linguistic form.* Weinheim–New York: Dahlem Workshop, Verlag Chemie, 1980.

Bladon, R. A. W., & Nolan, F. J. A video-fluorographic investigation of tip and blade alveolars in English. *Journal of Phonetics*, 1977, 5, 185–193.

Brodda, B. Något om de Svenska Ordens Fonotax och Morfotax. *Papers from the Institute of Linguistics, University of Stockholm*, 1979, *38*.

Carlsöö, S. Nervous coordination and mechanical function of the mandibular elevators. *Acta Odontologica Scandinavica*, 1952, *10* (Suppl. 11), Stockholm.

Carlsöö, S. *Människans Rörelser.* Stockholm: Personaladministrativa rådet, 1968.

Cavagna, G. A., Heglund, N. C., & Taylor, C. R. Mechanical work in terrestrial locomotion: Two basic mechanisms for minimizing energy expenditure. *American Journal of Physiology*, 1977, *233*(5), R243–R261.

Chapman, M. W., & Ralston, H. J. Effect of immobilization of the back and arms on energy expenditure during level walking. Unpublished report summarized by Carlsöö, 1964.

Chomsky, N. *Problems of knowledge and freedom: The Russell lectures.* London: Fontana, 1972.

Crothers, J. Typology and universals of vowel systems. In J. H. Greenberg (Ed.), *Universals of human language* (Vol. 2). Stanford, Cal.: Stanford University Press, 1978.

Donegan, P. J. *On the natural phonology of vowels*. Unpublished doctoral dissertation, Ohio State University, 1978.

Elert, C. -C. *Ljud och Ord i Svenskan*. Stockholm: Almqvist & Wiksell, 1970.

Gay, T. Effect of speaking rate on vowel formant movements. *Journal of the Acoustical Society of America*, 1978, *63*(1), 223–230.

Gay, T., Ushijima, T., Hirose, H., & Cooper, F. S. Effect of speaking rate on labial consonant–vowel articulation. *Journal of Phonetics*, 1974, *2*, 47–63.

Granit, R. *The basis of motor control*. London and New York: Academic Press, 1970.

Granit, R. *The purposive brain*. Cambridge, Mass.: MIT Press, 1977.

Grillner, S. Locomotion in vertebrates: Central mechanisms and reflex interaction. *Physiological Review*, 1975, *55*, 247–304.

Halle, M. Confessio grammatici. *Language*, 1975, *51*(3), 525–535.

Hooper, J. B. *An introduction to natural generative phonology*. New York: Academic Press, 1976.

Jakobson, R. *Kindersprache, Aphasie und Allgemeine Lautgesetze*. Uppsala, 1941. Reprinted in *Selected Writings* (Vol. 1). The Hague: Mouton, 1962.

Jespersen, O. *Lehrbuch der Phonetik*. Leipzig and Berlin: Teubner, 1926.

Kawasaki, H., & Ohala, J. J. Acoustic basis for universal constraints on sound sequences. *Journal of the Acoustical Society of America*, 1980, *68*(S1), T14(A).

Kiparsky, P. Historical linguistics. In J. Lyons (Ed.) *New horizons in linguistics*. Harmondsworth, Mx, England: Penguin, 1970.

Kiparsky, P. Comments on the role of phonology in language. In J. F. Kavanagh & J. E. Cutting (Eds.), *The role of speech in language*. Cambridge, Mass.: MIT Press, 1975, 271–280.

Kiritani, S., Miyawaki, K., & Fujimura, O. A computational model of the tongue. *Annual Bulletin, Research Institute of Logopedics and Phoniatrics (University of Tokyo)*, 1976, *10*, 243–252.

Kuehn, D. P. *A cinefluorographic investigation of articulatory velocities*. Unpublished doctoral dissertation, University of Iowa, 1973.

Kuehn, D. P., & Moll, K. L. A cineradiographic study of VC and CV articulatory velocities. *Journal of Phonetics*, 1976, *4*, 303–320.

Lenneberg, E. H. *Biological foundations of language*. New York: Wiley, 1967.

Liljencrants, J., & Lindblom, B. Numerical simulation of vowel quality systems: The role of perceptual contrast. *Language*, 1972, *48*, 839–862.

Lindblom, B. *On vowel reduction*. (FL thesis, University of Uppsala). Royal Institute of Technology, Speech Transmission Laboratory Report No. 29, 1963. (a)

Lindblom, B. Spectrographic study of vowel reduction. *Journal of the Acoustical Society of America*, 1963, *35*, 1773–1781. (b)

Lindblom, B. Articulatory activity in vowels. *Speech Transmission Laboratory Quarterly Progress and Status Report*, 1964, *2*, 1–15.

Lindblom, B. *On the production and recognition of vowels*. Unpublished doctoral dissertation, Lund University, 1968.

Lindblom, B. Experiments in sound structure. Plenary address, 8th International Congress of Phonetic Sciences, Leeds, 1975.

Lindblom, B. Phonetic universals in vowel systems. In J. J. Ohala (Ed.), *Experimental Phonology*. New York: Academic Press, 1982.

Lindblom, B., Lubker, J., & Gay, T. Formant frequencies of some fixed-mandible vowels and a model of speech motor programming by predictive simulation. *Journal of Phonetics*, 1979, *7*, 147–161.

Lindblom, B., Lyberg, B., & Holmgren, K. Durational patterns of Swedish phonology: Do they reflect short-term motor memory processes? 1976. Also reproduced by the Indiana University Linguistics Club, Jan. 1981.

Lindblom, B., Pauli, S., & Sundberg, J. Modeling coarticulation in apical stops. In G. Fant (Ed.), *Proceedings of the Speech Communication Seminar (Speech Communication*, Vol. 2). Stockholm: Almqvist & Wiksell, 1974.

Lindblom, B., & Sundberg, J. Acoustic consequences of lip, tongue, jaw and larynx movement. *Journal of the Acoustical Society of America*, 1971, *50*, 1166–1179.

Lyberg, B. *Temporal properties of spoken Swedish*. Unpublished doctoral dissertation, Stockholm University, 1981.

Nartey, J. N. A. A study in phonemic universals, especially concerning fricatives and stops. *UCLA Working Papers in Phonetics*, 1979, *46*.

Ohala, J. J. *On the origin of sound patterns in language*. (forthcoming).

Öhman, S. E. G. Coarticulation in VCV utterances: Spectrographic measurements. *Journal of the Acoustical Society of America*, 1966, *39*(1), 151–168.

Perkell, J. S. *A physiologically oriented model of tongue activity during speech production*. Unpublished doctoral dissertation, Massachusetts Institute of Technology, 1974.

Pike, K. L. *Phonetics*. Ann Arbor: University of Michigan Press, 1943.

Sedlak, P. Typological considerations of vowel quality systems. *Working Papers on Language Universals (Stanford University)*, 1969, *1*, 1–40.

Sigurd, B. *Phonotactic structures*. Lund: Berlingska, 1965.

Sorokin, V. N., Gay, T., & Ewan, W. G. Some biomechanical correlates of jaw movement. *Journal of the Acoustical Society of America*, 1980, *68* (S1), S32(A).

Stevens, K. N. The quantal nature of speech: Evidence from articulatory–acoustic data. In E. E. David & P. B. Denes (Eds.), *Human communication: A unified view*. New York: McGraw-Hill, 1972.

Stevens, K. N., & House, A. S. Perturbation of vowel articulations by consonantal context: An acoustical study. *Journal of Speech and Hearing Research*, 1963, *6*, 111–128.

Wilson, E. *Sociobiology*. Cambridge: Belknap Press, 1975.

Chapter 11
Design Features of Speech Sound Systems

KENNETH N. STEVENS

I. Introduction

A fundamental premise in the study of speech is that an utterance can be represented as a sequence of underlying segments. The evidence for this premise is primarily linguistic, and this evidence is derived from the fact that a wide variety of phonological regularities in language appear to operate over the domain of the segment.

Each underlying segment in an utterance of a language can be described in terms of a set of features or natural classes (Jakobson, Fant, & Halle, 1963). The hypothesis on which the discussion in this chapter is based is that each feature is represented in the sound wave as a unique acoustic property to which the auditory system responds in a distinctive way. The production of a segment is organized in such a way as to achieve the desired acoustic goals or properties that identify the features of the segment. A consequence of this strategy is that the articulatory structures are programmed to achieve an appropriate sequence of target configurations or states. There appear to be 15–20 features that describe the phonetic contrasts in all languages, and any one language selects a subset of 10–15 of these.

Situations often arise in which a particular feature does not play a role in signaling a phonetic contrast in a certain context in a language. In this case, a speaker of the language may have some freedom in actualizing some attributes of the segment, and this freedom or variability is often determined by the phonetic context in which the segment occurs. The ways in which such segments are to be produced in different contexts are usually specified in terms of a set of rules, some of which may be optional.

Our principal concern in this chapter is with the following question: What are the constraints that the speech production and perception systems impose on the selection of the features? That is, what are the factors governing the selection of acoustic properties that form the building blocks for speech sound systems in language? A subsidiary question that will also be addressed is: Given that these acoustic properties are present in the speech signal for an utterance in a given language, but do not constrain all aspects of the signal, what is the nature of the additional constraints that are imposed on the pattern of sound that is generated for the utterance?

With regard to the factors governing the selection of features, we will argue that one or possibly both of the following conditions should be met:

1. The sound output for a particular target configuration or state of the articulatory structures should be distinctive in the sense that it has acoustic properties that are significantly different from the properties associated with some other configuration. For small perturbations of the configuration, parameters of the sound resulting from the articulatory configuration should be relatively stable. When the perturbation is sufficiently large, then the acoustic properties change abruptly. Ranges of articulatory parameters within which the acoustic properties are relatively insensitive to articulatory perturbations seem to be preferred in selecting or delimiting an inventory of speech sounds for use in language (Stevens, 1972).
2. For a group of speech sounds forming a particular natural class, the sound output has a well-defined property that produces a distinctive response in the auditory system. As perturbations in the physical characteristics of the sound are made, a listener cannot easily discriminate these changes over some regions of the physical parameters, but can readily discriminate changes of similar magnitude over some other regions. That is, the auditory system does not discriminate these acoustic differences in a continuous fashion, but rather in a quantal manner (Liberman, Harris, Hoffman, & Griffith, 1957). This property of the auditory system is exploited in designing sound systems for use in language (Stevens, 1971a).

As we search for examples to illustrate these points, we will be referring to three kinds of data or observations: (1) psychoacoustic data and data from auditory physiology to indicate the nature of the auditory response to different sound patterns; (2) experimental and theoretical studies of the speech production system to determine what patterns of articulatory configurations and movements give rise to sound outputs with distinctive properties; and (3) acoustic analysis studies in which one looks for the recurrence of the same acoustic property for the same feature occurring in a variety of contexts. From the 15–20 features that define natural classes in different languages, we have selected a few features for discussion, in order to illustrate the role of speech production and auditory perception in establishing these classes.

II. Examples of Features and Their Articulatory and Acoustic Correlates

A. Rapid versus Slow Spectrum Change

Some classes of speech sounds are produced with a narrow constriction in the oral cavity. These sounds are all consonants, and a consequence of the narrow constriction is that at the release of the consonant, and at the implosion if it follows a vowel, there is a rapid change in the spectrum of the sound over a brief time interval of 20-odd msec (Stevens, 1971b). This change occurs because the rapid opening of the constriction causes rapid movements of some of the natural frequencies of the vocal tract, and hence rapid movements of the spectral peaks. The change in spectrum shape could also occur as a consequence of a rapid shift in the location of the source of sound in the vocal tract. Significant differences can be observed in the rate of movement of the spectral peaks in syllables like [wa, ha, ʔa] (for which the movements are relatively slow) compared with that in syllables like [ta, ba, ma] (for which the movements are rapid).

Examples of short-time spectra sampled at about 8-msec intervals at the release of the syllables [bæ] and [ʔ æ] and at the time of maximum rate of movement of the formants for [wæ] are shown in Figure 11-1. The change in the overall spectrum shape is much greater for [b] than for [ʔ] and [w], and there is a greater movement of the first formant frequency for [b] within this brief time interval of about 16 msec.

There is some evidence from experiments in speech perception that changes in the rate of movement of the formants at the consonant–vowel boundary result in a relatively abrupt shift in perception from a glide (e.g., [wa]) to a stop (e.g., [ba]) as the rate changes from slow to fast (Liberman, Delattre, Gerstman, & Cooper, 1956). Although more perceptual experiments are needed to document this finding in a more detailed way, it does seem as though listeners are predisposed to divide sounds into two classes, depending on a property that describes the rate of the change of the spectrum.

B. Strident

In English the consonants [s š z ž č ǰ] are distinguished from other consonants by the fact that they contain substantial noise energy. These consonants are members of the class *strident*. Acoustic measurements show that the amplitude of the noise in the high-frequency region for these consonants exceeds the spectral amplitude of the adjacent vowel in the same frequency region. Thus as the ongoing sound pattern proceeds from the consonant to the next vowel there is a fall in the amplitude of the spectrum at high frequencies. On the other hand, in a syllable beginning with the nonstrident consonant [θ] (*th*in), the spectral amplitude in the consonant is lower than that of the vowel at all frequencies,

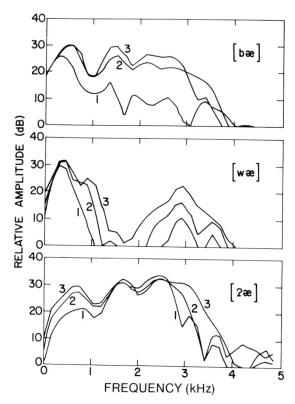

Figure 11-1. Short-time spectra sampled at about 8-msec intervals at the release of the consonants [b, w, ʔ] as indicated. The successive points in time at which the spectra are sampled are numbered. The duration of the time window is about 12 msec, and the speech is preemphasized at high frequencies. These examples are intended to show that there is a rapid change in the spectrum at the release of [b] but not for [w] and [ʔ].

including the high frequencies (except at frequencies above about 4.5 kHz, where the spectral amplitude of the consonant somewhat exceeds that of the vowel).

Examples of spectra of [s] and [θ], together with spectra sampled immediately after the vowel onset in the words *sin* and *thin* are shown in Figure 11-2. The spectrum for [s] has substantial high-frequency amplitude that exceeds the spectral amplitude for the adjacent vowel in the critical bands at high frequencies. Perceptual experiments with synthetic speech have verified in a qualitative way this finding that a fricative consonant is heard as being in one class (nonstrident) if the high-frequency spectral amplitude rises into the following vowel, and in another class (strident) if the amplitude in this frequency region falls (Stevens, 1981). This is intuitively a reasonable finding from the point of view of auditory psychophysics and physiology, since a rise in amplitude gives a response that is qualitatively different from a fall in amplitude.

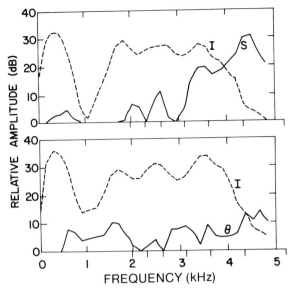

Figure 11-2. Short-time spectra sampled in the consonants [s] (upper panel) and [θ] (lower panel) in the words *sin* and *thin*. Also shown (dashed curves) are spectra of the vowel immediately following the onset of voicing. The frequency scale is linear, but it is also marked with ticks to indicate the frequency spans of critical bands in the high-frequency range. In the highest critical band in this frequency range, the spectral amplitude for [s] is well above that for the adjacent vowel, whereas for [θ] it is not. Spectra are calculated as in Figure 11-1.

From the point of view of articulation, strident consonants are produced by directing a rapid airstream against an obstacle (usually the lower teeth), giving rise to a significantly higher sound energy due to turbulence noise than the sound energy from turbulence in an unobstructed airstream. The noise generation process is qualitatively different in the two cases.

C. Place of Articulation for Consonants

One of the ways in which consonant sounds are classified is in terms of the place at which the constriction is made in the vocal tract. One such class is the coronal consonants, that is, consonants produced by forming a constriction with the tongue blade against the hard palate or teeth. These consonants appear to have a unique acoustic characteristic that can be described in terms of the gross shape of the spectrum sampled over a brief time interval in the vicinity of the consonantal release. This spectrum has energy in peaks that are distributed over a broad frequency region, and also has relatively high amplitude at high frequencies—a spectral amplitude that is equal to or greater than the spectral amplitude at high frequencies in the following vowel (Fant, 1973; Zue, 1976; Blumstein & Stevens, 1979).

An example of the spectrum sampled at the release for the consonant [d], together with the spectrum sampled near the beginning of the vowel, is shown in Figure 11-3a. The diffuse-rising shape, with substantial high-frequency energy, is evident in this example. The diffuse-rising spectrum shape is achieved by virtue of the fact that the natural frequencies of the vocal tract have a particular configuration when a constriction is made with the tongue blade—a configuration that gives rise to second and higher formants that are raised in frequency. The higher frequencies of these formants cause an increase in amplitude of the corresponding spectral peaks when there is a glottal source immediately following the consonantal release (Fant, 1960; Stevens & Blumstein, 1978). In stop and fricative consonants, the spectral amplitude at high frequencies is accentuated by the presence of a noise source at the constriction, and this noise is, in effect, filtered by the vocal tract to provide high-frequency energy in the sound. Experiments on the perception of synthetic consonant–vowel syllables in which the spectrum at onset is manipulated to give different spectrum shapes have shown that initial consonants are identified as coronals if the onset spectra have the attributes described above.

Other attributes of the onset spectrum appear to characterize other features that specify place of articulation for consonants. For example, for labial consonants spectral energy is also spread over a wide frequency range, but the spectrum is weak in high-frequency energy, in relation to the high-frequency spectral energy in the vowel. Velar consonants, on the other hand, have the property that the onset spectrum has a concentration of spectral energy within a limited range of middle frequencies (Fant, 1973; Blumstein & Stevens, 1979). Examples of spectra sampled at the release of a labial and a velar consonant are shown in Figure 11-3b, c.

D. Nasal

From the point of view of the speech production process, nasal segments are produced with the velopharyngeal port open, so that there is some acoustic coupling between the vocal tract proper and the nasal cavities. Acoustically, for a nasal consonant, this configuration results in a low-frequency spectral peak at about 250 Hz for adult speakers. This is a lower frequency than the first formant frequency for any vowel.

Perceptual experiments indicate that a consonant is heard as nasal if this low-frequency resonance is observed over at least a time interval of 20-odd msec in the vicinity of the consonant release, and if the amplitude of the spectral peak corresponding to this lowest resonance is at least as high as the spectral amplitude at about 250 Hz in the adjacent vowels (Stevens, 1981). If the spectral peak were of lower amplitude, the sound would be heard as a voiced

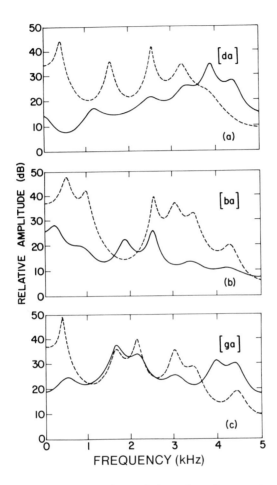

Figure 11-3. The solid lines in each panel show short-time spectra sampled at the onsets of [d], [b], and [g] in the syllables shown. The broken lines represent spectra sampled 15–20 msec after the onset of voicing for the vowel. The onset spectra are intended to show (a) a diffuse-rising shape for [d], with substantial high-frequency amplitude relative to the following vowel; (b) a diffuse-falling or flat shape for [b], with relatively low amplitude; and (c) a midfrequency spectral prominence for [g], with the spectral amplitude of this prominence being comparable to that in the following vowel. These spectra are obtained from the preemphasized speech wave, with a time window of about 26 msec, and are smoothed by using a linear prediction algorithm (Blumstein & Stevens, 1979).

stop consonant. Thus nasal consonants have rather well-defined acoustic properties that distinguish them from nonnasal consonants. The spectra in Figure 11-4 illustrate the low-frequency resonance for the nasal consonant in the utterance *a mail*, and show that the amplitude of this spectral peak is about equal to the spectral amplitude at this frequency at the beginning of the following vowel.

E. Obstruent

Another class of consonants, called *obstruent*, is defined in the articulatory domain by the presence of a pressure increase within the vocal tract during production of the consonant. This pressure increase occurs because a complete closure or a sufficiently narrow constriction is made within the vocal tract to contain the air. The acoustic consequence of this pressure increase is that turbulence noise is generated in the vicinity of the constriction at some point during production of the sound. This noise can occur either throughout the constriction interval (as in a fricative consonant) or at the release of a closure (as in a stop consonant), but in any case it will occur in the time interval in the vicinity of the region where the rapid spectrum change for the consonant occurs. Presumably a listener is sensitive to the presence or absence of this type of noise in the sound, and this attribute, then, defines the natural class of obstruent consonants.

F. Place of Articulation for Vowels

The acoustic information that distinguishes one vowel from another, and that can be used to classify vowels, resides in portions of the speech wave in which the spectrum is changing relatively slowly, and in which the amplitude of the sound within a syllabic nucleus is close to its maximum value. The spectrum shape for a vowel during such a time interval is determined primarily by the frequencies of the spectral peaks, or formants. These formants are directly related to the vocal-tract shape, as determined by the position and configuration of the tongue and lips (Fant, 1960).

An acoustic attribute that defines one of the vowel categories is the proximity of the first and second formants (F_1 and F_2). When F_1 and F_2 are within a few hundred hertz they form, in effect, a single broad energy concentration within the low-frequency region, and the spectral amplitude at high frequencies is relatively low. Vowels with this property are *back* vowels. When F_1 and F_2 are sufficiently far apart, there is a lack of spectral energy in the midfrequency region between the formants, and instead F_2 approaches F_3 and other higher formants. As a consequence, there is an increase in the spectral amplitude at these higher frequencies. These are called *front* vowels. Contrasting acoustic

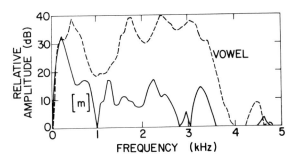

Figure 11-4. Short-time spectra sampled during the nasal murmur (solid line) and 20-odd msec after the release into the following vowel (broken line) in the utterance *a mail*. The procedure for obtaining the spectra is the same as for Figure 11-1. The intention here is to show that the spectral amplitude for the nasal murmur at the low-frequency peak is comparable to or slightly greater than that for the vowel immediately following the release.

spectra sampled in the middle of the vowels in the words *bet* and *but*, shown in Figure 11-5, illustrate the attributes that distinguish between these two classes of vowels. There is some evidence from psychoacoustic studies that a relatively sharp auditory distinction is made between a cluster of two formant peaks that are relatively close together (within 3–4 critical bands) and two formant peaks that are well separated in frequency (Chistovich & Lublinskaya, 1979). This experimental evidence suggests that for back vowels F_1 and F_2 form such a cluster of formants, whereas for front vowels F_1 and F_2 are well separated, and F_2 is clustered with F_3 (and possibly F_4). Thus it appears that one aspect of auditory processing of vowels favors a classification into these two categories. From the point of view of articulation, a vowel with closely spaced F_1 and F_2 is produced with the tongue body in a backed position, leading to a maximally low F_2, whereas a maximally high F_2 is produced with the tongue body in a fronted position (Fant, 1960; Stevens, 1972).

Another way in which vowels are classified is determined by the first formant frequency, independent of the frequencies of higher formants. If the lowest frequency peak in a vowel spectrum is within 3–4 critical bands of the low end of the frequency scale for audition, then the vowel falls into the class called *high* vowels. These vowels are produced with the tongue body raised as high as possible in the oral cavity without making too narrow a constriction. Spectrum envelopes for contrasting high and low vowels, shown in Figure 11-6, illustrate the low-frequency first-formant peak for the high vowel and the lack of spectral energy in the low-frequency region for the nonhigh vowel.

There are a number of other classes of vowels, in addition to the two just mentioned. Articulatory and perceptual bases for these vowel categories have not yet been quantified in detail, and must await a more thorough understanding of the auditory processing and production of vowels.

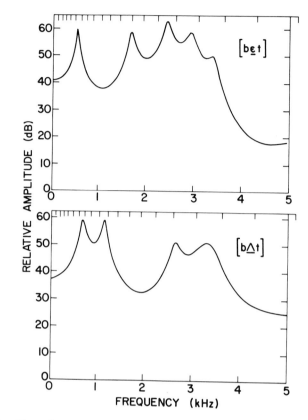

Figure 11-5. Short-time spectra for the front vowel [ɛ] and the back vowel [ʌ] in the words indicated. Spectra are obtained by using a linear prediction algorithm as in Figure 11-3. The ticks across the top of each panel delineate the widths of critical bands at different frequencies. For the back vowel [ʌ], the first and second formant peaks are separated by about 3 critical bands, whereas F_2 and F_3 are separated by less than 3 critical bands in the case of the front vowel [ɛ].

III. Constraints on Sound Patterns Other Than Those Described by Feature-Related Properties

In the discussion up to this point we have described some principles that appear to govern the design of sound systems for use in language, and we have given some examples of several features to illustrate how these principles might apply. Our view is that the speech stream can be characterized by sequences of segments, each of which is represented by a bundle of features. Associated with each feature there is an invariant acoustic property in the sound. The inventory of these acoustic properties and features is determined by the fact that the auditory system gives a distinctive response to sounds with these properties and

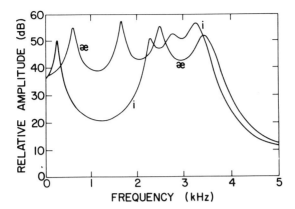

Figure 11-6. Examples of short-time spectra for a high vowel [i] and a low vowel [æ] showing that the high vowel has substantial low-frequency spectral amplitude (below about 400 Hz), whereas the low vowel does not.

the speech production system is capable of generating sounds with these properties.

When phonetic segments are concatenated to form syllables, words, and sentences, one often finds considerable variability in the sound pattern for a given segment, depending on the speaker, the phonetic context, and the speaking style and rate. This variability is governed by certain principles or rules, and the sound patterns that are used in language are determined both by principles specifying an inventory of invariant properties associated with features, as discussed earlier, and by principles that specify variable attributes of segments, particularly those that are influenced by phonetic context. We consider now some of these sources of variability.

There are, of course, times in the speech stream when the articulatory structures are in transition from one target configuration to the next. At these times, the attributes of the sound are influenced by the features of both of the adjacent segments. That is, there are points in time where the parameters of the speech signal do not have invariant properties determined by a particular feature, but are dependent on the features for at least two segments. An example is the transitions that occur in the second and higher formants following the release of a stop consonant in a consonant–vowel syllable. The time course of these transitions is determined both by the place of articulation of the consonant and by the vowel.

Another source of variability for a particular segment in a given language is that not all of the universal set of features specify oppositions in the language or are used to form natural classes in the language. As a consequence, those features that are nondistinctive often remain unspecified, and the acoustic properties associated with these features may show some variability. The variability often occurs because components of the speech production system that are not constrained by the features for a particular segment are free to be influenced by adjacent segments. In particular, these articulatory components are free to anticipate the configuration that is required for producing an upcoming segment, or to be influenced by a preceding segment.

For example, in English no words are distinguished solely on the basis of retroflexion of a stop consonant (although there are languages for which such a distinction does exist). Consequently, in producing the initial consonant cluster [tr], as in the word *trap*, American English speakers anticipate the [r] by producing a retroflex [ʈ]. Similar arguments can be used to explain several variants of the [t], all of which occur because the feature specification for this segment is, in a sense, incomplete. There are, however, certain acoustic properties that remain unchanged across all of these variants, since these are associated with features that are distinctive in the language. The feature *coronal*, for example, is one feature that all the [t]'s have in common. Examples of spectra sampled in the vicinity of the consonant release for [t] followed by two different vowels and by [r] are shown in Figure 11-7. While the major spectral peak is at different frequencies for these varieties of [t], all spectra have an overall diffuse-rising shape, at least up to about 2500 Hz. A more extensive discussion of the variants of stop consonants is given in Zue (1976).

Another example from English is the variation in the pronunciation of the back rounded vowel /u/ in different phonetic contexts. Spectrograms of the words *cube* and *boot* produced by an American English speaker are shown in Figure 11-8, together with spectra sampled in the middle of each vowel. The vowel in *cube* is produced with a relatively high F_2, characteristic of a front rather than a back vowel. The vowel is rounded, however, as evidenced by an F_3 value that is lower than F_3 for the unrounded front vowel [i]. Thus the rounding is preserved in the vowel of *cube*, although the front–back distinction is not preserved. In English, however, the front–back feature is not distinctive for high rounded vowels, and consequently it is not unreasonable for a speaker to exercise some latitude in actualizing this feature in this phonetic environment.

These contextual variations that occur in phonetic segments when certain

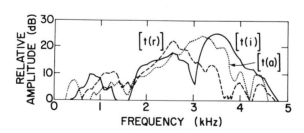

Figure 11-7. Spectra sampled at the release of the consonant [t] followed by three different segments: the front vowel [i], the back vowel [α], and the retroflex consonant [r]. The spectra have both similarities that are independent of context and differences that depend on the following segment.

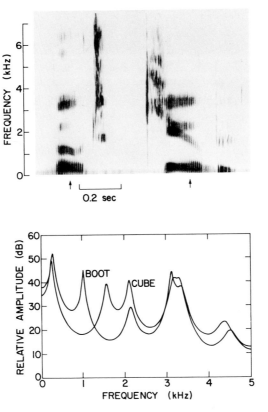

Figure 11-8. The upper panel shows spectrograms of the words *boot* (left) and *cube* (right) produced by a speaker of American English. Short-time spectra sampled within the two vowels, at the points indicated by the arrows, are displayed in the lower panel. The vowel in *cube* is produced with a more fronted tongue-body position (as evidenced by a higher F_2), but evidence for lip rounding remains.

features are not being utilized to specify contrasts appear to be of two kinds. There are some situations in which the feature in question gives rise to particular discrete acoustic properties depending on the context. Thus, for example, in English, the consonant [k] is consistently produced with a fronted constriction location before front vowels and a backed constriction before backed vowels, and these two versions have distinctive acoustic properties. On the other hand, there are other situations in which a continuous range of acoustic attributes can occur when a feature remains unspecified (as, e.g., in the case of /u/ discussed earlier).

In addition to the context-dependent influences on the acoustic manifestation of features that are not utilized to make distinctions in a language, there may be minor variations in the way a particular distinctive feature is implemented from one language to another. While the primary acoustic property identifying the feature remains invariant across languages, there may be secondary attributes that accompany the primary property and that vary from one language to another. Thus, for example, if a particular language tended to use a slightly more backed tongue-body position for producing coronal consonants, there could be an influence on the detailed acoustic spectrum of the consonants (cf. Figure 11-7) but not on the primary acoustic property that identifies coronal consonants as a class. The reasons for these cross-language variations in the detailed acoustic attributes that accompany the primary acoustic properties for certain features are not understood, and one can only make conjectures at this point as to the sources of these variations. These variations may, for example, be a consequence of an attempt to accentuate the perceptual contrast between phonetic categories (Liljencrants & Lindblom, 1972), or may result from a different "basis of articulation" or neutral vocal-tract posture from one language to another.

IV. Concluding Remarks

In conclusion, then, we can return to the question originally posed: What are the constraints that the speech production and perception systems impose on the sound patterns that are used in language?

On the one hand, the vocal tract as a generator of sound and the auditory system as a receiver of sound are structured in such a way that a limited set of acoustic properties is used to define the phonetic contrasts in language. Particular languages select from among these properties. We have given examples of properties that are acoustic correlates of the features consonantal, strident, nasal, and obstruent, and also certain features associated with place of articulation for consonants and vowels.

On the other hand, the strategy used by a speaker in achieving these acoustic properties or acoustic goals requires movement of the articulatory structures from one target configuration to another, and as a consequence, context-dependent acoustic attributes appear in the sound patterns. These context-dependent attributes are determined in part by the fact that some features do not play a role in defining phonetic contrasts for segments in some languages, and consequently some variation is permitted in the acoustic manifestation of these segments. The principles governing these variations depend on the language, the phonetic context, and the biomechanical properties of the speech production system, but at present these principles are not well understood.

Acknowledgments. This work was supported in part by grant NS-04332 from the National Institutes of Health. The contributions of Sheila Blumstein, Morris Halle, and Joseph Perkell in formulating the ideas presented in this chapter are gratefully acknowledged.

References

Blumstein, S. E., & Stevens, K. N. Acoustic invariance in speech production: Evidence from measurements of the spectral characteristics of stop consonants. *Journal of the Acoustical Society of America*, 1979, *66*, 1001–1017.

Chistovich, L. A., & Lublinskaya, V. V. The "center of gravity" effect in vowel spectra and critical distance between the formants: Psychoacoustical study of the perception of vowel-like stimuli. *Hearing Research* 1979, *1*, 185–195.

Fant, G. *Acoustic theory of speech production*. The Hague: Mouton, 1960.

Fant, G. *Speech sounds and features*. Cambridge, Mass.: MIT Press, 1973.

Jakobson, R., Fant, G., & Halle, M. *Preliminaries to speech analysis*. Cambridge, Mass.: MIT Press, 1963.

Liberman, A. M., Delattre, P. C., Gerstman, L. J., & Cooper, F. S. Tempo of frequency change as a cue for distinguishing classes of speech sounds. *Journal of Experimental Psychology*, 1956, *52*, 127–137.

Liberman, A. M., Harris, K. S., Hoffman, H. S., & Griffith, B. C. The discrimination of speech sounds within and across phoneme boundaries. *Journal of Experimental Psychology*, 1957, *54*, 358–368.

Liljencrants, J., & Lindblom, B. Numerical simulation of vowel quality systems: The role of perceptual contrast. *Language*, 1972, *48*, 839–862.

Stevens, K. N. Perception of phonetic segments: Evidence from phonology, acoustics, and psychoacoustics. In D. L. Horton & J. J. Jenkins (Eds.), *The perception of language*. Columbus, Ohio: Merrill, 1971, pp. 216–235. (a)

Stevens, K. N. The role of rapid spectrum changes in the production and perception of speech. In L. L. Hammerich, R. Jakobson, & E. Zwirner (Eds.), *Form and substance* (Festschrift for Eli Fischer-Jørgensen). Copenhagen: Akademsk Forlag, 1971, pp. 95–101. (b)

Stevens, K. N. The quantal nature of speech: Evidence from articulatory–acoustic data. In E. E. David and P. B. Denes (Eds.), *Human communication: A unified view*. New York: McGraw-Hill, 1972, pp. 51–66.

Stevens, K. N. Evidence for the role of acoustic boundaries in the perception of speech sounds. *Journal of the Acoustical Society of America*, 1981, *69* (Suppl. 1).

Stevens, K. N., & Blumstein, S. E. Invariant cues for place of articulation in stop consonants. *Journal of the Acoustical Society of America*, 1978, *64*, 1358–1368.

Zue, V. W. *Acoustic characteristics of stop consonants: A controlled study*. Unpublished doctoral dissertation, Massachusetts Institute of Technology, 1976. (Published as a research monograph by the University of Indiana Linguistics Club, 1980.)

Part III
Two Perspectives

Chapter 12

In Favor of Some Uncommon Approaches to the Study of Speech

M. Y. LIBERMAN

I. Introduction—Phonology vs. Phonetics

It is no secret that phonetics and phonology are two very different cultures, despite the close logical connection between their nominal aims. In education, in terminology, in research methods, in styles of argument, and in scientific journal and professional society allegiance, the divergence is striking.

When members of one group choose to take notice of work in the other camp, an undercurrent of something akin to ethnic prejudice is commonly quite plain. Most phonologists (at least unconsciously) subscribe to Trubetzkoy's dictum that phonetics is to phonology as numismatics is to economics. I do not know of an equally celebrated phrase to express the contrary prejudice; the phonetician's rejoinder might be that phonetics is to phonology as physics is to theology, except that theology is of insufficiently low academic status for this to have quite enough sting.

The editor of this volume has suggested that I play the role of phonologist among the phonetic lions. Such a role does not fit perfectly, but it offers me the opportunity to discuss this cultural divergence, which I think is becoming more and more harmful to work in both fields, and to describe some issues (in linguistics generally, and in speech production research in particular) where there is real promise for progress based on an approach that does not fit easily into the traditions of either group.

Justifying the Division of Labor

The notion of phonological analysis, in one form or another, underlies almost all work on human speech communication. This idea, in its basic form, holds that the sonic identity of the words of a given language can be expressed by combining elements drawn from a small set of semantically meaningless primitives. These primitives may be in the nature of phonemes, features, morae, or whatever, and the methods of combination range from simple concatenation to deployment in complex syllabic or even suprasyllabic structures.

In the two and a half millennia since Panini, in a dozen or so traditions around the world, those who have undertaken to study human speech and language have generally come to some form of this conclusion. Furthermore, each tradition of analysis seems to arrive fairly quickly at a particular hypothesis about the phonetic decomposition of the language or languages of local interest, a hypothesis that has what we might call "transcriptional adequacy." In other words, each such system of description offers a way to characterize the pronunciation of each word in the language, and perhaps goes on to differentiate some variant pronunciations, if this is desired. (In the case of Panini, it is at least etymologically misleading to call this representation a "transcription," since the Paninian tradition was apparently an oral one.) The discovery and codification of such a transcription system is always a big step forward, entirely apart from any practical use as an orthography, since it permits the collection of observations about spoken language and provides a common terminology for the discussion and elucidation of their meaning.

Once discovered, such descriptive systems are easily accepted and commonly used in the systematic study of speech; their fate as orthographic methods is more erratic, depending on cultural circumstances of a largely irrational nature. The success and usefulness of these descriptive systems cannot be solely attributed to the penchant of human rationality for analytic decomposition. There is an equally long tradition of attempts to reduce lexical semantics to the combination of elements drawn from a small set of primitives, and the results have never been very useful or very generally accepted.

The modern tradition of research in spoken language, of which we are all a part, assumes (informally) a system of description that reached essentially its current form in the work of Daniel Jones, for the case of English, and has been variously extended and modified to cover other languages. The originators of this descriptive system assumed that its categories were physically definable. To date, no attempts to redeem this assumption by construction of explicit algorithms (operating on either acoustic or articulatory measurements) have been successful. This failure to give objective status to such representations has caused a certain general nervousness, but has done little to change their usage in practice. If we leave aside the question of what such transcriptions really mean (i.e., how to reconstruct them theoretically), and if we permit typographical detail to count for nought, then there is an astonishing uniformity of practice in casual notation among researchers who otherwise agree on nothing. Almost no one accepts this style of transcription as a theoretical construct, but almost everyone uses it as a notational convenience.

Indeed, it is really much more than a convenience—it is to a large extent the unconscious object of our discourse, our initial method of organizing and characterizing the phenomena we intend to study. It is important to stress the pretheoretical and informal nature of this common description—any attempt to fix its details, or determine its exact status, would soon dissolve in a welter of recriminations. Nevertheless, we all rely on our own comfortable versions of this way of speaking about speech.

There are many approaches to phonetics, and many approaches to phonology, and the number of descriptions and justifications of the division of labor between the two fields is probably not much smaller than the Cartesian product of the two sets of schools. The general acceptance of the division between fields, and the cultural divergence that ensues, cannot easily be explained by reference to any particular instance of such theories. Instead, the foundation of the split is to be found in our common acceptance of the pretheoretical system of descriptive categories just discussed. Since everyone implicitly accepts this way of talking about the stuff of speech, it is perfectly natural for one group of researchers to concentrate on the relation of such descriptive categories to the physical realities of articulation and sound, while another group tries to understand the intricate patterning of the corresponding pretheoretical categories under morphological inflection and derivation, optional pronunciation, and so forth.

Most of the differences in style and method between the two fields then follow, as natural adaptations of the organism to its research environment. I will return to this point later, and argue that many of these divergences have become seriously counterproductive, at least in the study of some important questions in both fields.

To avoid misunderstanding, I hasten to add that I do not question the appropriateness of any division of labor in research on speech and language. Surely the study of Semitic morphology and the modeling of oronasal coupling require rather different knowledge and skills, and it would be unreasonable to insist that no one could undertake one of these who could not also handle the other.

II. Intonation: Where a Hybrid Approach Is Required

Much of my own research has dealt with English intonation. In this area, the comforting common ground of pretheoretical description is conspicuous by its absence. There is no generally accepted practice for notating, naming, or even categorizing intonations. A number of schools of description exist, but their systems are usually difficult for outsiders to learn, the completeness of their coverage is often suspect, the intersubjective reliability of their descriptions is generally dubious, and the basic categories employed have (at least super-ficially) very little similarity from school to school. The prospect facing a newcomer to the field is indeed depressing, unless he or she has a perverse taste for intellectual balkanization.

The situation improves slightly with time. Experience with the phenomena of intonation, and time spent poring over the examples in the literature, lead eventually to the suspicion that the various authorities are indeed talking about the same things in different ways, roughly in the sense that romaji and hiragana transcriptions both characterize the same Japanese language. But this suspicion does not, at least for me, develop into a comfortable pretheoretical description.

It is not clear whether these difficulties reflect a basic difference between intonation and "segmental" phonology. I suspect that they do. Some obvious symptoms of the difference are intonation's lack of referential meaning; its deficiency in the equivalent of "word constancy" (by which I mean the homely conviction that "rabbit" cooed and "rabbit" snarled are instances of the same word); and its preoccupation with apparently gradient distinctions.

I will not speculate here about the cause of these symptoms. All that matters to the present discussion is their effect, which is to make the usual phonetics–phonology distinction inapplicable. Regardless of background, all students of intonation must think for themselves about what the basic categorization of intonational phenomena should be before they can begin even an informal investigation. Their research is (or should be) constantly drawn back to this fundamental question: Each advance in the basic categories of description permits the interpretation of a broader range of data, which often suggests a new modification of the initial descriptive assumptions.

In the face of such a complex problem, it is natural to use the widest available set of methods; these tend to complement one another, allowing a clearer fix on the object of study than an approach from only one side would. In trying to puzzle out the nature of intonational patterns, I and various colleagues (principally Alan Prince, with whom I have worked on theories of stress, and Janet Pierrehumbert, who is responsible for much of the tonal theory sketched below) have used at least the following list of methods:

1. Reliance on linguistic theories of stress and phrasing, insofar as they are helpful, and revision of such theories where they are not;
2. Impressionistic categorization of intonations, based on progressive ear training, coupled with informal analysis of instrumental F_0 contours;
3. Construction of explicit models for the abstract representation of intonation, in which we try to be clear about what the primitive concepts are, how they can be combined, how they are related to other aspects of speech and language, and how they are to be used in accounting for our observations;
4. Perceptual experiments to test the distinctness of intonational types, their appropriateness to various contexts of utterance, and the dependence of subjective pitch height on phrasal position;
5. Testing of phonological descriptions of intonation by synthesis: Explicit

rules are used to construct F_0 contours from a "phonemic" representation, and the result is recombined with spectral parameters taken from a natural utterance, for evaluation by listening;

6. Modeling of the effects of length, order, and pitch-range variation on F_0 contours of the "same" intonational type.

The first three methods are typical of phonologists' practice; the last three methods are very much the sort of thing that phoneticians and psycholinguists do. I believe that we have made quite a bit of progress by using this combined approach; readers curious about details are referred to the bibliography. Our work would have had very little success, in my opinion, if we had taken either a purely phonological or a purely phonetic approach. Nor could we have succeeded by relying on the literature for either our phonological or our phonetic ideas—our results have depended on the interaction of new research in both areas.

Our conclusions have changed somewhat as the work has proceeded, and I am not yet confident that we have got the basic framework of description right. However, I have come to regard this feeling of uncertainty as a good thing, and would move on to new problems if it ever went away.

Of course, constant reevaluation of first principles in search of better theories is the normal method of science, and has been characteristic of most good work on language and speech. It is much less common to use a wide variety of methods, drawn from the traditions of both phonology and phonetics, in a concerted effort to clarify some aspect of human speech, considered simultaneously as a system of signs and as a signaling procedure.

The Hybrid Nature of the Resulting Theory

I have argued that some special properties of the field of intonation research make it appropriate to use hybrid methods in arriving at a theory. But it is interesting to note that the result is, in a sense, a hybrid theory. It is not that levels of analysis are inappropriate here—on the contrary, the theory proposes a rather clean and simple level of phonological analysis (involving sequences of high and low tones aligned with the stress pattern of the phrase), a few gradient "paralinguistic" dimensions (e.g., pitch range), and a small set of explicit principles for phonetic realization, which together are asserted to assign a (usually unique) description and derivation to every possible F_0 contour in the language. The division of the analysis into components is fairly traditional. However, the resulting theory can make sense of (even simple) examples only when all three aspects are brought into play at once.

The "phonetic realization principles" are very limited in power and scope—they work from left to right through the utterance, essentially one stress group at a time. However, they depend on local phonological structure, their local output usually depends on the pitch level assigned to a previous tone, and a certain amount of interpolation occurs across tonally unspecified material, so that the correspondence between tones and local F_0 levels or configurations becomes somewhat opaque. Therefore, the phonological analysis does not offer a convincing account of an F_0 contour without the help of the phonetic implementation principles, together with assignment of values to gradient parameters such as relative prominence and pitch range.

It also appears that the "phonetic implementation principles" for intonation differ somewhat from language to language, although too few languages are well described for this point to be compelling to a skeptic.

III. The Relevance of a Hybrid Approach to Segmental Problems

Most of the arguments for a hybrid approach to intonation research also apply to the traditional problems of segmental phonetics and phonology; the need is just a little less obvious. Authorities in the field disagree about the fundamental characterization of the phenomena to be explained, and there is always a value in trying to work toward the object of study from several directions at once. Furthermore, there is good reason to suppose that much of the traditional data in segmental phonetics and phonology requires an essentially hybrid explanation, in the sense previously suggested for the case of intonational data.

A. The Case of Phonology

Within and among the various schools of generative phonology, there is increasing uncertainty about the basic nature of phonological representation. This trend can best be understood in a historical perspective. In the beginning, generative phonology relied largely on data taken from its predecessors; in the Sound Pattern of English (SPE), the contents of Kenyon–Knott and of Trager–Smith were reanalyzed and explained in terms of feature theory, ordered values, the cycle, and so forth. An explicit analogy to the Copernican reanalysis of Ptolemaic data was noted. The output of the SPE phonology could be translated into the notation of Trager–Smith by simple substitution of symbols; the new theory explained the old data by direct generation. The main representational innovation was feature theory, which remains easily intertranslatable with segmental alphabet theories. The rest of the new explanation depended on innovations in the rule systems.

Over the last few years, a number of new representational devices have been introduced into the generative armamentarium, principally the constructs of so-called autosegmental and metrical theories. Various representations of syllabic and suprasyllabic structures have been suggested, and features are assumed to migrate about in a variety of trees and graphs defined as the need arises. Phonological rule systems can be simplified, almost trivialized, at the cost of such enrichment of the structures they modify, and typological properties of phenomena such as stress, vowel harmony, and vowel epenthesis are elucidated.

I am basically in favor of such approaches to phonology, but it must be admitted that they bring a new kind of uncertainty with them. In the context of SPE-era phonology, one end of the problem was essentially fixed. Everyone agreed about what the system was supposed to generate (aside from arguments about how to spell out phonetic symbols in featural terms); the only argument was about the nature of underlying representations and the intervening rules. Now that arbitrary new representational structures are up for consideration, the desired form of the system's output is much less well defined. The logic of the situation has not really changed at all, but as a practical matter, the uncertainty about representations is much greater than it was, and there is a greater need for phonetic or psychological evidence to help constrain the choices.

Few phonologists would argue about the benefits of converging evidence from other sources, but the next point will be more controversial. There is an increasing amount of evidence, I think, that much of the traditional domain of phonological data actually belongs to a component whose function is analogous to that of our intonational implementation principles. Specifically, phonologically transparent (not lexically governed) allophonic variation seems to belong with a larger class of phonetic regularities that are not well modeled as feature- or structure-changing rules. Such regularities are usually dependent on phonological environment, not just on the superficial physics of surrounding articulations, but their consequences are gradient, apparently linked to the inherent dimensions of articulation, and modulated by prosodic and paralinguistic parameters. These implementational regularities have language-particular and indeed dialect-particular aspects; this, along with their dependence on phonological environment, makes it seem unlikely that they can entirely be explained by reference to the physics and physiology of the vocal organs. If I am right about the characterization of these regularities, then it is plausible to suppose that they represent the higher level aspects of speech motor control.

This point of view raises serious questions about the types of regularities that ought to be expressed by manipulation of phonological representations. This is a more serious form of uncertainty than the one mentioned earlier, and it requires (rather than simply invites) investigation by hybrid methods. Out of historical necessity, phonology has assumed (at least in practice) that its task was to explain the patterning of information in a class of well-defined symbolic objects, namely, phonetic representations. This convenient fiction has become more and more counterproductive, and should be gradually abandoned, as opportunity permits.

B. The Case of Phonetics

The interpretation of segmentally related acoustic and articulatory measurements has a lot in common with the interpretation of F_0 contours; the main difference, as mentioned earlier, is that there is a generally accepted informal classification of segmental categories available to rationalize the task. Aside from this initial advantage, very similar problems arise. There are obvious effects of phonological environment, of prosodic and paralinguistic variation, and of physical coarticulation that collectively make the connection between phonetic category and physical measurement anything but transparent. There is no choice of unit, even up to the word or the phrase, that entirely avoids this problem. In particular, the consequences of rate, emphasis, and style of speech are complex and pervasive. Such variation prevents even phrase-level units for a single speaker from having a straightforward physical definition.

Furthermore, if I am right about the nature of the implementational regularities mentioned earlier, better theories of the physics and low-level physiology of speech, although obviously desirable, will by no means suffice to explain the complex relation between words and sounds. Such an explanation requires explicit modeling of the nature of an utterance plan and of the process by which it is spoken. If the phenomena of allophonic variation are (even in part) consequences of the realization process, then the utterance plan must be rather more abstract than the standard forms of phonetic representation would suggest, and must be sufficiently rich in structure to condition the relevant regularities. To have any value as predictors of real data, the realization model must allow for the effects of local environment (in the plan) on the units that are manipulated, whatever these are to be, and for the effects of stress pattern, phrasing, rate, and so forth on the realization of the plan as a whole. Obviously, the physics and low-level physiology of the vocal organs must be employed to explain what they can.

I do not believe that any observationally adequate models of this kind now exist. Speech synthesis systems are the closest overall approximation, but their treatment of the consequences of contextual, prosodic, and paralinguistic variation is a rather erratic fit to measurements of natural speech, in my experience, and their internal workings are generally determined more by engineering expediency than by any consideration of theory. The construction of a complete model in an entirely principled way will presumably not be possible for a long time. Many partial successes are possible in the interim, but I strongly suspect that progress depends on an approach that gives serious thought to representational issues, while using these representations in explicit modeling of appropriate measurements.

Historically, phonetics has generally assumed that its task is to explain the physical realization of a class of pretheoretically defined categories, which are essentially those implied by traditional phonetic representations. Phonetics' physicalist bias leads its practitioners (with some notable exceptions) to regard these phonetic categories as ontologically suspect entities, whose exact nature is not worth the courtesy of clear thought. Very often, hope is expressed that all such subjective categories can be replaced by physical predicates of some sort, for instance by finding neurological signals of a sufficiently digital kind. The history of such efforts is not a hopeful one—I suggest that they should be abandoned, and that abstract representations should be granted the kind of status in phonetics that they are given in phonology or in cognitive psychology.

IV. Conclusion

I have suggested that the plan for an utterance is perhaps rather more abstract than traditional forms of phonetic representation, and that the process of speaking should be taken to account for at least some of the traditional data of phonological alternation. It follows that the process of realizing an utterance plan has at least some language-particular aspects, and cannot be entirely attributed to physics and universally determined physiology. Also, the fact that the process of speaking integrates prosodic and paralinguistic variation cannot safely be ignored; indeed, the study of what remains invariant under such variation can provide invaluable clues about the realization process and its linguistic inputs.

My suggestions may well be wrong; the true nature of the representation that underlies speech is obviously to be determined by research, as is the nature of the speaking process. The research in question is not well served by the traditional concerns and methods of either phonology or phonetics, and would proceed faster if the two scientific cultures were a little more like one another.

References

Liberman, M. *The intonation system of English*. Ph.D. dissertation, M.I.T. New York: Garland Press, 1979.

Liberman, M., & Pierrehumbert, J. A metric for the height of certain pitch peaks in English. *Journal of the Acoustical Society of America*, 1979, *66*, Suppl. 1, S64.

Liberman, M., & Pierrehumbert, J. Intonational invariance under changes in pitch range and length.(to appear).

Liberman, M., & Prince, A. On stress and linguistic rhythm. *Linguistic Inquiry*, 1977, *8*, 249–336.

Liberman, M., & Sag, I. Prosodic form and discourse function. *CLS*, 1974, *10*, 416–426.

Pierrehumbert, J. The perception of fundamental frequency declination. *Journal of the Acoustical Society of America*, 1979, *66*, 363–369.

Pierrehumbert, J. *The phonology and phonetics of English intonation*. Ph.D. dissertation, M.I.T., 1979 (forthcoming from MIT Press).

Pierrehumbert, J. Synthesizing intonation. *Journal of the Acoustical Society of America*,1981, *70*, 985–995.

Pierrehumbert, J., & Liberman, M. Modeling the fundamental frequency of the voice. *Contemporary Psychology*, 1982, *27*(9), 690–692.

Sag, I., & Liberman, M. The intonational disambiguation of indirect speech acts. CLS, 1975, *11*, 487–498.

Chapter 13

Some Reflections on Speech Research

FRANKLIN S. COOPER

I. Introduction

It was a privilege indeed to give the introductory paper at the Conference on the Production of Speech on which this volume is based. The topic is an important one, at the cutting edge of present-day speech research, so it is not surprising that several divergent paths are being followed. The meeting gave us an opportunity not only to compare recent findings but also to reexamine our research goals—to ask again what it is we are looking for.

In his letter of invitation, Peter MacNeilage suggested that I include a retelling—for his students, since the rest of the participants knew the story—of how Haskins Laboratories became involved in speech research and how the initial work on perception developed into parallel research on speech production. Since the story starts from a conceptual context that is no longer familiar or is but dimly remembered, it seemed useful to go back to the still earlier events and ideas from which acoustic phonetics emerged some 30-odd years ago. So, in the first half of this chapter, I have tried to cover very briefly the contributions of linguists and of engineers to concepts of speech that were current at the beginning of the fifties, and then to turn to events at Haskins Laboratories as a case history of how those concepts continued to evolve.

Who would not be tempted to push on from history to prognostication? I have tried to avoid the trap in the second half of the chapter and, instead, to look at present-day research from a little distance—to reflect on where it seems to be going and how this follows from current concepts about the nature of speech. In doing so, I have found it instructive to think about the orientation of the research effort with respect to the processes by which speech flows from speaker to listener. But more of that later.

II. Retrospective: Speech Research to the 1960s

It is obvious, I suppose, that the topics we choose to discuss at conferences depend on what we currently know and believe about speech. It was always so, but what was known was different 20, or 50, or 100 years ago. Furthermore, what was known at any given time consisted of concepts as well as facts; indeed, only those facts agreeable to the concepts were likely to have been discovered or to have survived.

If, then, we want to understand the basis for our own research undertakings— the sometimes shaky ground on which we build—it may be better to trace back through the *ideas* that were held about speech rather than to try to find our way through the forest of facts that surrounded them. But first, some words of warning: The trip will be a sketchy one. You must expect gaps, biases, and disproportionate attention to personal experience, as well as less attention to credits and priorities than in a proper review.

A. Early Ideas about Speech

1. Linguistic and Phonetic[1] At any given time, ideas about speech depended on who held them. As of 100 years ago, linguists and phoneticians were about the only people interested in speech, and their concerns were with historical and family relationships among languages. Since they dealt mainly with written language, it is not surprising that the study of spoken language put emphasis on ways to "write" speech sounds. Thus, the IPA transcription system drew heavily on Henry Sweet's Broad Romic notation, which in turn was indebted to Melville Bell's Visible Speech, a system of descriptive symbols to show deaf students how to articulate the sounds of speech. So, very early—and even earlier for Sanskrit—speech came to be thought about as a string of symbols. This view followed naturally from the way phoneticians dealt with speech, that is, by listening carefully and discovering by trial and error how to produce acceptable imitations. Thus, perception and production shared about equally in shaping the phonetician's concept of speech: Perception gave irreducible units, production identified them with gestures, and the use of a notational system implied an underlying invariance, despite ubiquitous variation in the actual

---

[1] For a broad-ranging review of this topic, see D. B. Fry, Phonetics in the twentieth century. In T. A. Sebeok (Ed.), *Current Trends in Linguistics* (Vol. 12, Part 4). The Hague: Mouton, 1974, pp. 2201–2239.

sounds. There have, of course, been changes in emphasis and genuine refinements of these ideas, but the framework remains.

One of the refinements dealt with the problem of variability by distinguishing among the *kinds* of variability: those that were distinctive and so made a difference in meaning, those that were systematic but not distinctive, and those that seemed just to happen. But even within these categories there was further variation when one considered actual speech sounds, and this made it necessary to assume idealized entities, phonemic in nature, as counterparts of the erstwhile phonetic symbols. A further refinement attributed internal structure to the phoneme and came to characterize it as a bundle of distinctive features.

The interest of phoneticians and linguists in the production of speech very soon led to physiological experiments. These deserve our admiration for the ingenuity, even heroism, with which kymograph and tambours, Helmholtz resonators, and manometric flames were used to test and refine impressionistic ideas about specific sounds and how they were made. But the tools were then too crude to let experimental phonetics develop along lines of its own, and the better instruments that came with the 1920s and 1930s were mainly in the hands of engineers, who had quite different ideas about speech, as we shall see.

2. Communications Engineering[2] Let us turn to the years following the First World War and to the revolution in communications technology that occurred in the 1920s. Many things were new then that we now take for granted: radio broadcasting, talking movies, the rebirth of the phonograph, and even (albeit primitive) television. Much of this was due to the vacuum tube amplifier, for the ability to amplify signals as weak as speech had many practical consequences.

One consequence was that speech itself became of interest to engineers; that is, there was a practical need for telephone engineers to know more about speech as a signal, since that is what a telephone must transmit. At the beginning of the twenties, speech was commonly viewed as a kind of "acoustic stuff"—complex in detail but essentially homogeneous on average: "a continuous flow of distributed energy, analogous to total radiation from an optical source. This idea of speech is a convenient approximation, useful in the study of speech reproduction by mechanical means" (Crandall, 1917, p. 74).

But ideas changed as better tools became available. In the late twenties, a new high-speed oscillograph focused interest briefly on the *waveform* of speech (Fletcher, 1929). This soon gave way to interest in spectral representation and to the possibility that all speech sounds—not just vowels—could be described in terms of their "characteristic bands," that is, their prominent steady-state frequency components (Collard, 1930).

The conceptual shift from static components to a dynamically changing spectrum came rather slowly. In 1934, Steinberg published what is, in retrospect, the first speech spectrogram. But this one crude schematic "spectrogram"

---

[2]Condensed from a brief review presented at the 50th Anniversary Celebration of the Acoustical Society of America, June 12, 1979. See Cooper (1980).

of a single short sentence had required several hundred hours of hand measurement and computation, so it is easy to see why this way of representing speech—and of thinking about it—remained a curiosity for so long.

By the beginning of the next decade, a different way of thinking about speech—much closer to the views of phoneticians, but still rooted in engineering—was being proposed by Homer Dudley (1940). He explained speech by drawing an analogy with radio waves, which are not themselves the message, but only its carrier. So with speech: The message is the subaudible articulatory *gestures* that are made by the speaker; the sound stuff is only an acoustic carrier modulated by those gestures. This remarkable insight was obscured, for purely technical reasons, when it was embodied in hardware—voder and vocoder—since the gestural component became a set of fixed filters and the point of view shifted from gestures back to spectra.

The influence of instruments on ideas is nowhere better illustrated than by the unveiling of the sound spectrograph (Potter, 1946). Once spectrograms could be made in minutes, they had a profound effect on speech research. They provided, quite literally, a new way to look at speech, as well as new ways to think about it. One way, of course, was the familiar description in spectral terms, but with a new richness of detail. A second way was to view the spectrogram as a road map to the articulation. A third way was to view spectrograms simply as *patterns*. The richness of detail then became just a nuisance, since it obscured the underlying simpler design.

You will have noticed that engineering ideas about speech, as of the late forties, treated it as primarily an acoustic phenomenon, an ongoing stream that is complex, variable in structure, and continually changing. This contrasts with phonetic ideas, which viewed speech as a sequence of discrete entities. These phonetic units were of an ambivalent acoustic–articulatory nature, but they were unitary nevertheless, and their symbols stood for some kind of underlying idealized entities.

B. Acoustic Phonetics: The Forties and Fifties

This is about how things stood at the beginnings of the new science of acoustic phonetics. It is difficult to recapture either the conceptual currents or the sense of adventure of the late forties and early fifties. A few happenings from that period were the publication of *Visible Speech* with its catalog of spectrograms by Potter, Kopp, and Green (1947), and a classic interpretive account by Martin Joos (1948). At one of the early MIT speech conferences—happenings in their own right—Jakobson, Fant, and Halle (1951) circulated a draft of *Preliminaries to Speech Analysis*. This sought to round out the concept of distinctive features by showing their correlates in spectrographic as well as in articulatory and impressionistic terms. Then, too, there were new instruments, notably the speech synthesizers, and the ideas they fomented. More of this later.

First, who were the people at the speech conferences and what were their interests? Half at least came from engineering backgrounds and were interested in how speech signals could be manipulated for practial communications purposes. Experimental psychologists were becoming interested in the perception of speech. Phoneticians, the few there were, were of course very interested in the new possibilities for describing speech sounds, but most linguists, especially of the American School, found little that seemed relevant to their concerns with theory and formal structures. One result of the imbalance, especially between linguists and engineers, was that the term *phoneme* lost its precision in discussions of speech research and was misused more often than not. Another consequence was that almost everyone, but especially the engineers, adopted without reservation the view that speech by its very nature was a succession of unitary sounds and that the invariances implied by phonemic symbols were actually there in the acoustic signals, if only one could find them. This idea was implicit—often explicit—in most of the research of that period, and is not unfamiliar to this day.

There was also, in the research of the forties and fifties, a preoccupation with the acoustic and perceptive aspects of speech.[3] I recall rather little work, other than that of Stetson (1951), on physiological aspects of speech production, though there was much excellent research on the relationship of articulatory configurations to acoustic output (Fant, 1960; Stevens & House, 1955, 1956).

C. Perception to Production: A Case History

I should like now to abandon all attempts to trace the full range of ideas about speech into the sixties and seventies and turn to a more nearly personal account of how one sequence of ideas evolved—between the forties and sixties—from a nonspeech concern with sensory aids, via work on speech perception, to physiological research on speech production.

Alvin Liberman and I discovered speech shortly after World War II. We were trying to build a reading machine for blinded veterans by turning letter shapes into distinctive acoustic shapes. In fact, that was fairly easy. The resulting acoustic alphabets were learnable, but they were essentially useless because reading with them was intolerably slow (Cooper, 1950). The irony of the situation finally came home to us: In talking about our problem, we were using with great facility a complex, high-rate sound system to ask why it was so hard to make a simple sound system work at all, even at moderate rates. Maybe the real problem was to find out how *speech* is perceived, and why so fast? We

---

[3]Thus, Jakobson et al. (1951, p. 12) comment in their *Preliminaries . . .* that "the closer we are in our investigation to the destination of the message (i.e., its perception by the receiver), the more accurately can we gage the information conveyed by its sound shape. This determines the operational hierarchy of levels of decreasing pertinence: perceptual, aural, acoustical and articulatory (the latter carrying no direct information to the receiver). The systematic exploration of the first two of these levels belongs to the future and is an urgent duty."

did two things that proved to be important: We built a speech synthesizer, and with it we lured Pierre Delattre into working with us (Liberman & Cooper, 1972).

The Pattern Playback converted spectrograms back into sound—not quality speech but a fairly faithful rendering of the spectrum. The device was based on the very simple idea that spectrograms appeal to the eye because they reveal important spectral patterns in spite of a lot of acoustic clutter. So, if we could abstract the simple underlying patterns—by tracing them from spectrograms—and then play them back as sound, we could know by listening whether or not we had captured the essence of the speech. In the simplest case, the pattern elements that served as acoustic cues would be the invariants that correspond to the phonemes.

It was, in fact, possible to tease out sets of acoustic cues and even, by the mid-fifties, to use them in synthesizing speech "by rule" (from a phonemic text) rather than by copying spectrograms. But two things were puzzling: For one, the cues were rarely, if ever, truly invariant. For another, though they were indeed cues in the acoustic domain, they were not easy to describe or classify in conventional acoustic terms; rather, they seemed to fall naturally into arti-culatory categories. One reason why this might be so—an essentially trivial reason—is that the phonemic classification used in discovering the cues is itself based on articulation. Another more interesting reason could be that the perception of speech sounds is in fact based on the gestures by which speech is produced rather than on the sounds as acoustic entities (Liberman, Cooper, Shankweiler, & Studdert-Kennedy, 1967; Liberman & Studdert-Kennedy, 1978).

A variety of mechanisms can be imagined by which this might happen. The particular hypothesis that led the Haskins group into research on speech production had its roots in Donald Hebb's ideas about neural nets (Hebb, 1949) and possible interactions between sensory and motor networks, though precise mechanisms have not been a feature of what soon came to be called a motor theory of speech perception. Actually, neither the theory nor the possible mechanisms were directly involved in the rationale for the research on speech production—only the hypothesis that the underlying units of speech are articulatory in their natures. If they are, then the chances that these units will emerge in recognizable form get better and better the farther one can go experimentally toward the origins of the neuromotor signals that drive articulation.[4] This led us to use electromyography (EMG) for the study of muscle activity and to supplement it with analyses of movement (mostly by cine-radiography) and, of course, spectrographic analyses of the acoustic signal.

This was the rationale for our research. Actually, in its early stages when Katherine Harris and Peter MacNeilage joined in the work, the ideas we were

---

[4]This is just the opposite of the strategy described in the quotation from Jakobson et al. (Footnote 3). For an early account of the production-oriented strategy, see Cooper, Liberman, Harris, and Grubb (1958).

talking about were more concrete. The working hypothesis was that if things were really simple, then features and phonemes might be characterizable by motor commands to those particular muscles mainly involved in the respective articulations, and also that electromyographic signals would reveal those motor commands. Various qualifications were built into what we said about these expectations: Thus, no one could be sure about how much higher level restructuring there might be between linguistic unit and explicit neuromotor signal. For the very simple situation we first studied—lip closure for the bilabial stops—even the simple hypothesis seemed adequate; further studies, though, showed context dependence and the need for a less simplistic explanation (Cooper, 1966; Harris, 1974; MacNeilage, 1970; MacNeilage & DeClerk, 1969; MacNeilage & Sholes, 1964). Invariance, like the Holy Grail, seems always to remain just out of reach.

The experience of the Haskins group in studying speech *perception* explains one, though only one, of the reasons for a general shift toward research on speech *production* and particularly toward attempts to provide a basis in motor organization for understanding the communicative role of speech. It would be interesting, if time allowed, to review various models that have been proposed for speech perception and production and for the relationships between them. Fortunately, this is not necessary for production models, since an excellent review of just this topic has recently been published (Kent, 1976).

Let me say again that this brief look backward at speech research was not intended as a review of the subject, not even a sketchy one; rather, it is my impression of how some of the important ideas about speech developed and, especially, how a new interest in speech production developed out of research on speech perception. Other people would have other views, but I think we might agree in a general way as to where we stand now, at the beginning of the eighties.

III. Prospective: Concepts and Approaches

We have by now amassed much factual knowledge about speech production. We have developed the tools for learning even more. But we do not yet have a satisfactory model, or an understanding, of how speech conveys language. Why should this be? Do the difficulties and complexities inhere in the problem—that is, in the nature of speech processes—or rather in the ways in which we have chosen to think about the problem? The editor of this volume has given me leave to reflect on some of these basic issues—at my own peril, of course. One hazard is being dogmatic—which brings to mind the moral of Thurber's fable about a city dog who visited his cousin in the country. The city dog, know-it-all that he was, ignored his country cousin's willingness to answer questions about the animals of the forest. So, from a porcupine, he learned about guided missiles— though not about discretion—and he learned about chemical warfare from a little black and white animal that seemed only to be waving its tail in surrender.

The country dog reflected, as his city cousin limped back to the safety of the alleys, that "sometimes it is better to ask some of the questions than to know all of the answers" (Thurber, 1940).

Even questions, if they are about fundamental issues, may lead one into talking about things so familiar that they seem altogether obvious. But, the obvious—that which you see when you see it—can sometimes be that which you do *not* see, really see, until it jumps out at you. So perhaps there are insights to be had even from questioning things long familiar.

Let us look first at coarticulation—surely as familiar a topic as one could find; next, at some consequences of differing orientations to this problem; and then at the role of timing in speech.

A. Coarticulation: Problem or Pseudoproblem?

Coarticulation has been so much with us that it seems almost to have become an independent entity. Indeed, such comments as that certain speech behaviors "are due to coarticulation" seem even to imply that coarticulation *caused* them to happen. As a working definition, let us start with Hammarberg's view (1976) that "coarticulation is . . . a process whereby the properties of a segment are altered due to the influences exerted on it by neighboring segments." The central implication is that the successive segments intended by a speaker will reappear in the acoustic signal, but with their ideal acoustic shapes changed to adapt them to the local context. The adaptations are not trivial; they are not mere smoothings at the boundaries, but often amount to complete restructuring of segments and clusters of segments. So it is not surprising that much effort has gone into accounting for these effects, or that coarticulation is commonly regarded as a central problem for research in speech production.

But the explanations one has to contrive for his data, using coarticulation as a conceptual framework, are becoming ever more complex, and there has been a growing unease about this over the past several years. Are the difficulties of data interpretation due, perhaps, to faulty conceptions? If so, where did we go astray? There are several possibilities, some of which I should like to consider with you.

One view puts the blame on choosing the *wrong size* of linguistic unit as the input segments of speech production. Phonemes or bundles of features have been the usual choices. Perhaps larger units, such as the syllable or stress group, would allow more felicitous explanations, although this has yet to be demonstrated.

A second view also puts the blame on units—in particular, that the units chosen were *linguistic* units. Rather, according to this view, there is need for units of a different kind—for production units that are inherent in the articulatory process, just as comparable units inhere in other skilled motor behaviors. In this vein, MacNeilage and Ladefoged (1976) comment on the "inappropriateness of conceptualizing the dynamic processes of articulation itself in terms of discrete, static, context-free linguistic categories, such as 'phoneme' and 'distinctive features'." They go on to say that "there has arisen a need for new concepts to characterize articulatory function, concepts more appropriate to the description of movement processes than of stationary states."

Yet another view focuses on the *properties* of linguistic units, whether they be phoneme, feature bundle, or other canonical form. This view has been taken as a point of departure by Carol Fowler and her colleagues (Fowler, Rubin, Remez, & Turvey, 1980) in considering speech production in terms of coordinative structures. Although they do not challenge the use of units that are of the linguistic kind, they point out that the properties usually attributed to such units—that they are discrete and static—are in fact *irrelevant* to their linguistic function. This leaves the way open "to discover some way to characterize these units that preserves their essential linguistic properties, but also allows them to be actualized *unaltered* in a vocal tract and in an acoustic signal."

Let us, instead of following this line of argument, consider further the properties *discrete* and *static*. Even if we do not challenge the attribution of such properties to abstract linguistic units, should we not question the assumption that these properties will survive intact all the transformations that are involved in the act of speaking, and emerge at the end of that process as properties of the articulatory and acoustic entities? We know from experience that speech entities do not have these properties, but was there really any basis for supposing that they would? Or even that input units of whatever kind would reappear as output units of the same general size and kind?

Nevertheless, it is just these assumptions about the survival of segments that have trapped us into viewing speech as a succession of entities that *ought* to have retained their canonical forms, but *could not* for the merely practical reasons to which we give the name *coarticulation*.

B. Research Orientations and Their Consequences

A consequence of all the attention given to coarticulation has been to focus experimental work on the relationships between one stage and the next of the production process, that is, on successive causes and effects as one looks downstream, following the flow of messages from their inception by a speaker to their acoustic realization as speech and to their eventual assimilation by a listener. Thus, much attention is being given to careful measurement of forces, motions, mechanical linkages, and properties of the articulatory mechanism as a way to predict articulatory outcomes.

Such concerns have a long history, but it seems to me that the emphasis has shifted increasingly over the past several years toward this *downstream orientation* and away from an earlier *upstream orientation*. For that earlier orientation, that is, looking upstream, the problems were different and so were the experimental paradigms—necessarily so, since theoretical orientation affects what one looks for in Nature quite as much as observations about Nature affect theory. Looking upstream means trying to guess what causes were responsible for the effects that one is now observing; for example, what kind of neuromotor pattern would bring tongue tip to alveolar ridge regardless of jaw opening? And, for a longer leap, in what degree would such a neuromotor pattern reflect phonetic or phonemic units?

I am inclined to take seriously this distinction between upstream and downstream orientations toward speech research,[5] that is, to consider it a real dichotomy, since it has consequences for both theory and practice. Let us consider some of these consequences, but without making value judgments or disparaging one research orientation merely because another may be in fashion.

1. Differences of Method The obvious difference between the two orientations is one of method: Downstream, one works from known causes to predicted effect; upstream, from known effect to a plausible cause. Guessing at causes is much chancier than figuring out effects just as in football passing is more venturesome than linebucking, although it has more potential for yardage. The case can be made on historical grounds that upstream methods have contributed most of the advances to our knowledge of speech, although the method was most successful when the inferential leaps were small. The failures, when the attempted leap was all the way to a linguistic unit, were more spectacular, but even so they provoked good research and some careful thinking about theories and models.

2. Differences in Models and Theories The nature of theories and models about speech is in fact much affected by the upstream versus downstream orientation of the research. This is due in part to what we expect of a good model, in particular, the demand we make that it should have *both* predictive power and explanatory power. The former includes, of course, the capability to account for *all* effects in terms of their causes, not merely those more esteemed effects that were foretold. Also, predictive power implies an accounting that is as quantitative and as precise as may be—in the limit, a mathematical model.

Explanatory power seems intuitively desirable, though just what one means by "explanation" is not immediately evident. Perhaps the way Bridgman (1936) put it will meet our need: "Explanation consists merely in analyzing our complicated systems in such a way that we recognize in the complicated system the interplay of elements already so familiar to us that we accept them as not needing explanation."

Physics offers many examples of how models and theories differ in predictive and explanatory power: The Bohr atom was understandable, even believable, but in predictive power it was inferior to the much more opaque wave- and quantum-mechanical models. In optics, two distinct models were needed to achieve both prediction and explanation. Perhaps the classic extreme in

---

[5]The parallels with inductive and deductive inference will be obvious; however, these terms imply an emphasis on method per se, whereas I wish to stress the vector relationships betweeen method and process, that is, the orientation of research aims to speech flow.

predictive power is Einstein's formulation $E = mc^2$. It predicts with precision, and it is admirably simple and parsimonious as well, but it *explains* absolutely nothing about how or why energy and matter can be interconverted.

There is, it would seem, an inherent incompatibility—perhaps a trading relation—between predictive power and explanatory power. Moreover this characteristic of theories and models interacts with the orientation of research efforts. Thus, downstream efforts to account for effects and to do so reliably and accurately lead almost inevitably to models that predict, but are often wanting in explanatory power. Sometimes this imbalance results from devising rules or formulas without due concern for a rationalizing mechanism; sometimes it follows from complicating the mechanism past all understanding with more and more parameters and linkages. Of course, common sense should keep such efforts at realism from leading to a model so complex that it approximates the organism itself.

An upstream orientation is likely to depend heavily on analogies with known mechanisms for its inspired guesses, and so its models can be expected to explain better than they predict. But when rule systems are substituted for concrete mechanisms—a choice not excluded by upstream orientation—explanatory power is retained only to the extent that the rules are well motivated. A more serious hazard, judging from experience, is the "black box" model, usually a block diagram. Models of this kind can "explain" almost anything—so long as one does not enquire too closely into the inner workings of certain components.

If there is a moral to be drawn from these observations about models, I suppose it is that one should remember the biases inherent in his own research orientation and try a little harder for a reasonable balance between explanation and prediction; also, that one should try to accept philosophically that he cannot expect both virtues in full measure from either his own model or those of his colleagues.

C. The Problem of Relevance

The bias toward one or another kind of model is not the only consequence that follows from research orientation. Upstream from where we are now in studying speech production—and I take our present stance to be at the level of observing neuromuscular and movement events—there is not much room left for direct physiological assessment of the causes for the events we observe, and so we must fall back on behavioral indicators. True, there is much yet to be done in order to complete the representation of speech at the neuromuscular/movement level, especially when feedback loops are included. Nevertheless, the main upstream goal is to find out how neural signals are put together to drive the motor events of speech. This forces us, however reluctantly, to think about those patternings of neural activity in relation to the structure of the speech message. We are, after all, attempting to account for *purposeful* motor behavior, and that can hardly be done without taking account of the purpose, namely, to convey a message. It might help if we knew the nature and properties of the entities that make up a message—although we might then fall into the error of expecting these entities to survive the downstream transformations into neuromuscular, configurational, and acoustic representations of that message!

But if upstream research is obliged to be message oriented, that same compulsion keeps it from wandering away from the goal of understanding speech *as communication*. Does this restraint apply also to downstream research? Is it similarly constrained and guided? Not by its own nature, I think, since all manner of neuromuscular movement, and even acoustic events, challenge us to explore their cause–effect relationships. But only a limited set of these challenges lie on the critical path to an understanding of how speech conveys messages. It is no derogation of, say, motor behavior to assert that not all of it is relevant to speech, and especially to speech as communication.

Where can one find guidance? Probably not—as both logic and experience would warn us—by looking *within* a particular representation for entities and/or properties that properly belong to the message itself in its original form. Since this warning applies also to the terminal representation—the acoustic signal— all we have left are perceptual criteria; that is, if we wish to assess the relevance of a production event, we must ask a listener whether it does or does not make a difference in the message—a difference at some linguistic level. All this does not imply, of course, that perceptual tests should regularly be incorporated into production research; rather, that thinking about perceptual relevance when planning production experiments will help to keep the research on target. It may seem ironic that whether we try to go downstream or upstream we do not escape linguistic units, or some entities very like them. Perhaps we must learn to live with them.

Coarticulation Again . . . and Relevance It was, you may remember, coarticulation that led us into these reflections on research orientations and their consequences. Are there consequences for coarticulation itself? It had already been found suspect as a conceptual framework because it depended so heavily on the reincarnation of presumed input units, entities that were not themselves above suspicion. It now seems necessary to look carefully even at those phenomena that are loosely called *coarticulation effects*. To what extent are they still a central concern of speech research, or even relevant to it, if one hews to the line of communicative function? The intent of the question is not to imply a negative answer, but rather to suggest that such phenomena should be scrutinized as to relevance before they are investigated in detail, at least under the banner of speech research.

D. Timing of Speech Events

Let me turn to another topic—timing—in some of its several aspects. Relative timing is generally considered an important aspect of speech production.

Indeed, some of the recent approaches, such as action theory, give it a central place. Also, in some recent experiments—as well as in many older ones—we see anew how close is the relationship between production and perception.

1. Duration It is an easy step, by equally easy assumptions, from the relative timing of speech events to the *duration* of individual events. There is in fact a considerable literature about durations, much of it flawed by the easy assumptions I have just mentioned. The most transparently questionable one is that the durations of individual phones are to be found by subdividing the total duration of the string into successive intervals—which is the same as supposing that phones do not overlap along the time axis. To put the same point another way, paralleling questions about coarticulation: Is it reasonable to suppose that whatever inherent duration a phoneme might have would survive all the transformations between its central and its acoustic embodiments? Even if it did, could one expect that just those acoustic segments that are easiest to measure would be those that truly "belong" to the consonants and vowels?

2. Relative Timing But the *relative* times at which events are initialized is a feature of almost every model of speech production. Are there ways to observe what this initial timing might be? Could we, for example, get people to tell us when things happen? Some recent—and very neat—experiments follow from the observation of Morton, Marcus, and Frankish (1976) that listeners hear acoustically isochronous digit sequences as anisochronous. In these follow-on experiments, talkers were asked to *produce* isochronous sequences of syllables with the same, and also with alternating, initial consonants. Even though those sequences that were spoken with alternating initial consonants were *not* isochronous by acoustic measures, they were judged by *listeners* to be evenly paced. "The findings," to quote Carol Fowler and her colleagues (Fowler, 1979; Tuller & Fowler, 1980), "suggest that listeners judge isochrony on the basis of acoustic information about *articulatory* timing rather than on some articulation-free acoustic basis." It will not surprise you to hear that electromyographic measures support this idea. They show that talkers are indeed pacing their *gestures*, not the sounds they make.

Such use of electromyography to get at the *relative timing* of articulatory events has some noteworthy advantages as compared with measures of movement and acoustic output, although all these measures in combination are essential in order to fully specify an articulatory gesture. Arguments in support of electromyographic measures are that the onset of electrical activity in a muscle is usually easier to detect with precision than the onset of the consequent movement; also, the electrical activation of several different muscles that participate in a single movement can be sorted out and timed separately, and so more easily and accurately than the components of the movement can be timed. Acoustic events, although some due to occlusions and releases can be timed with precision, are a class only loosely coupled to the onsets of the motor events· of articulation, and so provide only indirect information about the organization of motor control.

There is, in addition to these pragmatic considerations, a persuasive rationale for the use of electromyography in studying the relative timing of articulatory events, namely, that electromyography marks rather directly the time of execution—though not the magnitude—of motor commands from which the happenings downstream eventuate. To put it another way, measures of timing that are taken downstream (on movement and acoustic events) will often be less reliable or interpretable since they are likely to be contaminated by factors that operate after—and so do not affect—electromyographic measures of timing.

Even so, it is sometimes argued that one cannot safely make inferences upstream without full knowledge of all downstream consequences because these consequences may affect what one is *observing* at any given level and attempting to *explain* from above. This is a very general, almost philosophical, point that one cannot totally reject—because sometimes it has merit—but cannot fully accept either, because it counsels the despair of indefinite delay: the dismal prospect that one cannot even look upstream until one has learned all about everything downstream. Perhaps a practical approach is to examine carefully how speech is represented at the particular level under study. Is the representation reasonably complete? Are its parts reasonably independent of each other, and of subsequent representations? For EMG, the relative timing part of the representation seems to meet these criteria—with one proviso— although the relative magnitude part often does not. The proviso has to do with feedback loops that might introduce differential delays between observed and presumed timing.

In commenting on timing as a part of action theory, I can be quite brief because that topic is dealt with in chapter 7. Let me mention only one point: If timing is taken to be an inherent part of the central representation of speech units—whatever they are—then the problem of serial ordering (as it was put by Lashley) simply disappears and with it the special machinery required to actualize the units on schedule. These issues are developed in an incisive way in a recent article in the *Journal of Phonetics* (Fowler, 1980). Even if that view of timing proves to have other, equally troublesome, problems, at least it is a move away from complex timing mechanisms as the stuff from which models of speech production are made.

Surely there are many other questions that ought to be asked about other topics, but let me bring to a close these reflections of an old country dog, and thank you for your attention.

References

Bridgman, P. W. *The nature of physical theory*. Princeton, N.J.: Princeton University Press, 1936, (N.Y.: Dover Publications, p. 63).

Collard, J. Calculation of the articulation of a. telephone circuit from the circuit constants. *Electronic Communication*, 1930, *8*, 141–163.

Cooper, F. S. Research on reading machines for the blind. In P. A. Zahl (Ed.),

Blindness: Modern approaches to the unseen environment. Princeton, N.J.: Princeton University Press, 1950.

Cooper, F. S. Describing the speech process in motor command terms. *Haskins Laboratories Status Report on Speech Research*, 1966, *SR-5/6*, 2.1–2.27.

Cooper, F. S. Acoustics in human communication: Evolving ideas about the nature of speech. *Journal of the Acoustical Society of America*, 1980, *68*, 18–21.

Cooper, F. S., Liberman, A. M., Harris, K. S., & Grubb, P. M. Some input–output relations observed in experiments on the perception of speech. In *Proceedings of the 2nd International Congress on Cybernetics*, 1958, pp. 930–941.

Crandall, I. B. The composition of speech. *Physical Review*, 1917, *10*, 74–76.

Dudley, H. The carrier nature of speech. *Bell System Technical Journal*, 1940, 19, 495–515.

Fant, C. G. M. *Acoustic theory of speech production.* The Hague: Mouton, 1960.

Fletcher, H. *Speech and hearing.* New York: Van Nostrand, 1929.

Fowler, C. "Perceptual centers" in speech production and perception. *Perception & Psychophysics*, 1979, *25*, 375–388.

Fowler, C. Coarticulation and theories of extrinsic timing control. *Journal of Phonetics*, 1980, *8*, 113–133.

Fowler, C., Rubin, P., Remez, R., & Turvey, M. T. Implications for speech production of a general theory of action. In B. Butterworth (Ed.), *Language production.* London: Academic Press, 1980.

Fry, D. B. Phonetics in the twentieth century. In T. A. Sebeok (Ed.), *Current Trends in Linguistics* (Vol. 12, Part 4). The Hague: Mouton, 1974, pp. 2201–2239.

Hammarberg, R. The metaphysics of coarticulation. *Journal of Phonetics*, 1976, *4*, 353–363.

Harris, K. S. Physiological aspects of articulatory behavior. In T. A. Sebeok (Ed.), *Current Trends in Linguistics* (Vol. 12, Part 4). The Hague: Mouton, 1974, pp. 2281–2302.

Hebb, D. O. *The organization of behavior.* New York: Wiley, 1949.

Jakobson, R., Fant, C. G. M., & Halle, M. Preliminaries to speech analysis: The distinctive features and their correlates. Cambridge, Mass.: MIT Press, 1951.

Joos, M. Acoustic phonetics. *Language Monograph No. 23*, 1948, *24* (Suppl).

Kent, R. D. Models of speech production. In N. J. Lass (Ed.), *Contemporary issues in experimental phonetics.* New York: Academic Press, 1976.

Liberman, A. M., & Cooper, F. S. In search of the acoustic cues. In A. Valdman (Ed.), *Papers in linguistics and phonetics to the memory of Pierre Delattre.* The Hague: Mouton, 1972.

Liberman, A. M., Cooper, F. S., Shankweiler, D. P., & Studdert-Kennedy, M. Perception of the speech code. *Psychological Review*, 1967, *74*, 431–461.

Liberman, A. M., & Studdert-Kennedy, M. Phonetic perception. In R. Held, H. Leibowitz, & H. L. Teuber (Eds.), *Handbook of sensory physiology* (Vol. 8). Heidelberg: Springer-Verlag, 1978.

MacNeilage, P. F. Motor control of serial ordering of speech. *Psychological Review*, 1970, *77*, 182–196.

MacNeilage, P. F., & DeClerk, J. On the motor control of coarticulation in CVC monosyllables. *Journal of the Acoustical Society of America*, 1969, *45*, 1217–1233.

MacNeilage, P. F., & Ladefoged, P. The production of speech and language. In E. Carterette & M. P. Friedman (Eds.), *Handbook of perception* (Vol. 7): *Language and perception.* New York: Academic Press, 1976.

MacNeilage, P. F., & Sholes, G. N. An electromyographic study of the tongue during vowel production. *Journal of Speech and Hearing Research*, 1964, *7*, 209–232.

Morton, J., Marcus, S., & Frankish, C. Perceptual centers (P-centers). *Psychological Review*, 1976, *83*, 405–408.

Potter, R. K. Introduction to technical discussions of sound portrayal. *Journal of the Acoustical Society of America*, 1946, *18*, 1–3. See also the five related articles that follow this introduction.

Potter, R. K., Kopp, G. A., & Green, H. C. *Visible speech*. New York: Van Nostrand, 1947.

Steinberg, J. C. Application of sound measuring instruments to the study of phonetic sounds. *Journal of the Acoustical Society of America*, 1934, *6*, 16–24.

Stetson, R. H. *Motor phonetics*. Amsterdam: North-Holland, 1951.

Stevens, K. N., & House, A. S. The development of a quantitative description of vowel articulation. *Journal of the Acoustical Society of America*, 1955, *27*, 484–493.

Stevens, K. N., & House, A. S. Studies of formant transitions using a vocal tract analog. *Journal of the Acoustical Society of America*, 1956, *28*, 578–585.

Thurber, J. The scottie who knew too much. In *Fables for our time and famous poems illustrated*. New York: Harper, 1940.

Tuller, B., & Fowler, C. Some articulatory correlates of perceptual isochrony. *Perception & Psychophysics*, 1980, *27*, 277–283.

Author Index

Subject Index

Language Index